1992
YEAR BOOK OF
INFECTIOUS DISEASES®

The 1992 Year Book® Series

Year Book of Anesthesia and Pain Management: Drs. Miller, Kirby, Ostheimer, Roizen, and Stoelting

Year Book of Cardiology®: Drs. Schlant, Collins, Engle, Frye, Kaplan, and O'Rourke

Year Book of Critical Care Medicine®: Drs. Rogers and Parrillo

Year Book of Dentistry®: Drs. Meskin, Currier, Kennedy, Leinfelder, Matukas, and Rovin

Year Book of Dermatologic Surgery: Drs. Swanson, Salasche, and Glogau

Year Book of Dermatology®: Drs. Sober and Fitzpatrick

Year Book of Diagnostic Radiology®: Drs. Federle, Clark, Gross, Madewell, Maynard, Sackett, and Young

Year Book of Digestive Diseases®: Drs. Greenberger and Moody

Year Book of Drug Therapy®: Drs. Lasagna and Weintraub

Year Book of Emergency Medicine®: Drs. Wagner, Burdick, Davidson, Roberts, and Spivey

Year Book of Endocrinology®: Drs. Bagdade, Braverman, Horton, Kannan, Landsberg, Molitch, Morley, Odell, Rogol, Ryan, and Sherwin

Year Book of Family Practice®: Drs. Berg, Bowman, Davidson, Dietrich, and Scherger

Year Book of Geriatrics and Gerontology®: Drs. Beck, Abrass, Burton, Cummings, Makinodan, and Small

Year Book of Hand Surgery®: Drs. Amadio and Hentz

Year Book of Health Care Management: Drs. Heyssel, Brock, King, and Steinberg, Ms. Avakian, and Messrs. Berman, Kues, and Rosenberg

Year Book of Hematology®: Drs. Spivak, Bell, Ness, Quesenberry, and Wiernik

Year Book of Infectious Diseases®: Drs. Wolff, Barza, Keusch, Klempner, and Snydman

Year Book of Infertility: Drs. Mishell, Paulsen, and Lobo

Year Book of Medicine®: Drs. Rogers, Bone, Cline, Braunwald, Greenberger, Utiger, Epstein, and Malawista

Year Book of Neonatal and Perinatal Medicine®: Drs. Klaus and Fanaroff

Year Book of Nephrology®: Drs. Coe, Favus, Henderson, Kashgarian, Luke, Myers, and Strom

Year Book of Neurology and Neurosurgery®: Drs. Currier and Crowell

Year Book of Neuroradiology: Drs. Osborn, Harnsberger, Halbach, and Grossman

Year Book of Nuclear Medicine®: Drs. Hoffer, Gore, Gottschalk, Sostman, Zaret, and Zubal

Year Book of Obstetrics and Gynecology®: Drs. Mishell, Kirschbaum, and Morrow

Year Book of Occupational and Environmental Medicine: Drs. Emmett, Brooks, Harris, and Schenker

Year Book of Oncology: Drs. Young, Longo, Ozols, Simone, Steele, and Weichselbaum

Year Book of Ophthalmology®: Drs. Laibson, Adams, Augsberger, Benson, Cohen, Eagle, Flanagan, Nelson, Reinecke, Sergott, and Wilson

Year Book of Orthopedics®: Drs. Sledge, Poss, Cofield, Frymoyer, Griffin, Hansen, Johnson, Simmons, and Springfield

Year Book of Otolaryngology–Head and Neck Surgery®: Drs. Bailey and Paparella

Year Book of Pathology and Clinical Pathology®: Drs. Gardner, Bennett, Cousar, Garvin, and Worsham

Year Book of Pediatrics®: Dr. Stockman

Year Book of Plastic, Reconstructive, and Aesthetic Surgery: Drs. Miller, Cohen, McKinney, Robson, Ruberg, and Whitaker

Year Book of Podiatric Medicine and Surgery®: Dr. La Porta

Year Book of Psychiatry and Applied Mental Health®: Drs. Talbott, Frances, Freedman, Meltzer, Perry, Schowalter, and Yudofsky

Year Book of Pulmonary Disease®: Drs. Bone and Petty

Year Book of Speech, Language, and Hearing: Drs. Bernthal, Hall, and Tomblin

Year Book of Sports Medicine®: Drs. Shephard, Eichner, Sutton, and Torg, Col. Anderson, and Mr. George

Year Book of Surgery®: Drs. Schwartz, Jonasson, Robson, Shires, Spencer, and Thompson

Year Book of Transplantation: Drs. Ascher, Hansen, and Strom

Year Book of Ultrasound: Drs. Merritt, Mittelstaedt, Carroll, and Nyberg

Year Book of Urology®: Drs. Gillenwater and Howards

Year Book of Vascular Surgery®: Dr. Bergan

Roundsmanship '92–'93: A Year Book® Guide to Clinical Medicine: Drs. Dan, Feigin, Quilligan, Schrock, Stein, and Talbot

Editor

Sheldon M. Wolff, M.D.

Endicott Professor and Chairman, Department of Medicine, Tufts University School of Medicine; Physician-in-Chief, New England Medical Center, Boston

Associate Editors

Michael J. Barza, M.D.

Professor of Medicine, Tufts University School of Medicine; Attending Physician, Division of Geographic Medicine and Infectious Diseases, and Head of Epidemiology, Department of Medicine, New England Medical Center, Boston

Gerald T. Keusch, M.D.

Professor of Medicine, Tufts University School of Medicine; Chief, Division of Geographic Medicine and Infectious Diseases, Department of Medicine, New England Medical Center, Boston

Mark S. Klempner, M.D.

Professor of Medicine, Tufts University School of Medicine; Division of Geographic Medicine and Infectious Diseases, Department of Medicine, New England Medical Center, Boston

David R. Snydman, M.D.

Professor of Medicine and Pathology, Tufts University School of Medicine; Director, Clinical Microbiology, New England Medical Center, Boston

1992

The Year Book of INFECTIOUS DISEASES®

Editor

Sheldon M. Wolff, M.D.

Associate Editors

Michael J. Barza, M.D.
Gerald T. Keusch, M.D.
Mark S. Klempner, M.D.
David R. Snydman, M.D.

Mosby
Year Book

St. Louis Baltimore Boston Chicago London Philadelphia Sydney Toronto

Editor-in-Chief, Year Book Publishing: Kenneth H. Killion
Sponsoring Editor: Linda Steiner
Manager, Medical Information Services: Edith M. Podrazik
Senior Medical Information Specialist: Terri Strorigl
Senior Medical Writer: David A. Cramer, M.D.
Assistant Director, Manuscript Services: Frances M. Perveiler
Associate Managing Editor, Year Book Editing Services: Elizabeth Fitch
Production Coordinator: Max F. Perez
Proofroom Manager: Barbara M. Kelly

Mosby-Year Book, Inc.
11830 Westline Industrial Drive
St. Louis, MO 63146

Editorial Office:
Mosby-Year Book, Inc.
200 North LaSalle St.
Chicago, IL 60601

International Standard Serial Number: 0743-9261
International Standard Book Number: 0-8151-9382-3

Table of Contents

The material in this volume represents literature reviewed up to February 1991.

Journals Represented

Mosby–Year Book subscribes to and surveys nearly 850 U.S. and foreign medical and allied health journals. From these journals, the Editors select the articles to be abstracted. Journals represented in this YEAR BOOK are listed below.

American Journal of Diseases of Children
American Journal of Epidemiology
American Journal of Medicine
American Journal of Obstetrics and Gynecology
American Journal of Public Health
American Journal of Surgery
American Review of Respiratory Disease
Annals of Internal Medicine
Annals of Surgery
Annals of Thoracic Surgery
Archives of Internal Medicine
Archives of Neurology
Archives of Ophthalmology
Archives of Otolaryngology–Head and Neck Surgery
Archives of Surgery
Arthritis and Rheumatism
Blood
British Medical Journal
Cancer
Cell
Chest
Clinical Orthopaedics and Related Research
Clinical and Experimental Dermatology
Critical Care Medicine
European Journal of Cancer and Clinical Oncology
European Journal of Obstetrics, Gynecology and Reproductive Biology
European Respiratory Journal
Hepatology
Human Pathology
Intensive Care Medicine
Journal of Clinical Investigation
Journal of Clinical Microbiology
Journal of Clinical Oncology
Journal of Clinical Pathology
Journal of Infectious Diseases
Journal of Parenteral and Enteral Nutrition
Journal of Pediatrics
Journal of Trauma
Journal of the American College of Cardiology
Journal of the American Geriatrics Society
Journal of the American Medical Association
Lancet
Laryngoscope
New England Journal of Medicine
Obstetrics and Gynecology
Ophthalmology
Pediatric Infectious Disease Journal
Pediatric Neurology

Pedatrics
Presse Medicale
Proceedings of the National Academy of Sciences
Radiology
Reviews of Infectious Diseases
Scandinavian Journal of Infectious Diseases
Southern Medical Journal
Transplantation
Transplantation Proceedings

Standard Abbreviations

The following terms are abbreviated in this edition: acquired immunodeficiency syndrome (AIDS), central nervous system (CNS), cerebrospinal fluid (CSF), computed tomography (CT), electrocardiography (ECG), human immunodeficiency virus (HIV), and magnetic resonance (MR) imaging (MRI).

Introduction

As I review this year's selection of articles, I am struck not only by the continued growth of research pertaining to human immunodeficiency virus, but also newer presentations of old diseases such as toxic-shock-like illness with group A, β-hemolytic streptococcal infection, and *Legionella* sternal wound infections. This volume contains a number of notable papers from the past year's literature concerning infectious diseases, including what will be the classic descriptions of 6-month chemotherapy for pulmonary and extrapulmonary tuberculosis, controlled trials comparing vidarabine to acyclovir for neonatal herpes simplex infection, fluconazole compared with amphotericin B for cryptococcal meningitis, and zidovudine for asymptomatic HIV infection. In addition, descriptions of newly recognized clinical entities such as bacillary peliosis hepatis in association with HIV are provided.

This year we have reinstated the section on pediatrics, although a number of other papers related to pediatric infections can be found throughout the volume under their appropriate general headings. The section on AIDS continues to expand in conjunction with our growth regarding knowledge and therapy for this disease.

I am indebted to the associate editors for their willingness to continue to share a large portion of the burden of bringing this volume to life. I want to express my gratitude to them.

Sheldon M. Wolff, M.D.

1 Bacterial Infections

Sepsis, Endocarditis, and Vascular

An Acquired Chemotactic Defect in Neutrophils From Patients Receiving Interleukin-2 Immunotherapy

Klempner MS, Noring R, Mier JW, Atkins MB (New England Med Ctr, Boston; Tufts Univ)

N Engl J Med 322:959–965, 1990 1–1

Bacteremia occurs frequently in patients given interleukin-2 (IL-2) treatment with lymphokine-activated killer cells. Neutrophil function was evaluated in 31 such patients, most of whom had metastatic melanoma or renal cell carcinoma. None of the patients received concomitant chemotherapy. Maximum tolerated doses of IL-2 were given, alone or in conjunction with lymphokine-activated killer cells and/or interferon-alfa. Seven patients had bacterial sepsis and 1 died as a result.

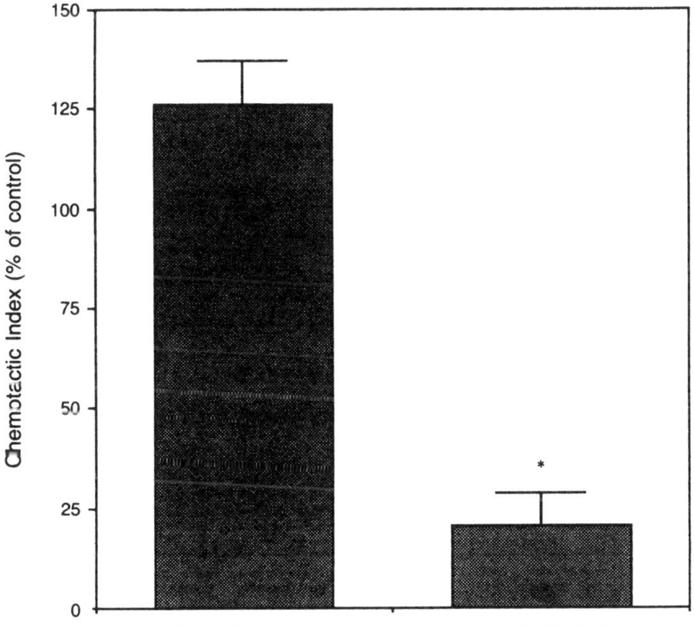

Fig 1–1.—Effect of IL-2 therapy on the chemotactic response of neutrophils to 10% zymosan-activated serum. Results are expressed as mean ± 1 SEM percentage of the chemotactic index in normal subjects (control) in neutrophils from 8 patients studied before and after IL-2 therapy. The *asterisk* indicates a significant difference ($P < .001$) in response at the end of the first course of IL-2 as compared with the pretreatment response. (Courtesy of Klempner MS, Noring R, Mier JW, et al: *N Engl J Med* 322:959–965, 1990.)

No patient was markedly neutropenic during the study. Initially, patient neutrophils were normal in assays of migration and chemotaxis and also with respect to superoxide production, phagocytosis, and bactericidal activity. Chemotaxis became significantly impaired by the end of the first course of IL-2 therapy (Fig 1–1). Chemotactic function improved after treatment but worsened again during a second course. Superoxide production and bactericidal activity remained normal.

Chemotactic activity is markedly but reversibly impaired by high-dose IL-2 treatment in patients with metastatic malignancy. This effect may contribute to morbidity from bacterial infection and, if this is the case, prophylactic antibiotics may well be beneficial. Antibiotics directed chiefly against *Staphylococcus aureus* and *Staphylococcus epidermidis* would be indicated.

▶ The high frequency of bacterial sepsis in patients receiving interleukin-2 (IL-2) therapy with or without lymphokine-activated killer cells was reported in the 1991 YEAR BOOK (1). In approximately 20% of all patients sepsis develops, usually catheter associated and Gram positive. These elegant studies by Klempner et al. document at least one important polymorphonuclear leukocyte defect in patients receiving IL-2. Although the mechanisms of this defect are not clear, clinicians need to be aware of this complication. Furthermore, presumably because of the acquired chemotactic defect, these patients have very high-grade bacteremia and require prolonged antibiotic therapy. Look for studies of antibiotic prophylaxis for these patients in the future. A high frequency of nonopportunistic bacterial infections has also been reported in patients with AIDS who receive IL-2 (2).—D.R. Snydman, M.D.

References

1. 1991 YEAR BOOK OF INFECTIOUS DISEASES, pp 271–273.
2. 1990 YEAR BOOK OF INFECTIOUS DISEASES, pp 213–214.

Treatment of Endocarditis Caused by Relatively Resistant Nonenterococcal Streptococci: Is Penicillin Enough?

DiNubile MJ (Univ of Medicine and Dentistry, Camden, NJ; Cooper Hosp/Univ Med Ctr, Camden)

Rev Infect Dis 12:112–117, 1990 1–2

In most patients with native valve and late prosthetic valve streptococcal endocarditis, infection is caused by nonenterococcal streptococci that are exquisitely responsive to short-term monotherapy with penicillin. Some nonenterococcal streptococci are relatively resistant to penicillin, as indicated by minimum inhibitory concentrations (MICs) of more than .1–.2 μg/mL but less than 1 μg/mL. Several have suggested that endocarditis caused by relatively resistant streptococci should be treated with a drug regimen similar to that used in patients with enterococcal endocarditis. These regimens, which involve administration for at least 4

Suggested Regimens for Treatment of Streptococcal Endocarditis

Cause of endocarditis	Antibiotic	Duration of therapy (w)
Nonenterococcal streptococci with MICs of <0.2 μg of penicillin/mL	Penicillin/aminoglycoside	4/2
	Penicillin/aminoglycoside	2/2
	Penicillin	4
All enterococci and those nonenterococcal streptococci with MICs of ⩾0.2 μg of penicillin/mL	Penicillin/aminoglycoside	4–6/2–6

(Courtesy of DiNubile MJ: *Rev Infect Dis* 12:112–117, 1990.)

weeks of both an aminoglycoside and high-dose penicillin, are potentially more toxic than the more flexible regimens used to treat exquisitely sensitive streptococci (table). However, data to support that recommendation are limited and inconclusive.

A review of the literature yielded 5 patients with endocarditis caused by relatively resistant nonenterococcal streptococci, with MICs of penicillin ranging between .19 and .63 μg/mL, who were treated successfully with short-term β-lactam antibiotics. Another 5 patients with endocarditis caused by nonenterococcal streptococci with MICs of between .19 and .78 μg of penicillin per mL were cured with a short-term penicillin and streptomycin regimen.

Because no conclusive reports of failures with penicillin monotherapy for relatively resistant streptococcal endocarditis were found in the literature, it is suggested that the standard regimens recommended for the treatment of endocarditis caused by exquisitely sensitive streptococci may also be effective for endocarditis caused by relatively resistant streptococci. However, all patients with streptococcal endocarditis are not alike, and no treatment can be expected to be universally successful.

▶ This is an excellent and balanced review of a difficult topic. The author recommends penicillin alone for most cases of native valve endocarditis caused by relative resistant streptococci (MIC, .1–.2 μg/mL). The duration of treatment suggested is that for highly susceptible strains, i.e., 4 weeks of penicillin alone. However, the author is careful to acknowledge that the database is extremely small, and that the decision to use the regimen must be individualized.—M.J. Barza, M.D.

Staphylococcus aureus **Bacteremia in Patients With Hickman Catheters**

Dugdale DC, Ramsey PG (Univ of Washington)

Am J Med 89:137–141, 1990 1–3

The long-term use of indwelling catheters has made delivery of medications and nutrition easier, but up to 30% of patients with Hickman catheters have infectious complications. Treatment strategies have been developed that are effective against *Staphylococcus epidermidis*, but there have been no studies to determine whether the same treatments will have the same effect against *S. aureus*. The charts of 37 patients with indwelling Hickman catheters and *S. aureus* bacteremia were studied and infections were classified according to whether they were cured without catheter removal, cured with catheter removal, progressed to death or relapse after initial "cure," or had indeterminate outcomes.

Three of the 6 deaths were caused by progressive catheter-related sepsis. The other 3 were not directly related to the catheter. Twenty-two episodes of *S. aureus* bacteremia were cured with antibiotics and removal of the catheter. Eighteen catheters were removed initially; 4 were removed only after relapse of bacteremia. Eight episodes of *S. aureus* bacteremia were cured without removal of the catheter.

Overall, only 18% of all Hickman-catheter-associated *S. aureus* bacteremias and only 10% of cases with exit-site infections were cured without removing the catheter. Seventeen percent of episodes ultimately resulted in bacteremic relapse or death. Patients most likely to have a satisfactory outcome had infections with a low blood culture colony count of less than 1 colony per mL. In the table the results of this study are compared with those of an earlier study by Press et al.

Hickman-catheter-associated bacteremias caused by *S. aureus* have a less favorable prognosis than do other bacteremias associated with this

Complication and Cure Rates Found Previously and in Current Study

	Type of Infection				
Outcome	**Tunnel**	**Exit Site**	**Catheter-Associated Bacteremia**	**BUO**	**Total**
[13]					
Catheter removed	2	1	2	0	5
Recurrence	0	0	0	0	0
Death	0	0	0	0	0
Cured without catheter removal	2	2	0	23	27
Total	4	3	2	23	32
Current study (indeterminate outcomes excluded)					
Catheter removed	9	6	6	0	21
Recurrence	0	3	0	1	4
Death	0	0	0	3	3
Cured without catheter removal	0	1	0	5	6
Total	9	10	6	9	34

Abbreviation: BUO, bacteremia of unknown origin.
Notes: Previous study shown at top of table. Figures represent number of cases.
(Courtesy of Dugdale DC, Ramsey PG: *Am J Med* 89:137–141, 1990.)

catheter. Clinicians should consider early removal of the catheter unless the focus of infection is remote and not catheter related, or there are no catheter-related physical signs and blood culture colony counts are less than 1/mL.

▶ Although this study may be cited as a reason to remove catheters associated with *S. aureus* bacteremia, I would hesitate to draw any firm conclusions. The investigation was retrospective, and there was no treatment protocol; therefore, the description of outcomes can be misleading. Of 37 patients, 22 were cured by catheter removal plus antibiotics, but in 18 of the 22 patients the catheter was removed as part of the initial treatment. This is hardly proof that the catheter had to be removed! Eight of the 18 catheters were removed because of the finding of tunnel infection: Such infections have been reported to respond poorly without catheter removal but, again, removal at the outset becomes self-justifying.—M.J. Barza, M.D.

Prevention of Bacteremia Attributed to Luminal Colonization of Tunneled Central Venous Catheters With Vancomycin-Susceptible Organisms

Schwartz C, Henrickson KJ, Roghmann K, Powell K (Univ of Rochester, NY)

J Clin Oncol 8:1591–1597, 1990 1–4

Bacteremias associated with the use of tunneled central venous catheters in immunocompromised patients with oncologic or hematologic disorders are a significant clinical problem. Bacteremia can be attributed either to dissemination of bacteria from cellulitis at the exit site into the bloodstream or to luminal colonization by commensal organisms from normal skin. In a double-blind, randomized study conducted to determine whether the addition of vancomycin to heparinized saline catheter flush solution would prevent bacteremia from luminal colonization of tunneled central venous catheters, 45 children (median age, 46 months) who required such catheters in the treatment of oncologic or hematologic disorders were randomly allocated to catheter flush solution containing heparin and vancomycin (21 children) or heparin (24 children) alone (Table 1). The total number of days of tunneled central venous catheter use

TABLE 1.—Patient Characteristics

	H-V	H	Total
No. of patients	21	24	45
No. of catheters	24	29	53
Median age in months (range)	46 (4-205)	46 (2-227)	46 (2-227)
Girls/boys	12/9	13/11	25/20
Total catheter days	4,792	6,303	11,095
Catheter days/patient (±SD)	228 ± 129	262 ± 150	247 ± 140

(Courtesy of Schwartz C, Henrickson KJ, Roghmann K, et al: *J Clin Oncol* 8:1591–1597, 1990.)

TABLE 2.—Bacteremia Attributed to Luminal Colonization

Bacteria Isolated	H-V	H
SSCN	0	5
Corynebacterium	0	1
K pneumoniae	1	0
E coli	0	1
Total	1	6*

*There were 6 episodes of bacteremia attributed to luminal colonization in 5 patients; 1 episode was a mixed infection with coagulase-negative *Staphylococcus* species *(SSCN)* and *Escherichia coli.*

(Courtesy of Schwartz C, Hendrickson KJ, Roghmann K, et al: *J Clin Oncol* 8:1591–1597, 1990.)

was 11,095 days, with an average of 247 catheter days per patient. The patients given heparin and vancomycin had a total of 24 catheter insertions during the course of the study; the patients allocated to receive heparin alone had 29 catheter insertions.

The patients who received heparin plus vancomycin underwent evaluation for suspected sepsis on 56 occasions, compared with 71 evaluations in the patients given heparin alone. The difference was not statistically significant. None of the patients receiving heparin plus vancomycin had bacteremia attributable to luminal colonization with vancomycin-susceptible organisms. In contrast, 5 patients receiving heparin alone had 6 bacteremic episodes in the course of the study. One patient treated with heparin alone had 2 episodes of bacteremia with a vancomycin-susceptible organism (Table 2). None of the patients with bacteremia had evidence of an exit-site infection. Bacteremias not attributable to luminal colonization, systemic fungal infections, exit-site cellulitis, and contaminated blood specimens occurred with equal frequency in both groups. None of the patients experienced vancomycin-related toxicity. The use of a heparin-vancomycin catheter flush solution in immunocompromised patients can decrease the frequency of bacteremia attributed to luminal colonization of tunneled central venous catheters with vancomycin-susceptible organisms.

▶ This provocative study is likely to be influential and may lead to the common use of vancomycin flushes for prophylaxis in patients with central venous catheters. It would be desirable to see other studies of the issue before the practice becomes widespread. A criticism of this study is that it was small. The authors argue that their approach is not likely to foster the emergence of resistant organisms because the drug is applied locally and in a high concentration rather than in the subtherapeutic concentrations that seem most prone to lead to resistance. Whether the drug actually prevented colonization of the catheter or simply suppressed bacterial growth to the point of minimizing infectious consequences was not answered by this study: too few catheters were cultured to allow a conclusion.—M.J. Barza, M.D.

Perivalvular Extension of Infection in Patients With Infectious Endocarditis

Carpenter JL (Univ of Texas, Dallas)

Rev Infect Dis 13:127–138, 1991 1–5

Perivalvular extension of infection (PVEI), a potentially fatal complication of bacterial endocarditis, causes difficulties in diagnosis. A selective review of published literature was carried out to assess the value of various diagnostic modalities (table).

The easiest diagnostic tool to use is the ECG. This method is readily available and is particularly valuable in detecting extension of the infection past the valve annulus into the myocardium or aorta. But ECG appears to be less sensitive than other modalities, except in detecting septal extension of infection.

Transthoracic 2-dimensional echocardiography, transesophageal echocardiography, and color-flow Doppler echocardiography are the most practical and useful echocardiographic techniques to apply to PVEI. The most invasive test used to diagnose PVEI is cardiac catheterization with angiography. This method can detect aneurysms (primarily of the sinus of Valsalva), valve dehiscence, and annular and periannular abscesses. But cardiac catheterization is more specific than sensitive and complications may occur. The utility of CT in the diagnosis of PVEI is not known;

Comparison of Utility of Different Diagnostic Modalities in the Detection of PVEI

Total no. of cases	No. with positive result/no. tested				
	ECG	2-D echocardiogram	Transesophageal echocardiogram	Cardiac catheterization	MRI
22	9/22	20/22			
9	5/9	9/9		5/6	
4	3/4	4/4		2/3	
5	2/5	5/5		3/3	
20		14/20		7/9	
14		11/14		4/6	
6		3/6		3/3	
3	3/3	3/3			
17		3/17	13/17		
3		0/3	3/3		
6	5/6			5/6	
4		0/3		4/4	
19	11/19			14/19	
6	1/6			5/6	
13	10/13			9/9	
3		0/3		0/3	
3		0/3		1/1	3/3

(Courtesy of Carpenter JL: *Rev Infect Dis* 13:127–138, 1991.)

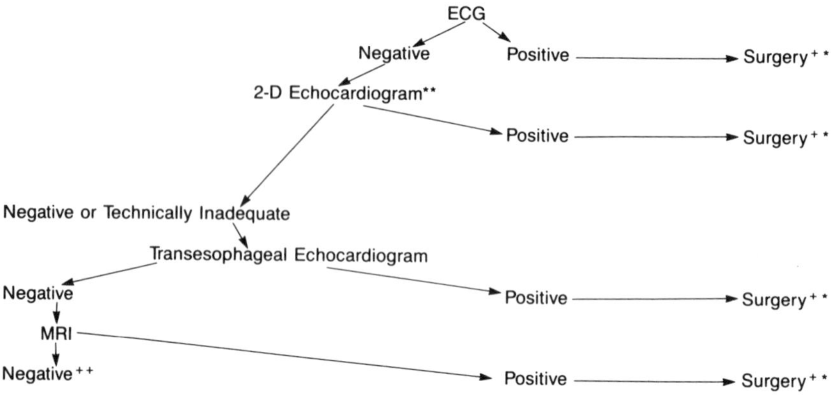

Fig 1–2.—Proposed approach to diagnosis of PVEI. +, if surgery is not elected, patient should be treated as though perivalvular abscess is definitely present; *, cardiac catheterization may be desired by cardio-vascular surgeon before surgery; **, ideally with Doppler, color Doppler, contrast 2-D echocardiogram; ++, medical therapy or cardiac catheterization. (Courtesy of Carpenter JL: *Rev Infect Dis* 13:127–138, 1991.)

studies on the use of MRI appear encouraging. Data on radionuceotide imaging with either gallium or indium are as yet inconclusive.

The optimal approach to the diagnosis of PVEI has not been determined, yet the various available studies do offer a reasonable approach. An initial ECG is recommended for all patients with endocarditis. Serial ECGs should be performed if prosthetic valve endocarditis occurs. Another standard procedure in the patient with endocarditis is the 2-D echocardiogram. Greater sensitivity is achieved with Doppler, color Doppler, or contrast echocardiography. Transesophageal echocardiography should be performed if other types of echocardiography yield negative results. If these studies are inconclusive, the next option to consider is MRI. Cardiac catheterization can be performed if the issue of PVEI is still unresolved after MRI (Fig 1–2).

▶ As we refine imaging techniques, one of the first infectious disease applications is to see whether the technique will better resolve the question of the presence of endocarditis and/or its applications. Carpenter reviews the diagnostic approach to patients with perivalvular extension of their endocarditis. The review, however, may already be somewhat dated, because a recent paper by Daniel et al. in the *New England Journal of Medicine* (1) enforces the growing impression that the transesophageal echocardiogram is an excellent diagnostic technique to detect this complication. In this most recent study, the positive and negative predictive values for transesophageal echo were 90.9% and 92.1%, respectively. As with all evolving technologies, these numbers are highly dependent on the skill of the operator, and this test will probably not perform as well in the hands of inexperienced investigators.—M.S. Klempner, M.D.

Reference

1. Daniel WG, et al: *N Engl J Med* 324:795, 1991.

Initial Evaluation of Human Monoclonal Anti-Lipid A Antibody (HA-1A) in Patients With Sepsis Syndrome

Fisher CJ Jr, Zimmerman J, Khazaeli MB, Albertson TE, Dellinger RP, Panacek EA, Foulke GE, Dating C, Smith CR, LoBuglio AF (Case Western Reserve Univ; Baylor College of Medicine, Houston; Univ of California, Davis Med Ctr, Sacramento; Univ of Alabama, Birmingham; Centocor, Malvern, Pa)

Crit Care Med 18:1311–1315, 1990 1–6

A human monoclonal IgM antibody that binds specifically to the lipid A domain of endotoxin is known as HA-1A. Its immunogenicity and safety were examined in septic patients highly suspected of having gram-negative bacterial infection. Thirty-four patients received an infusion of 25, 100, or 250 mg of HA-1A in .3 M saline solution with sodium phosphate and were followed for 2 to 3 weeks.

The patients were severely ill, and nearly 60% were found to have gram-negative bacterial infection. Treatment was well tolerated, with no evidence of toxicity at any dose level. Serum binding activity did not change significantly after administration of HA-1A. The pharmacokinetics were well described by a single compartment model with a mean serum half-life of 16 hours. Neither the serum clearance of HA-1A nor the volume of distribution changed significantly according to the dose administered or the presence of gram-negative bacterial infection. Administration of HA-1A to severely septic patients is safe and nonimmunogenic.

▶ Ever since the initial studies of Ziegler and his colleagues (1) showing that a polyclonal antiserum to the J-5 mutant of *Escherichia coli* was effective in reducing mortality from gram-negative sepsis, we have awaited a monoclonal antibody. These initial studies suggest that the monoclonal antibody is safe. Large-scale trials have been finished, and I am sure they will be reviewed in the 1993 YEAR BOOK.—S.M. Wolff, M.D.

Reference

1. Ziegler EJ, et al: *N Engl J Med* 307:1225, 1982.

Elevated von Willebrand Factor Antigen Is an Early Plasma Predictor of Acute Lung Injury in Nonpulmonary Sepsis Syndrome

Rubin DB, Wiener-Kronish JP, Murray JF, Green DR, Turner J, Luce JM, Montgomery AB, Marks JD, Matthay MA (Univ of California, San Francisco; Rush Presbyterian-St Luke's Med Ctr, Chicago; Northwestern Univ)

J Clin Invest 86:474–480, 1990 1–7

Endotoxemia and bacteremia cause injury to endothelial cells, and von Willebrand factor antigen (vWf-Ag) is a sensitive marker of endothelial cell injury. To determine whether markedly elevated levels of plasma vWf-Ag in patients with nonpulmonary sepsis syndrome might predict the occurrence of acute lung injury, 45 patients with sepsis syndrome who had no evidence of lung injury were tested. The assessment of acute

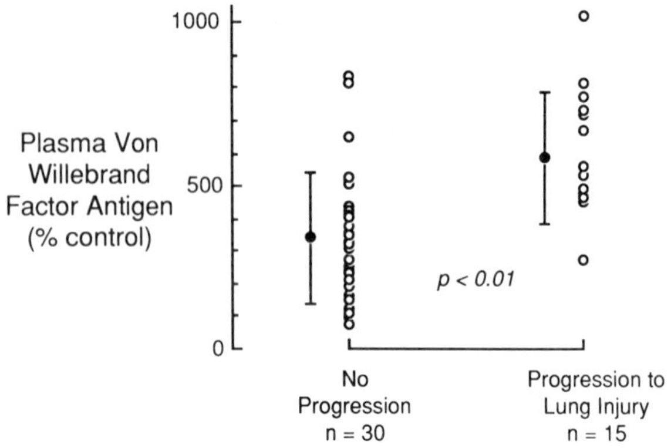

Fig 1–3.—Individual data points represent plasma level of vWf-Ag (percentage of control) measured at time of entry into study. Thirty patients who did not have lung injury comprised group I and 15 patients who did have lung injury made up group II. (Courtesy of Rubin DB, Wiener-Kronish JP, Murray JF, et al: *J Clin Invest* 86:474–480, 1990.)

lung injury was based on a composite 4-point scoring system for rating chest radiographs, arterial oxygenation, compliance of the respiratory system, and positive end-expiratory pressure in intubated and mechanically ventilated patients. Plasma levels of vWf-Ag were expressed as a percentage of control values.

Acute lung injury occurred in 15 patients with nonpulmonary sepsis syndrome. The mean plasma level of vWf-Ag in these 15 was 588 (percentage of control), compared with a mean plasma level of vWf-Ag of 338 in the 30 patients who did not have lung injury (Fig 1–3).

When a plasma level of vWf-Ag of 450 or greater was used as the cutoff, the test had an 87% sensitivity and a 77% specificity for predicting the occurrence of acute lung injury in patients with nonpulmonary sepsis. The combination of a plasma level of vWf-Ag of more than 450 and nonpulmonary organ failure at the time of entry into the study had a positive predictive value of 80% for acute lung injury. The test was also significantly predictive of mortality when the same plasma level of vWf-Ag was used as the cutoff level. In patients with nonpulmonary sepsis, an elevated plasma level of vWf-Ag has predictive value for the occurrence of acute lung injury and prognostic value for survival.

▶ Defining predictive markers of upcoming morbid events is important for studies of interventions to avert these events. For example, many of the ongoing studies in AIDS patients are predicated on events that are predicted to occur on the basis of CD4 cell counts. In patients with sepsis, there have not been good predictors of those who will progress to acute respiratory distress syndrome and lung injury. Von Willebrand factor is produced by endothelial cells in response to noxious stimuli. In this paper, the authors demonstrate that the combination of a high plasma level of vWf and failure of at least 1 nonpulmonary organ is a good positive predictor of the development of lung injury (>80% positive predictive value). If acute lung injury did develop in patients with another organ failure and a high level of vWf, all of the patients died. Further refinements in this test may make it clinically useful, and I suspect it will be helpful as intervention studies are planned.—M.S. Klempner, M.D.

Blood Culture Phlebotomy: Switching Needles Does Not Prevent Contamination
Krumholz HM, Cummings S, York M (Univ of California, San Francisco)
Ann Intern Med 113:290–292, 1990 1–8

Needle-stick injuries are an important source of infection in health care workers. Because recapping needles is the most common cause of accidental puncture, many institutions presently urge health care workers not to recap needles. However, the technique for blood culturing still requires changing to a sterile needle after venipuncture and before inoculating culture media to avoid contamination with the patient's skin flora.

To determine the validity of switching needles after venipuncture for blood culture, 34 experienced phlebotomists were randomly assigned to use the conventional needle-switching technique and 38 to use inoculated culture media without switching to a sterile needle. A total of 917 blood cultures were collected, 462 by the conventional needle-switching technique and 451 by the no-switch technique. More than 90% of the cultures in each group were collected from arm venipuncture sites.

Twenty-nine of 462 cultures obtained with the switch technique (18%) were positive and 6 (1.30%) were considered to be skin flora contaminations. Forty-one of 451 cultures obtained by the no-switch technique (23%) were positive and 7 (1.55%) were skin flora contaminations. The difference was not statistically significant.

Switching needles after venipuncture for blood culture does not reduce the rate of skin flora contamination. In view of the increased risk for needle-stick injury associated with switching needles in the conventional blood culture technique, this practice should be abandoned.

▶ This is an important and well-done study. The result is persuasive. The authors make the unqualified recommendation that the technique of switching needles should be abandoned because it has no advantages and is more expensive, more time consuming, and more likely to lead to a needle-stick injury.—M.J. Barza, M.D.

Prolonged Bacteremia With Catheter-Related Central Venous Thrombosis
Rupar DG, Herzog KD, Fisher MC, Long SS (St Christopher's Hosp for Children, Philadelphia; Temple Univ)
Am J Dis Child 144:879–882, 1990 1–9

Venous thrombosis with infection is a rarely recognized complication of the use of central venous catheters in children. Data were reviewed on 7 children with central venous catheters in whom serious catheter-related infections developed.

All 7 children had signs and symptoms of persistent bacteremia or candidemia, but only 1 had clinical evidence of venous obstruction. Bacteremia or candidemia persisted for 6–35 days (median, 8 days). Blood cultures remained positive for a median of 6 days after beginning appropri-

Microbiologic and Imaging Data, Treatment, and Outcome of Patients

Patient No./ Organism	No. of Positive Blood Cultures	Days of Bacteremia, Total*/ Antibiotic Therapy†/ Catheter Removal‡	Results of Ultrasound of Thrombus, Day§/ Site or Outcome	Antibiotic Therapy (No. of Days)	Outcome
1/*Candida albicans*	6	6/6/5	13/IVC; 33/decreased	Amphotericin B (35) and flucytosine (28)	Recovered
2/*Enterococcus* species	8	8/5/0	7/SVC; 17/unchanged	Ampicillin (33) and gentamicin sulfate (27)	Recovered
3/*Staphylococcus aureus*	4	8/8/8	3/SVC	Vancomycin hydrochloride (28)	Heparin therapy; thrombectomy on day 23; died on day 66
4/*Enterococcus* species	7	9/9/5	2/SVC	Vancomycin/ampicillin (23) and gentamicin (23)	Died on day 23
5/*Candida tropicalis*	6	6/3/6	5/Internal jugular vein	Amphotericin B (27)	Venogram showed SVC, subclavian, internal jugular vein obstruction; heparin therapy; recovered
6/*C albicans*	5	7/3/7	9/SVC into the atrium; 19/Unchanged; 36/Unchanged	Amphotericin B (32) and flucytosine (28)	Recovered
7/*Corynebacterium* species	11	35/32/0	2/SVC into the atrium	Vancomycin (62)	Recovered

Abbreviations: IVC, inferior vena cava; *SVC,* superior vena cava.
*Time from first to last positive blood culture.
†Time from starting appropriate antibiotic therapy to last positive blood culture.
‡Time from removal of catheter to last positive blood culture.
§Time after removal of catheter.
(Courtesy of Rupar DG, Herzog KD, Fisher MC, et al: *Am J Dis Child* 144:879–882, 1990.)

ate antimicrobial therapy and for a median of 5 days after removal of the catheter (table). Central venous thrombosis was demonstrated by ultrasonography in all patients after removal of the catheter. Antibiotics were administered parenterally for longer than 28 days to 6 patients, and heparin was administered to 3. Although 2 patients died, neither death was attributed to infection.

Venous thrombosis with infection should be suspected in children with central venous catheters and persistent bacteremia. Clinical clues to the diagnosis of catheter-related complications are frequently subtle or absent, but ultrasonography may prove helpful in the diagnosis. The optimal treatment of prolonged bacteremia with catheter-related central venous thrombosis is not yet known.

▶ The major message of this article is that thrombosis of the central veins in pediatric patients with catheter-related infections not only predisposes to more prolonged bacteremia or fungemia than in patients without thrombosis, but may be otherwise occult, i.e., there may be no malfunction of the catheter. The diagnosis can be made by ultrasound. The optimum treatment, including the use of anticoagulants, is not clear. There is currently a tendency to try to preserve the catheter in patients with catheter-related infections (not recommended for fungal or gram-negative bacillary infections). The authors endorse this approach but suggest that, if the clinical signs do not resolve and blood cultures become negative within 3 days of the beginning of antimicrobial treatment, the catheter should be removed. If bacteremia persists for another 3 days after catheter removal, the authors recommend ultrasonography to detect thrombosis of the great vessels. If the ultrasound is positive, they treat the patient for at least 2 weeks after removal of the catheter and sterilization of the blood stream on the assumption that the infection is akin to endocarditis.—M.J. Barza, M.D.

Gastrointestinal Tract

Empiric Antimicrobial Therapy of Domestically Acquired Acute Diarrhea in Urban Adults

Goodman LJ, Trenholme GM, Kaplan RL, Segreti J, Hines D, Petrak R, Nelson JA, Mayer KW, Landau W, Parkhurst GW, Levin S (Rush-Presbyterian-St Luke's Med Ctr, Chicago; Grant Hosp, Chicago; MacNeal Hosp, Berwyn, Ill)
Arch Intern Med 150:541–546, 1990 1–10

Empirical antimicrobial therapy for acute diarrhea is generally limited to patients with signs of invasive pathogens (e.g., fever and moderate to severe illness). Because empirical antibiotic therapy shortens the duration and severity of diarrhea in patients with traveler's diarrhea, it was postulated that the same treatment would likewise be useful in patients with domestically acquired acute diarrhea. To test this hypothesis, 202 adult non–travelers with acute diarrhea received ciprofloxacin (500 mg), sulfamethoxazole and trimethoprim (160 mg/800 mg), or placebo in a randomized, double-blind fashion. Treatment was started on the day of presentation and given twice daily for 5 days.

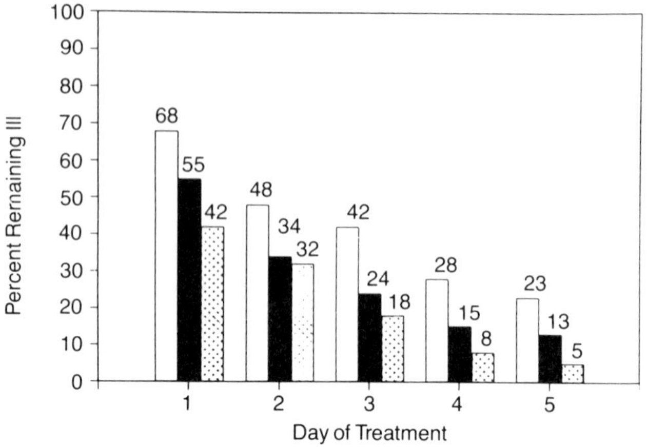

Fig 1–4.—Percentage of patients remaining ill on treatment days 1 through 5 among those who received ciprofloxacin *(speckled bars)*, sulfamethoxazole and trimethoprim *(filled bars)*, and placebo *(open bars)*. Percentage of patients remaining ill excludes those who were well or improved. Differences between placebo and ciprofloxacin were significant on days 1, 3, 4, and 5. (Courtesy of Goodman LJ, Trenholme GM, Kaplan RL, et al: *Arch Intern Med* 150:541–546, 1990.)

The most common pathogens were *Campylobacter, Shigella,* and *Salmonella.* Figure 1–4 shows the clinical response to therapy for all 173 assessable patients based on information collected from patient diaries and from physician evaluation. Ciprofloxacin was significantly more effective than sulfamethoxazole and trimethoprim or placebo in eradicating these pathogens from the stools (table). Compared with placebo-treated patients, those who received ciprofloxacin had a significant shorter duration of illness and better clinical response (cured or improved) by days 1, 3, 4, and 5 of treatment. These differences were not apparent in the sulfamethoxazole and trimethoprim-treated group.

Ciprofloxacin shortens the duration of illness in adult non–travelers with acute diarrhea and is more effective than trimethoprim and sul-

Microbiologic Response to Therapy for 61 Bacterial Enteric Pathogens

		Treatment Group*		
Pathogen	**No. of Isolates**	**Ciprofloxacin**	**Sulfamethoxazole and Trimethoprim**	**Placebo**
Campylobacter	32	8/2	7/7	2/6
Shigella	16	4/1	4/3	1/3
Salmonella	13	2/0	1/3	1/6
Total	**61**	**14/3†**	**12/13**	**4/15**

*Number cured vs. number failed or relapsed.

†$P < .001$ when compared with sulfamethoxazole and trimethoprim group and with placebo group.

(Courtesy of Goodman LJ, Trenholme GM, Kaplan RL, et al: *Arch Intern Med* 150:541–546, 1990.)

famethoxazole in eradicating the most common bacterial pathogens from the stool. Further studies in a broader population group are necessary to define the role of empirical antibiotic treatment in domestically acquired acute diarrhea.

▶ The results of this study are likely to be applicable to adult ambulatory patients in urban areas of the United States. Patients with known HIV infection were excluded. It is noteworthy that only 68 of 134 patients (51%) had infection caused by *Salmonella, Shigella,* or *Campylobacter* sp. Most of the others had diarrhea of unknown cause. Patients from whom 1 of these 3 bacterial species was isolated had fecal leukocytes significantly more often (77% vs 37%; $P < .001$) and had a higher diarrheal index score than other patients had, but they could not be identified on other grounds. Moreover, it was difficult to distinguish among the "big 3" bacterial pathogens except by culture results. Overall, ciprofloxacin was significantly beneficial in reducing the duration of diarrhea and, importantly in some situations, eliminating the bacterial pathogens from the stool. Interestingly, attempts to find subsets of patients who would benefit particularly from the treatment (e.g., those with fecal leukocytes) were unsuccessful. Despite these findings, the authors do not recommend treatment for all patients with diarrhea but restrict the indication to those with signs of an invasive pathogen, i.e., with fever, fecal leukocytes, and moderate to severe illness.—M.J. Barza, M.D.

Failure of Ciprofloxacin to Eradicate Convalescent Fecal Excretion After Acute Salmonellosis: Experience During an Outbreak in Health Care Workers

Neill MA, Opal SM, Heelan J, Giusti R, Cassidy JE, White R, Mayer KH (Brown Univ; Hosp of Rhode Island, Pawtucket; Ctrs for Disease Control, Atlanta)
Ann Intern Med 114:195–199, 1991 1–11

Enteric infection with nontyphoidal salmonellae is increasing in the United States. Convalescent fecal excretion of nontyphoidal salmonellae may last for several weeks after acute infection. The effectiveness of ciprofloxacin treatment in eradicating such excretion was determined in 15 health care workers with acute *Salmonella java* infection. Eight patients were randomly asigned to receive ciprofloxacin, 750 mg, and 7 were given placebo beginning on the ninth day after infection. Both ciprofloxacin and placebo were given orally twice a day for 14 days. Stool cultures were obtained every 3 days initially, then weekly for 3 weeks.

All 8 patients in the treatment group had eradication of *S. java* from stool cultures within 7 days of beginning treatment, compared with only 1 of the 7 placebo recipients. Stool cultures in the treatment group remained negative up to 14 days after treatment was discontinued. However, 4 patients relapsed. Their stool cultures became positive 14–21 days after therapy. Also, all 3 hospitalized patients treated with ciprofloxacin who did not participate in the trial relapsed. The total relapse rate was therefore 64%. In 4 of the 7 patients who relapsed, the relapse was associated with a longer duration of fecal excretion of salmonellae than in placebo recipients. Relapse could not be attributed to noncompliance, development of resistance, or the presence of biliary disease.

Despite its excellent antimicrobial activity against salmonellae and its favorable pharmacokinetic profile, ciprofloxacin at the dosage given in this trial has an unacceptably high failure rate in patients with acute salmonellosis. It may prolong fecal excretion of salmonellae. The late occurrence of relapses indicates the need for stool culture follow-up for 21 days after therapy.

▶ This small study of convalescent excretors should serve as a caution that treatment with ciprofloxacin may produce a high bacteriologic relapse rate and prolonged excretion of salmonellae. In other studies of patients with acute salmonellosis, bacteriologic relapse has occurred in 4 of 16 patients and 2 of 9 patients treated with ciprofloxacin. Taken together, these data suggest that ciprofloxacin, like other antimicrobial agents, should be used selectively in patients with acute *Salmonella* gastroenteritis because of the risk of relapse and prolonged excretion of the organisms. In contrast to the results of the present study, at least 2 other small studies have shown an excellent ability of ciprofloxacin to eradicate chronic carriage of *Salmonella typhi*. Further investigations of the issue are needed to discern the reasons for these apparent differences in outcome.—M.J. Barza, M.D.

Quinolone Antibiotics in the Treatment of *Salmonella* Infections

Asperilla MO, Smego RA Jr, Scott LK (Albany Med College, NY)

Rev Infect Dis 12:873–889, 1990 1–12

Salmonella infections have commonly been treated with ampicillin, chloramphenicol, and trimethoprim-sulfamethoxazole. However, the increasing incidence of drug-resistant and multiresistant *Salmonella* isolates led to the search for newer agents having clinical activity against these resistant organisms. Fluoroquinolones are potent synthetic antimicrobials with proved in vitro efficacy against enteric pathogens. To assess the clinical efficacy of fluoroquinolone antibiotics in the treatment of *Salmonella* infections, studies that evaluated these antibiotics were identified with a computerized MEDLINE search. Patients were included if they had invasive *Salmonella* infection or chronic intestinal carriage of *Salmonella* and had been treated with fluoroquinolone antibiotics, including norfloxacin, ofloxacin, pefloxacin, fleroxacin, or ciprofloxacin.

Analysis of the data confirmed the clinical efficacy of the fluoroquinolones against drug-sensitive and multiresistant strains of *Salmonella*. Although the older antimicrobials generally had little impact on the duration of symptomatic illness in *Salmonella* enterocolitis, the fluoroquinolones alleviated and shortened the course of clinical disease and terminated excretion of organisms in stool. Furthermore, the fluoroquinolones eradicated biliary and fecal reservoirs of infection in chronic *Salmonella* carriers more effectively than did conventional antimicrobials. In both immunocompetent and immunocompromised patients with bacteremia and metastatic infections caused by *Salmonella,* treatment with a fluoroquinolone antimicrobial was more effective and better tolerated than treatment with conventional antimicrobials. The optimal dose and duration of treatment for fluoroquinolone antimicrobials need to be determined in controlled clinical trials.

▶ A thorough review of this subject. The authors speculate, as others have speculated, that the good efficacy of the fluoroquinolones in *Salmonella* infections may relate to their excellent penetration of phagocytic cells in which these intracellular pathogens reside. Their enthusiasm may be tempered by the article by Neill et al. (see Abstract 1–11).—M.J. Barza, M.D.

Characterization and Description of *"Campylobacter upsaliensis"* Isolated From Human Feces

Goossens H, Pot B, Vlaes L, van den Borre C, van den Abbeele R, van Naelten C, Levy J, Cogniau H, Marbehant P, Verhoef J, Kersters K, Butzler J-P, Vandamme P (St Pieters Univ Hosp, Brussels; Rijksuniversiteit, Gent, Belgium; Univ of Utrecht, The Netherlands)

J Clin Microbiol 28:1039–1046, 1990 1–13

A catalase-negative or weakly positive strain of *Campylobacter,* named *Campylobacter upsaliensis,* was first isolated from dogs in 1986. Hybridization of DNA showed that these organisms represented a new *Campylobacter* species. However, neither the species name nor the type strain has standing in the literature as its description was not published in a peer-reviewed journal. *Campylobacter upsaliensis* has since been recovered from adults and children in the United States, Canada, and Australia.

During a 3-year period, 15,185 stool specimens were cultured for *Campylobacter* species. *Campylobacter* isolates that were catalase-negative or weakly positive, or that could not be identified by biotyping, were further characterized phenotypically and were finally identified by protein electrophoresis. Organisms resembling *Campylobacter* strains were isolated from 802 patients, 753 of which could be identified further, including 99 isolates identified as *C. upsaliensis.*

Phenotypic characterization and computerized numerical analysis of the protein electrophoregrams showed that *C. upsaliensis* is a distinct *Campylobacter* species with unique characteristics (table). In vitro antibiotic susceptibility testing of these strains showed that *C. upsaliensis* is generally susceptible to ampicillin, gentamicin, chloramphenicol, and tetracycline. Ten strains were resistant to erythromycin. Plasmid DNA was detectable in 89 of the 99 strains. Sixteen plasmid profiles were identified. Bactericidal assay and phagocytosis studies of 8 representative strains of *C. upsaliensis* showed that this strain has activity similar to that of *Campylobacter jejuni.*

▶ In this report, weakly catalase-positive *Campylobacter* species were characterized and found to be biochemically similar and consistent with a distinct spe-

Phenotypic Characteristics of 99 "*C. upsaliensis*" Strains Isolated From Human Feces and *Campylobacter* Reference and Type Strains*

Characteristic	% of the 99 tested "*C. upsaliensis*" strains that were positive	"*C. upsaliensis*" LMG 8850†	*C. jejuni* subsp. *jejuni* LMG 6444^T	*C. jejuni* subsp. *doylei* LMG 8843^T	*C. coli* LMG 6440^T	*C. laridis* LMG 8846^T	*C. hyointestinalis* LMG 7817^T	*C. fetus* subsp. *fetus* LMG 6442^T
Oxidase	100	+	+	+	+	+	+	+
Catalase	100‡	+‡	+	+	+	+	+	+
Urease	0	−	−	−	−	−	−	−
Nitrate reduced to nitrite	100	+	+	−	+	+	+	+
H_2S production								
TSI slant	0	−	−	−	+	−	+	−
FBP agar	0	−	−	−	−	+	+	−
Growth at:								
25°C	0	−	−	−	−	−	+‡	+
42°C	81	+	+	+	+	+	+	+
Growth in:								
1% Glycine	61	+	+	+	+	+	+	+
1% Oxgall	80	−	+	+	+	+	+	+
3.5% NaCl	2	−	−	−	−	−	−	−
1.5% NaCl	0	−	−	−	−	+	−	−
Growth on 0.04% TTC	0	−	+	−	+	−	−	−
Anaerobic growth in 0.1% TMAO	0	−	−	−	−	+	+	−
Hippurate hydrolysis	0	−	+	+	−	−	−	−
Susceptibility § to:								
Nalidixic acid	100	S	S	S	S	R	R	R
Cephalothin	100	S	R	S	R	R	S	S
DNase	0	−	−	−	−	−	−	−
Indoxyl acetate hydrolysis	100	+	+	+	+	−	−	−

*Type strains are indicated by a superscript T.
†Reference strain from Sandstedt K, Ursing J, Walder M: *Curr Microbiol* 8:209–213, 1983.
‡Weak reaction.
§*Abbreviations: S,* susceptible; *R,* resistant.
(Courtesy of Goossens H, Pot B, Vlaes L, et al: *J Clin Microbiol* 28:1039–1046, 1990.)

cies previously proposed as *C. upsaliensis*. The data in this paper substantiate that proposal and should lead to acceptance of *C. upsaliensis* as a distinct species. It appears to be associated with human diarrhea; however, the epidemiology and clinical significance remain to be fully described. This will, no doubt, be easier with defined criteria for identification.—G.T. Keusch, M.D.

Toxin A of *Clostridium difficile* Is a Potent Cytotoxin

Tucker KD, Carrig PE, Wilkins TD (Virginia Polytechnic Inst and State Univ, Blacksburg)

J Clin Microbiol 28:869–871, 1990 1–14

Clostridium difficile causes antibiotic-associated colitis in humans. The organism produces 2 toxins, A and B. Toxin B is one of the most potent cytotoxins known, but it is not thought to be responsible for most of the symptoms of pseudomembranous colitis. Toxin A, reported to have slight cytotoxic activity and generally known as the enterotoxin, appears to cause the diarrhea and destruction of the colonic mucosa that is characteristic of the disease. Some cell lines are much more sensitive to toxin A than those that have been tested previously.

Clostridium difficile VPI 10463 was grown in brain heart infusion dialysis flasks. Purification of toxin A was performed by affinity chromatography that used immobilized bovine thryoglobulin. Toxin B was purified by ion-exchange chromatography on DEAE-Sepharose CL-6B and immunoadsorption. Cell lines that expressed the trisaccharide to which toxin A binds would, it was hypothesized, be more sensitive to the toxin than other cell lines.

This hypothesis was supported by results of the experiments. Cell lines (F9, OTF9-63, and P19), which express the toxin A receptor, are more sensitive to the toxin. The cytotoxic responses of cells to toxin A appear to be almost identical to the responses to toxin B. The cytotoxicity assay, when performed with any of these 3 cell lines, is the most sensitive test for the toxin so far reported.

These cell lines should be of use to physicians seeking to determine levels of biologically active toxin A. The standard to which other methods of diagnosis of *C. difficile* colitis are compared is the cytotoxicity assay for toxin B in feces. If it could be shown that levels of active toxin A correlate better with the clinical course of the patient than levels of toxin B, then assays for toxin A could be developed for routine use.

▶ The state of the art of *C. difficile* colitis is that the toxicity assayed in routine cell culture, toxin B, is not the toxicity responsible for antibiotic colitis; rather, it serves as a surrogate marker. Presumably, it is for this reason that false negative stool toxin assays are obtained, and a simple assay for toxin A has been sought. In this study, Tucker et al. colected tissue culture cell types expressing the receptor trisaccharide for toxin A, Galα1->3Galβ1->4GlcNAc, and found that the cytotoxicity of toxin A was 100-fold increased compared to its effects in CHO cells. With the greater sensitivity of the assay using the described cell lines, and the inclusion of antibody to neutralize toxin B, a toxin A specific cell culture assay is quite feasible. Studies to determine whether this test correlates better with clinical events in antibiotic colitis than the standard tissue culture assay will be the obvious clinical payoff, and I would be very surprised if this were not in fact being done by the authors. If this proves to be the case, a very useful and simple test will be available to the clinician.—G.T. Keusch, M.D.

Escherichia coli O157:H7 and the Hemolytic Uremic Syndrome: Importance of Early Cultures in Establishing the Etiology

Tarr PI, Neill MA, Clausen CR, Watkins SL, Christie DL, Hickman RO (Univ of Washington; Children's Hosp and Med Ctr, Seattle; Brown Univ)

J Infect Dis 162:553–556, 1990 1–15

Escherichia coli capable of producing Shiga-like toxins (SLT) have recently been identified as etiologic agents in most patients with hemolytic uremic syndrome (HUS). The most common serotype of SLT-producing *E. coli* isolated from stools of patients with HUS with antecedent diarrhea in the United States is *E. coli* O157:H7, although the rate of its recovery has varied considerably. *Escherichia coli* O157:H7 has been found in stools of 58% of patients from Seattle, but in only 7.5% of patients from Toronto.

To determine the cause of HUS, studies were made in 52 patients (mean age, 14 years) with HUS and antecedent diarrhea. The HUS was diagnosed an average of 6.5 days after the onset of diarrhea. Most patients (77%) received erythrocyte or platelet transfusions, and more than half (58%) required dialysis because of acute renal failure; 4 patients died.

There were 33 positive and 4 probable *E. coli* O157:H7 infections. Culture-positive patients were significantly more likely than culture-negative patients to have had bloody diarrhea or fecal leukocytes, or to have required blood transfusions during their episode of HUS. *Escherichia coli* O157:H7 was isolated from stools collected significantly earlier in the ill-

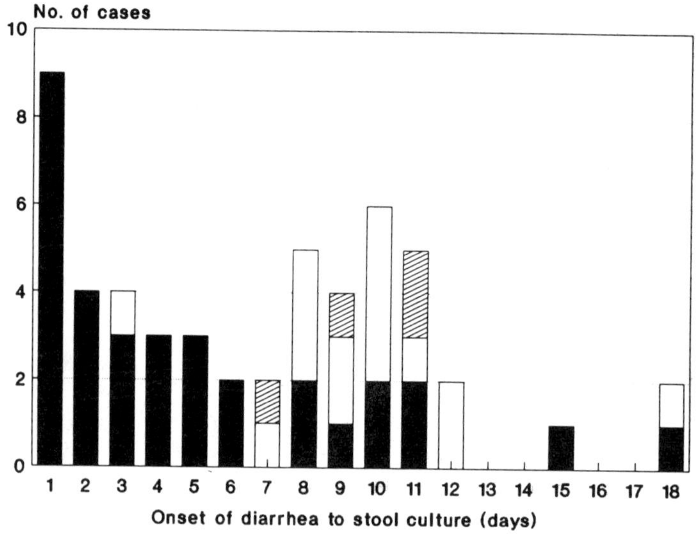

Fig 1–5.—Recovery of *Escherichia coli* O157:H7 by days between onset of diarrhea and collection of stool for culture in 52 patients with HUS. *Filled bars* indicate culture-positive; *open bars*, culture-negative; *hatched bars*, culture-negative patients with HUS previously in group setting with culture-positive patients with HUS. (Courtesy of Tarr PI, Neill MA, Clausen CR, et al: *J Infect Dis* 162:553–556, 1990.)

ness (Fig 1–5). When stools were collected within 2 days of the onset of diarrhea, the isolation rate of *E. coli* O157:H7 was 100%.

In this series, *E. coli* O157:H7 appeared to be the predominant cause of HUS preceded by diarrhea. Stool cultures of all patients with acute bloody diarrhea should be cultured for this organism to identify those at risk for the development of HUS. For the pathogen to be recovered, stool cultures should be obtained within 6 days of diarrhea.

▶ The leading cause of acute renal failure in children in the United States has become HUS, caused almost exclusively by *E. coli* producing Shiga-like toxins. Although it is not yet established that early treatment and eradication of the causative organism reduce the incidence (or possibly the severity) of HUS by interrupting the production of the toxins believed to be involved in pathogenesis, this is a major presumption underlying the desire for early diagnosis. This paper demonstrates that culture methods for *E. coli* O157:H7 are most efficient within the first few days of diarrhea, several days before HUS develops, and that the yield of positive cultures for this organism diminishes thereafter. Because O157:H7 is not the only serotype involved in pathogenesis of HUS but is the most readily diagnosed in the routine microbiology laboratory, early diagnosis may be difficult. This would be facilitated by the use of gene probes for virulence factors or methods to detect the toxins themselves. It should also be mentioned that some workers have suggested that the use of certain antibiotics (in particular, trimethoprim-sulfamethoxazole) in treatment of the diarrhea preceding HUS may actually be a risk factor for the disease. However, the more logical explanation at this time is that patients receiving antibiotics are more severely ill and therefore at greater risk of complications.—G.T. Keusch, M.D.

Genitourinary

Asymptomatic Bacteriuria in Patients With Diabetes Mellitus

Zhanel GG, Harding GKM, Nicolle LE (Univ of Manitoba; St Boniface Gen Hosp, Winnipeg, Man)

Rev Infect Dis 13:150–154, 1991 1–16

The prevalence of asymptomatic bacteriuria is threefold higher among diabetic than among nondiabetic women, but rates among diabetic and nondiabetic men are comparable. The prevalence of asymptomatic bacteriuria is not affected by the type or duration of diabetes or the quality of diabetic control. The microorganisms that cause asymptomatic bacteriuria in persons with diabetes are similar to those that cause it in nondiabetic persons. Upper urinary tract involvement occurs in more than half of the diabetic patients with asymptomatic bacteriuria.

The long-term consequences of asymptomatic bacteriuria in diabetic persons have not been well documented. Clinical trials suggest that a 2-week course of treatment is equivalent to a 6-week course for the initial eradication of bacteriuria. After treatment, reinfection rather than relapse usually occurs.

Many important questions remain about asymptomatic bacteriuria in patients with diabetes. The appropriate management of this problem is not clear. Further research is needed to determine whether and when antimicrobial treatment should be given and to characterize the natural history of untreated asymptomatic bacteriuria in this patient population.

▶ This "meta-analysis" shows an increased rate of asymptomatic bacteriuria among diabetic women. As in most bacteriuric populations, the indications for treatment are obscure. Given that about half of the patients have microbiological evidence of upper tract involvement, my inclination would be to treat patients, especially younger ones, with 1 course of treatment. It may not be worth further efforts at treatment in patients who have a recurrence soon after initial therapy. Other studies, not focusing on diabetic patients, have suggested that in older patients, especially debilitated ones, asymptomatic bacteriuria does not have significant consequences and the rate of reinfection after treatment is very high. Therefore, I would be less prone to treat older, debilitated diabetic patients with asymptomatic bacteriuria.—M.J. Barza, M.D.

Postcoital Antimicrobial Prophylaxis for Recurrent Urinary Tract Infection: A Randomized, Double-Blind, Placebo-Controlled Trial

Stapleton A, Latham RH, Johnson C, Stamm WE (Univ of Washington; Vanderbilt Univ)

JAMA 264:703–706, 1990 1–17

Because studies have shown an apparent association between sexual intercourse and urinary tract infections (UTIs), postcoital antimicrobial prophylaxis has been suggested as an alternative to continuous treatment. To study the efficacy of postcoital antimicrobial prophylaxis in sexually active young women with a history of frequent UTIs, data were obtained from 16 patients randomized to receive postcoital trimethoprim-sulfamethoxazole and 11 patients who received postcoital placebo. The 2 groups were similar with respect to the use of a diaphragm, history of

Relationship of Frequency of Intercourse to Efficacy of Prophylaxis With Trimethoprim-Sulfamethoxazole or Placebo

Intercourse Frequency, Episodes per Week*	Trimethoprim-Sulfamethoxazole		Placebo	
	No. of Patients	Infections per Patient-Year	No. of Patients	Infections per Patient-Year
<2	6	0	4	1.8
2-3	4	0.6	3	4.3
>3	4	0.6	3	15.0†

*Data on frequency of intercourse were unavailable for 2 patients who took postcoital trimethoprim-sulfamethoxazole and 1 placebo-treated patient whose diaries were not returned.

†$P = .004$, $r = .80$ for relationship of increased frequency to increased infection rate.

(Courtesy of Stapleton A, Latham RH, Johnson C, et al: *JAMA* 264:703–706, 1990.)

lifetime UTIs, overall frequency of intercourse, and number of lifetime sexual partners.

After 6 months of observation only 2 of the 16 patients who used postcoital trimethoprim-sulfamethoxazole became infected. In contrast, UTIs occurred in 9 of the 11 patients who received placebo. Treatment was effective for patients with both low and high intercourse frequencies (table). There were few side effects with trimethoprim-sulfamethoxazole and compliance was excellent. The drug had little impact on vaginal, urethral, or rectal colonization with *Escherichia coli.*

Postcoital trimethoprim-sulfamethoxazole was highly effective in preventing recurrent UTIs in young women with a history of frequent UTIs. This prophylaxis compares favorably with the regimen of continuous antibiotic therapy. Because the use of a diaphragm predisposes to UTI, postcoital prophylaxis may make it possible for infection-prone women to continue to use this contraceptive method.

▶ The data presented in this paper found, in a double-blinded, placebo-controlled, randomized trial, that one of our standard practices of advising postcoital antibiotics in young women with recurrent UTIs is an effective strategy. There are now 3 effective, well-studied approaches to these women: continuous prophylaxis with trimethoprim-sulfamethoxazole and postcoital or intermittent self-administered antimicrobials. These authors recommend that postintercourse prophylaxis be used in women who report that their infections are temporally related to intercourse. Other women who report infection rates of 3 or more per year should receive continuous prophylaxis.—M.S. Klempner, M.D.

Bacterial Vaginosis: Treatment With Topical Intravaginal Clindamycin Phosphate

Livengood CH III, Thomason JL, Hill GB (Duke Univ, Durham, NC; Univ of Wisconsin at Milwaukee)

Obstet Gynecol 76:118–123, 1990 1–18

The safety and efficacy of topically applied intravaginal clindamycin phosphate as treatment for bacterial vaginosis were investigated in a randomized, double-blind, placebo-controlled trial of 62 women. The women were randomized to receive a standard 5-g vaginal applicator and tubes of a cream-based vehicle with added clindamycin phosphate at either .1%, 1%, or 2%, or no clindamycin (placebo).

Patients were instructed to inject 5 g of cream high into the vagina in the morning and at bedtime for 5 consecutive days. They were also told not to douche or use other intravaginal or systemic antibacterial agents, to use condoms during coitus, and to notify investigators of any adverse effects. Patients were interviewed and examined clinically 4–7 days after completion of treatment. Those considered cured were evaluated again 1 month later. Patients whose treatment failed were offered entry into an open-label trial of 1% clindamycin cream, 5 g daily for 5 days; otherwise, these patients received the same follow-up protocol as cured patients.

Within 4–7 days after therapy, blinded intravaginal clindamycin phosphate treatment had cured bacterial vaginosis in 93.5% of patients. In contrast, 25% of those receiving placebo were cured in that time. At 1 month of follow-up, 89.7% of those who initially responded to clindamycin phosphate treatment remained cured. There were no significant side effects. These data strongly support the use of topically applied clindamycin phosphate in the treatment of symptomatic bacterial vaginosis. The treatment is safe and highly effective, and it has the advantage of local application.

▶ This is an impressive study. My only question is why the authors used 3 clindamycin concentrations (.1%, 1%, and 2%); it seems that either the 1% or the 2% concentration could have been eliminated. In any event, the outcomes were striking, a high cure rate being achieved with all 3 clindamycin concentrations. The high rate of improvement was seen in terms of symptoms, elimination of clue cells, and elimination of *Mobiluncus* on culture; the decrease in vaginal pH was less striking. One caution: Rare instances of pseudomembranous colitis have been recorded among patients applying clindamycin topically.—M.J. Barza, M.D.

Prevention of Catheter-Associated Urinary Tract Infection With a Silver Oxide-Coated Urinary Catheter: Clinical and Microbiologic Correlates

Johnson JR, Roberts PL, Olsen RJ, Moyer KA, Stamm WE (Univ of Washington; Univ of Minnesota)

J Infect Dis 162:1145–1150, 1990 1–19

Recent studies have suggested that the use of catheters coated with silver or silver oxide appears to be protective against urinary tract infection (UTI) in high-risk patients. In a prospective study of an unselected general hospital population the use of a newly developed silver oxide-coated urinary catheter during acute bladder catheterization was evaluated, as well as the clinical and microbiologic correlates of catheter-associated UTI in this setting. Among 482 hospitalized patients, 207 received the silver oxide-coated catheters (silver catheter) and 275 received silicone control catheters.

Urinary tract infection developed in 10% of patients, and incidence was similar among silver catheter recipients (9%) and control catheter recipients (10%). Multivariate regression analysis showed that antimicrobial use, female sex, and an increased serum concentration of creatinine were associated with UTI. However, after stratification by sex and antimicrobial use, the silver catheter significantly reduced the incidence of UTI among women who were not receiving an antimicrobial agent; the incidence of UTI was 0% among the silver catheter recipients, compared to 19% among the control catheter recipients (Fig 1–6). The protective

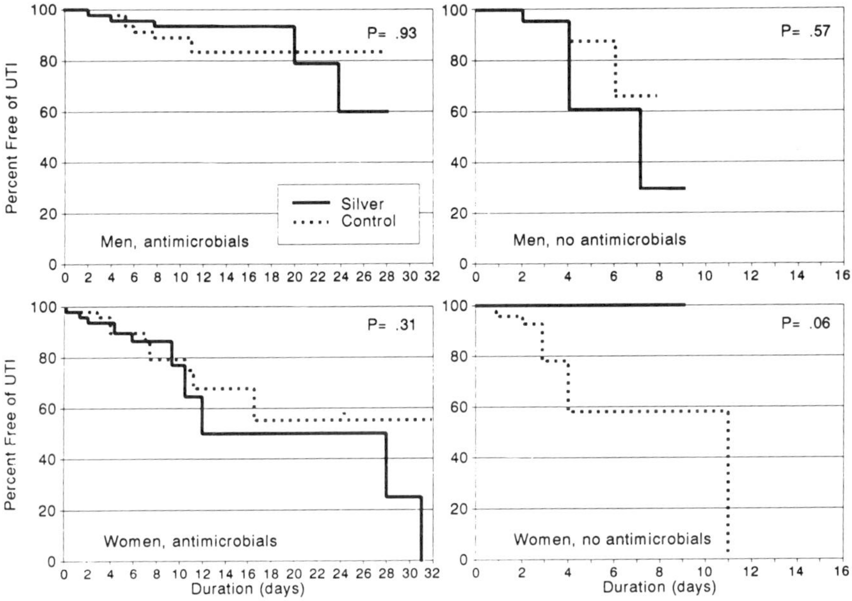

Fig 1–6.—Survival curves showing proportion of patients with control or silver catheter remaining free or UTI during catheterization. *P* values (by generalized Savage test) are for comparisons of curves for control catheter and silver catheter groups within each subset. (Courtesy of Johnson JR, Roberts PL, Olsen RJ, et al: *J Infect Dis* 162:1145–1150, 1990.)

effect of the silver catheter was not evident in other subgroups studied.

Organisms that caused UTI included gram-positive cocci, gram-negative rods, and yeast. Gram-positive UTIs were associated with the absence of antimicrobial use, use of a control catheter, and violations of catheter care. Gram-negative and candidal UTI occurred more often after 7 days of catheterization, whereas candidal UTI occurred more often in women and with antimicrobial use.

The use of silver oxide-coated urinary catheters provides a protective effect against UTI in a defined subset of patients: women not receiving antimicrobials. These findings suggest that several clinical variables influence the incidence and microbiology of catheter-associated UTI that should be taken into consideration when evaluating the efficacy of measures to prevent UTI.

▶ This study, in contrast to previous studies, found a beneficial effect of the silver-impregnated catheter only in the subgroup of women not receiving an antimicrobial agent. As with all subgroup analyses that are established in retrospect, as I believe this one was, one must be skeptical of the interpretation. I am even more skeptical in this case because there is no obvious reason why this subgroup should differ from other subgroups. I would interpret this study as a negative one for the utility of silver-impregnated urinary catheters.—M.J. Barza, M.D.

Skin, Soft Tissue, Bone, and Joint

The Nonpuerperal Breast Infection: Aerobic and Anaerobic Microbial Recovery From Acute and Chronic Disease

Edmiston CE Jr, Walker AP, Krepel CJ, Gohr C (Med College of Wisconsin, Milwaukee)

J Infect Dis 162:695–699, 1990 1–20

The microbiology of nonpuerperal breast infection was studied to identify the role played by aerobes and anaerobes in 60 breast culture specimens obtained from 54 women and 2 men using needle aspiration. Cultures were positive in 52 specimens. Analysis of the 221 microbial isolates obtained from these samples showed that 11 cultures were positive for aerobes only and 5 were positive for anaerobes only (table). There were mixed aerobic and anaerobic flora in 36 patients in whom anaerobic gram-positive cocci were the predominant isolates. Patients with an acute abscess had a mean microbial recovery of 2.9 isolates and patients with chronic infections had a mean microbial recovery of 5. Anaerobic populations outnumbered facultative isolates 2 to 1; 34% of anaerobic isolates were recovered from subcultures.

These results indicate that nonpuerperal breast infection is a mixed in-

Microbial Recovery From Acute and Chronic Nonpuerperal Breast Infections

	Acute patients (n = 19)	Chronic patients (n = 33)
Aerobic and facultative		
Gram-positive cocci		
Staphylococcus aureus	10	1
Staphylococcus epidermidis	3	12
Coagulase-negative staphylococci	2	14
Streptococcus milleri group	–	6
α-hemolytic streptococci	–	4
Enterococcus faecalis	–	1
Gram-positive bacilli		
Actinomyces israelii	–	2
Actinomyces meyeri	2	–
Actinomyces odontolyticus	–	3
Actinomyces species	–	3
Bacillus species	1	–
Corynebacterium species	–	1
Lactobacillus species	3	5
Gram-negative bacilli		
Escherichia coli	1	–
Proteus mirabilis	–	2
Pseudomonas cepacia	1	2
Total	23	56

(cont'd on p 27)

Anaerobic		
Anaerobic cocci		
Peptostreptococcus anaerobius	1	2
Peptostreptococcus asaccharolyticus	4	8
Peptostreptococcus magnus	7	16
Peptostreptococcus micros	2	7
Peptostreptococcus prevoti	3	11
Peptostreptococcus species	3	4
Veillonella parvula	–	3
Gram-positive bacilli		
Clostridium species	–	5
Eubacterium species	–	10
Propionibacterium species	6	12
Gram-negative bacilli		
Bacteroides bivius	–	1
Bacteroides disiens	1	1
Bacteroides distasonis	1	–
Bacteroides pneumosintes	1	1
Bacteroides ureolyticus	–	7
Bacteroides vulgatus	–	1
Bacteroides species	3	10
Fusobacterium species	–	6
Mitsuokella multiacidus	1	–
Mobiluncus curtisii holmesii	–	1
Porphyomonas asaccharolyticus	–	2
Porphyomonas endodontalis	–	1
Total	33	109

Note: Data are number of strains isolated; *n* indicates number of specimens from which organisms were isolated.

(Courtesy of Edmiston CE Jr, Walker AP, Krepel CJ, et al: *J Infect Dis* 192:695–699, 1990.)

fection with a major anaerobic component. There appears to be no one cause of nonpuerperal breast infection.

► These authors describe 3 presentations of nonpuerperal breast infections. The first is the acute presentation of erythema and induration in the breast without fluctuance. There is no abscess, and most of these infections are caused by *Staphylococcus aureus*, but some are mixed infections containing aerobes and anaerobes. Antimicrobial therapy alone is sufficient in this group of patients. In the second form of acute presentation there is inflammation with suppuration, and a tender fluctuant subaereolar mass is present. These patients require surgical drainage and antimicrobial therapy against both aerobic and anaerobic organisms. The third group of patients has multiple recurrent infections over a few months to a few years, and they present with multiple sinus tracts. The predominant organisms here are anaerobic, and therapy should include aggressive surgical management. Overall, this is a well-done study that calls attention to organisms other than *S. aureus* as important agents of nonpuerperal breast infections.—M.S. Klempner, M.D.

Results of Treatment of Tibial and Femoral Osteomyelitis in Adults

Kelly PJ, Fitzgerald RH Jr, Cabanela ME, Wood MB, Cooney WP, Arnold PG, Irons GB (Mayo Clinic and Mayo Found, Rochester, Minn)

Clin Orthop 259:295–303, 1990 1–21

In a previous report (1970), 50.9% of patients treated for chronic osteomyelitis of the femur or tibia had a successful outcome. However, 425 patients seen between 1971 and 1985 (the subjects of the present study) had a success rate of 84.4%.

Common organisms isolated were gram-negative bacilli in pure or mixed cultures. *Staphylococcus aureus* in mixed cultures was also a frequent isolate. The increase in isolation of *Pseudomonas aeruginosa,* beginning in 1978, necessitated the use of more toxic agents for antimicrobial therapy. Although *S. aureus* was only occasionally susceptible to penicillin, most isolates have remained susceptible to the semisynthetic penicillinase-resistant penicillins.

Most patients (73%) had chronic osteomyelitis after fracture of the tibia or femur, with or without union. A total of 470 procedures was performed. Débridement of soft tissue and dead bone was the first stage of treatment in all patients. A few days later patients underwent delayed closure with suction drainage alone, or irrigation and suction with use of a muscle flap or a free tissue transfer. Bone grafts were used either to fill in a saucerized cavity or to repair a nonunion. Free microvascular osseous grafts have permitted more aggressive resection of the involved osseous tissue in those treated recently. Muscle flaps and free tissue transfers were performed more frequently (Fig 1–7).

Metallic internal fixation devices had to be removed in all patients

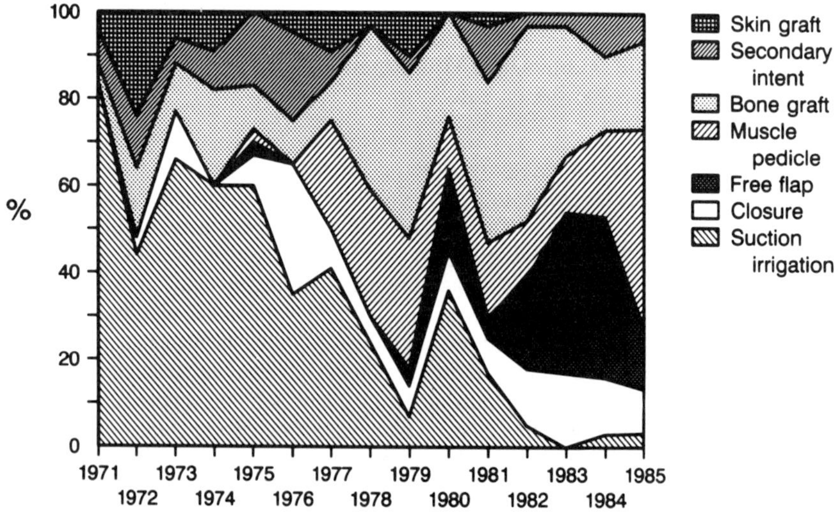

Fig 1–7.—Use of various forms of soft tissue closure by year (470 procedures in 425 patients). (Courtesy of Kelly PJ, Fitzgerald RH Jr, Cabanela ME, et al: *Clin Orthop* 259:295–303, 1990.)

Closure in 124 Infected Tibial Nonunions and 60 Infected Femoral Nonunions

Closure	*Total*	*Success*	*Failure*	*Success Rate (%)*
Tibial nonunion				
Delayed	44	35	6	85
Split-thickness skin graft	22	19	3	86
Second intention	23	21	2	91
Cross-leg	1	1	0	100
Free flap	20	17	3	85
Local muscle pedicle	14	11	2	85
Femoral nonunion				
Delayed	39	32	7	82
Second intention	12	9	2	82
Free flap	8	8	0	100
Local muscle pedicle	1	1	0	100

(Courtesy of Kelly PJ, Fitzgerald RH Jr, Cabanela ME, et al: *Clin Orthop* 259:295–303, 1990.)

whose osteomyelitis resulted from a fracture or open reduction. The most complex problem in the management of patients with chronic osteomyelitis is infected nonunion. External fixation, wound débridement, and bone-grafting procedures have improved the outcome in such patients. Wound closure was more complex in infected tibial nonunion than in infected femoral nonunion (table).

▶ The main message of this paper is that the rate of cure of chronic osteomyelitis of the tibia and fibula is now in the 85% range. There are so many differences in the management of these infections between the current era (1971–1985) and the earlier one that it is difficult to know which aspects are the most important. The paper is included mainly as a reference for those readers who want some guidelines for the likelihood of cure in this type of osteomyelitis.—M.J. Barza, M.D.

▶ ↓ We generally think of *Pseudomonas aeruginosa* causing osteomyelitis from puncture wounds of the foot. These cases expand the list of organisms one should consider.—D.R. Snydman, M.D.

Serratia **Osteochondritis After Puncture Wounds of the Foot**

Murray MM, Welch DF, Kuhls TL (Univ of Oklahoma)

Pediatr Infect Dis J 9:523–525, 1990 1–22

Instances of osteochondritis after puncture wounds of the foot are most commonly caused by *Pseudomonas aeruginosa* and *Staphylococcus aureus*. *Serratia* osteochondritis developed in 2 children after foot puncture wounds.

Case 1.—Boy, 16 years, had a small puncture wound to the foot. Six weeks after the initial injury, he returned with a nontender, nonerythematous wound with purulent discharge. A radiograph revealed a radiolucent area within the cuboid. The patient underwent surgical débridement and a 3-week course of intravenous antibiotics. *Serratia liquefaciens* was isolated from the bone specimens. A second surgical débridement was necessary 2 weeks after discontinuation of intravenous therapy. Trimethoprim/sulfamethoxazole was given orally for a total of 8 weeks.

Case 2.—Boy, 5 years, stepped on a nail and was seen 3 weeks later with a swollen, tender foot. Radiography revealed a radiolucent area in the calcaneus and a partial loss of the adjacent cortical margin. The patient was treated with surgical débridement and a 10-day course of intravenous antibiotics. *Serratia marcescens* was grown from cultures of the débrided bone. After discharge, he was treated at home with trimethoprim/sulfamethoxazole orally for 4 weeks.

These are the first reported pediatric cases of *Serratia* osteochondritis complicating common plantar foot punctures. *Serratia liquefaciens* and *S. marcescens* should be added to the list of organisms causing osteochondritis after puncture wounds of the foot in children. Treatment consists of aggressive surgical débridement and appropriate antibiotic therapy.

Puncture Wound Osteochondritis of the Foot Caused by *Pseudomonas maltophilia*

Baltimore RS, Jenson HB (Yale Univ)
Pediatr Infect Dis J 9:143–144, 1990 1–23

Osteochondritis of the small bones of the foot is most commonly associated with infection by *Pseudomonas aeruginosa* after a puncture wound. Another organism, *Pseudomonas maltophilia,* also was implicated in the development of osteochondritis.

Boy, 11 years, stepped on a rusty nail that penetrated the sole of his shoe and punctured his foot near the head of the fifth metatarsal bone. Three days later, the boy was treated by the family physician for intense pain, swelling, and erythema. Dicloxacillin, warm soaks, and elevation were prescribed. The symptoms subsided but recurred with swelling extending over the dorsum of the foot. At presentation, the swollen foot had lymphangitic streaks extending from the medial surface of the foot to the ankle. Plain roentgenograms were normal except for soft tissue swelling. After empiric microbial therapy, symptoms subsided except for point tenderness at the puncture site. Both ^{99m}Tc and ^{67}Ga scans showed accumulation in the proximal end of the fifth metatarsal bone. The patient underwent open exploration and biopsy of the metatarsal bone. The sinus tract was excised, all softened cartilage and bone were débrided, and the wound was packed. There was no gross pus. Culture of the excised tissue revealed *P. maltophilia* and *Staphylococcus epidermidis.* The *P. maltophilia* was susceptible only to trimethoprim/sulfamethoxazole and ciprofloxacin. A regimen of orally administered trimethoprim/sulfamethoxazole was prescribed. After 2 weeks, the patient had a pruritic maculopapular rash, and trimethoprim/sulfamethoxazole was discontinued in favor of ciprofloxacin for an additional 2 weeks. In a follow-up of 1 year, the patient had no recurrence of symptoms or signs of infection.

The principal clinical importance of *P. maltophilia* is its resistance to aminoglycosides, penicillins, cephalosporins, imipenem, and aztreonam. It is variably susceptible to quinolone antimicrobials. In this case, the isolate was susceptible only to trimethoprim-sulfamethoxazole and ciprofloxacin. Despite broad antimicrobial resistance, mortality from *P. maltophilia* infections is low.

▶ Puncture wounds of the foot are classic epidemiologic settings for *P. aeruginosa* osteomyelitis. In this case report, after ineffective antistaphylococcal therapy, bone biopsy was done and culture revealed the presence of *P. maltophilia.* This case is presented to alert infectious disease clinicians to the possibility that non–*aeruginosa* pseudomonads may also be associated with the classic nail in the foot osteomyelitis, and that biopsy, culture, and determination of antibiotic sensitivity remain the first line strategy for management.— G.T. Keusch, M.D.

Respiratory Tract, Eye, Ear, Nose, and Throat

Hospitalization Decision in Patients With Community-Acquired Pneumonia: A Prospective Cohort Study

Fine MJ, Smith DN, Singer DE (Massachusetts Gen Hosp, Boston; Univ of Pittsburgh)

Am J Med 89:713–721, 1990 1–24

Adult community-acquired pneumonia accounts for more than 500,000 hospital admissions each year. Because the criteria for admission appear to vary considerably throughout the United States, some patients who could safely be treated in an ambulatory setting may be incurring the greater costs of hospitalization. This low-risk subset of patients with community-acquired pneumonia was identified.

During the 10-month study period, 280 cases of confirmed pneumonia met the entry criteria. Of this group, 110 patients had an indication for admission based on a modified version of the Appropriateness Evaluation Protocol. These indications include a severe vital sign abnormality, altered mental status, arterial hypoxemia, a suppurative pneumonia-related infection, a severe electrolyte, hematologic, or metabolic laboratory abnormality, or an acute coexistent medical condition. The remaining 170 patients had no indication for admission. All but 2 of the patients with an indication for admission were hospitalized. Seventy-six patients with no such indication were treated as inpatients.

The overall mortality was 12.6%. More than one third (38%) of the patients with no indication for admission had a complicated course, and 55 of these patients were hospitalized for more than 3 days. Logistic regression identified 5 independent predictors of a complicated course (ta-

Independent Predictors of a Complicated Course in Patients Without an Indication for Admission at Presentation

Predictor	Odds Ratio	95% CI*
Age > 65 years	2.7	1.4–4.1
Comorbid illness†	3.2	1.4–7.5
Temperature > 38.3°C (101°F)	4.1	1.8–9.2
Immunosuppression‡	12.0	1.1–132.9
High-risk etiology§	23.3	2.7–200.7

**Abbreviation:* CI, confidence interval.

†Comorbid illness was defined as a history of diabetes mellitus, renal insufficiency, or congestive heart failure or a hospitalization within 1 year of the pneumonia presentation.

‡Immunosuppression was defined as the use of systemic corticosteroids or systemic chemotherapy for a malignant neoplasm within 6 months of the pneumonia presentation.

§High-risk etiology was defined as staphylococcal, gram-negative rod, aspiration, or postobstructive pneumonia.

(Courtesy of Fine MJ, Smith DN, Singer DE: *Am J Med* 89:713–721, 1990.)

ble); the factors most strongly predictive were high-risk pneumonia etiology and immunosuppression. An increase in the number of independent risk factors was associated with an increased number of complicated outcomes (Fig 1–8).

Admitting physicians who completed a questionnaire cited the severity

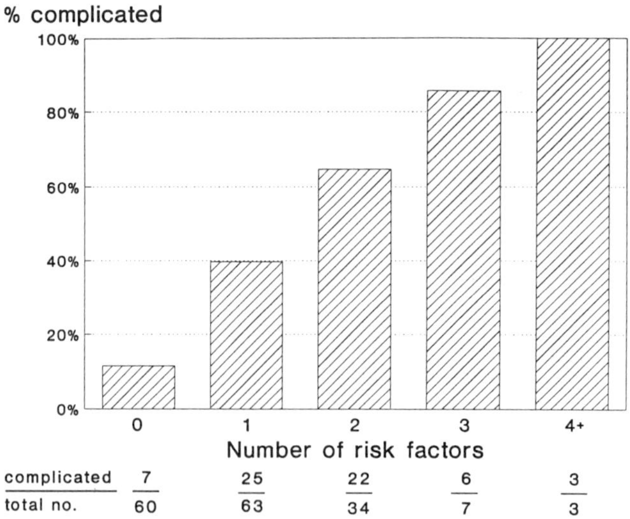

Fig 1–8.—Occurrence of a complicated outcome according to number of risk factors at presentation. The risk factors included age older than 65 years, immunosuppression (recent systemic corticosteroid use or cancer chemotherapy), temperature more than 38.3° C (101° F), comorbid illness (diabetes mellitus, congestive heart failure, renal insufficiency, or hospitalization within 1 year of the pneumonia episode), and a high-risk pneumonia etiology (staphylococcal, gram-negative rod, aspiration, or postobstructive pneumonia). The χ^2 test for trend in proportions was significant ($P < .001$). The denominator equals 167 because of missing data in 2 patients and absence of follow-up in 1 patient. (Courtesy of Fine MJ, Smith DN, Singer DE: *Am J Med* 89:713–721, 1990.)

of current illness and underlying medical problems as the most important factors considered in the decision to treat in the ambulatory settings. Based on the results of this study, patients without an indication for admission and with 2 or fewer risk factors for a complicated course might safely be treated as outpatients.

▶ The bottom line of this study is that even among patients who do not meet the criteria used widely by quality assurance and utilization review committees for hospital admission for pneumonia, there is a high (38%) incidence of a complicated course. Many of those with a complicated course could be identified because of the risk factor of immunosuppression or a "high-risk etiology" of the pneumonia (defined as staphylococcal, gram-negative rod, aspiration, or postobstructive pneumonia).—M.J. Barza, M.D.

Primary Meningococcal Conjunctivitis: Report of 21 Patients and Review

Barquet N, Gasser I, Domingo P, Moraga FA, Macaya A, Elcuaz R (Hosp Infantil Vall d'Hebron, Barcelona, Spain; Ciutat Sanitaria Vall d'Hebron; Autonomous Univ of Barcelona)

Rev Infect Dis 12:838–847, 1990 1–25

Neisseria meningitidis is an uncommon cause of acute bacterial conjunctivitis. Primary meningococcal conjunctivitis was treated in 21 children in a 5-year period. Data on these patients and 63 others reported in the literature were reviewed.

The 21 children with primary meningococcal conjunctivitis were among 1,030 children with acute bacterial conjunctivitis seen during the study period, for an overall incidence of 2.04%. Among all 84 patients with meningococcal conjunctivitis were 9 neonates, 55 children, and 20 adults. The male to female ratio was 1.76:1. Conjunctivitis was unilateral in 66.3% of the patients.

Gram-stain of the conjunctival exudate showed gram-negative diplococci in all 50 patients in whom the testing was done. Culture of the conjunctival exudate showed *N. meningitidis* in all patients; 44% of the isolated meningococci belonged to serogroup B and 34.9% belonged to serogroup A. Initial treatment consisted of topical therapy alone in 41 patients, usually sulfonamides; 42 patients received systemic therapy, either sulfonamides of β-lactam antibiotics; and treatment was combined with topical therapy in 29 patients.

Ocular complications occurred in only 15.5% of patients, and the most frequent were corneal ulcers. Systemic meningococcal disease occurred in 17.8% of patients at a mean interval of 41.3 hours after the appearance of ocular symptoms. Systemic meningococcal disease was more frequent in patients who received topical therapy alone (31.7%) than in those treated with systemic therapy (2.9%). The risk of systemic meningococcal disease when topical therapy alone was used was 19.03 times greater than with systemic therapy. Overall mortality for patients with systemic meningococcal disease was 13.3%. There were no permanent ocular sequelae.

Because of the high risk of systemic disease, systemic antibiotic therapy should be mandatory for all patients with primary meningococcal conjunctivitis. Gram stain of the conjunctival exudate is a rapid and extremely useful method in guiding the initial therapy. The prognosis is favorable.

▶ Systemic infection arising from bacterial conjunctivitis is a very rare occurrence and has been reported almost exclusively with meningococcal infection. There is not much of a take-home lesson here. The paper has been included mainly for those who collect unusual tidbits in infectious disease.—M.J. Barza, M.D.

Acute Bacterial Sialadenitis: A Study of 29 Cases and Review
Raad II, Sabbagh MF, Caranasos GJ (Univ of Florida)
Rev Infect Dis 12:591–601, 1990 1–26

Acute bacterial parotitis was described in the 1950s and 1960s as a nosocomial postoperative infection with a high mortality rate. Since then, several reports have suggested a change in the etiology and management of acute bacterial parotitis. Data on the microbiologic and clinical patterns of acute bacterial sialadenitis of the submandibular and parotid glands seen in a university hospital since 1970 were reviewed.

From 1970 to 1988, 17 patients with acute bacterial parotitis and 12 patients with acute bacterial submandibular sialadenitis were hospitalized. Underlying conditions that predisposed to xerostomia were found in 53% of patients with acute bacterial parotitis and 42% of patients with acute bacterial submandibular sialadenitis, particularly diuretic therapy and hypovolemia. During the 18-year period there were only 6 patients with nosocomial parotitis among the 289,234 hospital admissions and 3 with postoperative parotitis among the 119,342 major surgical procedures. *Staphylococcus aureus* was the most frequently isolated organism in the patients with nosocomial infections. All patients responded to antimicrobial therapy; none required surgical drainage, and none died.

Acute bacterial sialadenitis is becoming a community-acquired disease, with dehydration, diuretics, and other drugs acting as major risk factors. The prognosis is often favorable with appropriate antimicrobial therapy. In contrast to this, a review of data on 15 studies before 1970 showed that acute bacterial parotitis is mainly a nosocomial postoperative complication associated with mortality rates of 10% to 50% (table). It appears that advances in antimicrobial drug therapy and fluid management of hospitalized patients have improved the outcome of this disease and reduced the need for surgical intervention. *Staphylococcus aureus* remains the most common pathogen causing acute bacterial parotitis.

▶ It is puzzling that salivary sialadenitis is usually caused by *S. aureus,* in contrast to most other infections that begin within the oral cavity. Interestingly, in

Comparison of Acute Bacterial Parotitis Studies Completed Before 1970 With Those Completed After 1970

	Data for indicated period	
Parameter	1911-1969*	1970–1988†
No. of studies	15	2
No. of patients	722	44
Organisms frequently isolated	*S. aureus* Viridans streptococci	*S. aureus* Viridans streptococci
Epidemiology	Mostly nosocomial	Mostly community-acquired
Common underlying factors	Surgery Dehydration Poor oral hygiene Elderly Dry mouth Diuretics and other drugs	Dehydration Ductal obstruction Sjogren's syndrome Diuretics
Type of therapy	Surgery Antibiotics Rehydration Irradiation	Antibiotics Rehydration
Related mortality (%)	10-50‡	0

(Courtesy of Raad II, Sabbagh MF, Caranasos GJ: *Rev Infect Dis* 12:591–601 1990.)

this study, only 53% of infections yielded *S. aureus* and 31% were caused by viridans streptococci. The authors point out that recent reports of *Pseudomonas aeruginosa* causing this infection have dealt with critically ill patients in whom nasopharyngeal colonization by gram-negative species would be expected. M.J Barza, M.D.

Conservative Management of Adult Epiglottitis

Wolf M, Strauss B, Kronenberg J, Leventon G (Tel-Aviv Univ, Israel)

Laryngoscope 100:183–185, 1990 1–27

Acute epiglottitis is considered a mainly pediatric emergency, but recent reports have suggested an increasing incidence among adults. Some authors have reported a rapid and aggressive course in adults with epiglottitis, whereas others have reported a more benign outcome. Furthermore, there is controversy over the need for intubation, tracheotomy, or both. A study was done to identify any specific risk factors that may contribute to the development of a compromised airway in adult epiglottitis.

During a 10-year period, 30 adults were seen with acute epiglottitis. At presentation, all patients had pain, 28 had dysphagia, 8 complained of hoarseness, and 6 were dyspneic. Three of the latter had experienced dyspnea of sudden onset. Two patients had hemoptysis. The onset of epiglottitis was gradual in 15 patients, abrupt in 8, and unclear in 7. Acute disease developed, either gradually, usually beginning as an upper respiratory tract infection, or abruptly, within hours.

Eight patients had epiglottic abscesses, 3 on the free edge of the epiglottis, 1 on the laryngeal surface, and 4 on the lingual surface of the epiglottis. All patients were treated by intravenous antibiotics, and 15 patients were given steroids. None of the patients required intubation or tracheotomy. No age-related or sex-related differences in symptoms and signs were noted; patients with dyspnea had no characteristic features.

The course of epiglottitis in adults differs from that usually seen in children. In contrast to the interventionist approach in children, a noninterventionist and conservative approach is recommended for adults with acute epiglottitis.

▶ There are a number of important differences between acute epiglottitis in adults and children. First, the course is relatively benign in adults. None of the 30 patients reported in this study required intubation. The authors make an extremely convincing case for a conservative approach with antibiotics alone. Second, bacteremia was not observed in any of the patients, unlike the relatively high incidence in pediatric patients with *Hemophilus influenzae*. Third, most of the cultures from these adult patients with acute epiglottitis were negative, and those that were positive were mostly positive for *Streptococcus veridans* or *Streptococcus hemolyticus*. Fourth, steroids (which were administered to half of the patients) had no benefit. All of these points are worth keeping in mind when treating adult patients with epiglottitis.—M.S. Klempner, M.D.

Lack of Impact of Early Antibiotic Therapy for Streptococcal Pharyngitis on Recurrence Rates

Gerber MA, Randolph MF, DeMeo KK, Kaplan EL (Univ of Connecticut, Framington)

J Pediatr 117:853–858, 1990 1–28

The development of type-specific immunity to group A β-hemolytic streptococcal (GABHS) pharyngitis has been considered a major protection against subsequent GABHS infections. Inhibition of the development of this type-specific immunity has been thought to arise from the widespread use of immediate antibiotic therapy for pharyngitis. A prospective study was undertaken to test whether a 48-hour delay in antibiotic therapy would reduce the number of recurrences of GABHS by allowing the development of type-specific immunity.

A total of 113 patients with GABHS were assigned randomly to receive penicillin V treatment at the time of diagnosis or to begin therapy after 48 hours. Serotyping of all isolates was performed to distinguish between recurrences with homologous or heterologous serotypes.

There was no significant difference between recurrence rates in the 2 groups. Of the 50 patients in the immediate treatment group, 6 (12%) had homologous serotypes of GABHS isolated on a follow-up throat culture. Of 63 patients in the delayed treatment group, 9 (14%) had homologous serotypes of GAHBS on follow-up. Delaying therapy for 48 hours in a patient with documented GABHS pharyngitis does not promote a better immune response.

▶ It is reassuring to know that an issue that most of us would never have worried about is not an issue after all. The study shows that the relapse rate in streptococcal pharyngitis is not higher when treatment is initiated promptly (resulting in some decrease in antibody production to the organism) than when there is a delay of 48 hours before treatment is started. On most other grounds, early rather than delayed treatment would be recommended, so the results of this study are appealing.—M.J. Barza, M.D.

Lack of Influence of Beta-Lactamase-Producing Flora on Recovery of Group A Streptococci After Treatment of Acute Pharyngitis

Tanz RR, Shulman ST, Stroka PA, Marubio S, Brook I, Yogev R (Children's Mem Hosp, Chicago; Northwestern Univ; Naval Med Research Inst, Bethesda, Md)

J Pediatr 117:859–863, 1990 1–29

The effects of anaerobic and aerobic β-lactamase-producing bacteria on bacteriologic outcome in acute group A β-hemolytic streptococcal (GABHS) pharyngitis were studied in a randomized, single-blind study of 89 patients aged 2–16 years. The patients received either phenoxymethyl penicillin or amoxicillin-clavulanic acid orally for 10 days.

After completion of therapy, throat cultures were positive for GABHS in 3 of 46 patients (6.5%) treated with amoxicillin-clavulanic acid and 4 of 43 patients (9.3%) treated with penicillin. The initial GABHS T type persisted in all 3 patients given amoxicillin-clavulanic acid and in 1 given penicillin; the difference was not significant. Beta-lactamase-producing organisms were isolated in 63% of patients treated with amoxicillin-clavulanic acid and in 67% of those treated with penicillin before therapy and in 66% of those treated with amoxicillin-clavulanic acid and in 31% of those treated with penicillin after treatment. Bacteriologic treatment failure was not related to the recovery of β-lactamase-producing bacteria before or after treatment.

These findings indicate that penicillin treatment failure in patients with acute streptococcal pharyngitis cannot be attributed to the production of β-lactamase by pharyngeal organisms. Using an antibiotic effective against β-lactamase-producing bacteria will not eliminate the problem of bacteriologic treatment failure.

▶ The hypothesis that failures of treatment of streptococcal pharyngitis with penicillin might be related to degradation of the drug in the oropharynx by β-lactamase-producing microorganisms is an old one. A number of recent studies comparing agents not susceptible to β-lactamases (e.g., cephalosporins, clindamycin, amoxicillin with clavulanic acid) with penicillin V have shown superiority of the former in eradicating streptococci from the throat, which is in accord with the hypothesis. Interestingly, this study found no lower a failure rate with amoxicillin-clavulanic acid than with penicillin V. Moreover, bacteriologic treatment failure was not asociated with the recovery of β-lactamase-producing bacteria before or after treatment. Further, more than a third of the patients were not compliant in taking their medication, but they were eliminated from the analysis.

The reason for failure of penicillin V to eradicate streptococci from the nasopharynx of compliant patients remains unclear. Although the benefit of a β-lactamase-resistant drug for this purpose remains controversial, my interpretation is that the bulk of the data indicate slightly higher cure rates with such drugs than with penicillin V. Nevertheless, penicillin V remains the mainstay of primary empiric treatment for streptococcal pharyngitis.—M.J. Barza, M.D.

Association of Group C β-Hemolytic Streptococci With Endemic Pharyngitis Among College Students

Turner JC, Hayden GF, Kiselica D, Lohr J, Fishburne CF, Murren D (Univ of South Carolina; Univ of Virginia)

JAMA 264:2644–2647, 1990 1–30

A clear causative role for non–group-A β-hemolytic streptococci in endemic pharyngitis has yet to be demonstrated. Previous studies have failed to show consistent differences in isolation of these organisms in symptomatic and asymptomatic groups. To determine whether non–group-A β-hemolytic streptococci can be detected more frequently in the throats of students with symptomatic pharyngitis than in throats of healthy age-matched controls, throat cultures were obtained from 232 college students who had symptomatic pharyngitis and 198 students with noninfectious problems during 2 school years. Duplicate throat swabs were inoculated onto plates that contained sheep blood agar. One plate was incubated in a 5% carbon dioxide (CO_2) atmosphere and the other was incubated in an anaerobic environment.

Among the non–group-A β-hemolytic streptococci, only those from group C were isolated significantly more often among patients (26%) than among controls (11%). Almost half of the group C β-hemolytic streptococci isolates from patients (47%) were detected in both the CO_2-enriched and anaerobic atmospheres. In contrast, 86% of the group C isolates from the controls were detected only in the anaerobic atmosphere. Quantitative colony counts of these isolates were generally higher among patients than controls. Fever, exudative tonsillitis, and anterior cervical adenopathy occurred significantly more often in patients with group C β-hemolytic streptococci than in patients whose throat cultures were negative for these organisms.

In this population of college students, group C β-hemolytic streptococci were epidemiologically associated with endemic pharyngitis. The rate of colonization in healthy controls (11%) suggests that some strains of group C β-hemolytic streptococci may represent normal oropharyngeal flora.

▶ It appears that group C streptococci are, at least sometimes, a cause of pharyngitis indistinguishable from that produced by group A streptococci. However, the results should not be considered conclusive. Other studies, many of them using less rigorous microbiological methods, have shown conflicting results. The differences may be related to the microbiological techniques used or to differences in the populations studied or to other factors. In this population of college students, group C streptococci were isolated on throat culture from 26%, whereas group A organisms were isolated from only 6%. About half of the isolates of group C streptococci from patients were isolated in the CO_2 atmosphere, whereas 86% of the isolates from controls were detected only in an anaerobic atmosphere. This finding, if it can be reproduced, puts a high predictive value on the finding of group C streptococci in the usual CO_2 atmosphere.—M.J. Barza, M.D.

A Mutation in the *mip* Gene Results in an Attenuation of *Legionella pneumophila* Virulence

Cianciotto NP, Eisenstein BI, Mody CH, Engleberg NC (Univ of Michigan)

J Infect Dis 162:121–126, 1990 1–31

Although much information has been gathered about *Legionella pneumophila* pathogenesis from the host cell standpoint, little is known about the bacterial factors responsible for intracellular infection and virulence. Several lines of evidence, however, suggest that infection by *L. pneumophila* depends on its ability to multiply within host alveolar macrophages. A mutant defective in this function may be attenuated in virulence for animals. The abilities of the mutant and its isogenic parent to cause lethal infection were compared in an animal model.

The mutated gene was designated as *mip* for macrophage infectivity potentiator. The constructed mutant demonstrated an 80-fold loss of infectivity for both U937 cells and explanted human alveolar macrophages. Guinea pigs underwent intratracheal inoculation to compare strain AA105, the *mip* mutant, and strain AA103, its isogenic parent.

Six of 8 animals that received the parent strain had signs of illness by day 2, and 4 died within 5 days of inoculation. No guinea pig inoculated with the mutant strain died, although 7 had transient signs of illness. At higher doses, 7 of 9 animals that received strain AA103 died within 3 days; in contrast, only 3 of the AA105-inoculated animals died. Overall, the mutant strain produced fewer illnesses, slower-progressing disease, and fewer lethal infections than either the parent strain or a derivative of the mutant strain with the wild-type *mip* gene reintroduced.

Macrophage infectivity potentiator is necessary for full virulence of *L. pneumophila* and may represent the first genetically defined virulence factor in this species. The fact that illness was delayed with the mutant strain suggests that a longer time is required for the attainment of an illness-producing load of bacteria when intracellular replication is impaired.

▶ The investigators identified an *L. pneumophila* gene associated with the initial stage of multiplication within macrophages and showed that mutations in this gene attenuate the infection in an in vivo model in guinea pigs. This provides further evidence of the importance of intracellular infection of macrophages in the pathogenesis of legionellosis. The gene is peculiar to the genus and encodes a unique basic protein on the surface of the organism. Its precise function is unknown. However, this system will provide an interesting contrast to *Salmonella* in future studies to define the molecular basis and mechanism of virulence and the basis for intracellular parasitism.—G.T. Keusch, M.D.

Intra-Abdominal

Peritoneal Lavage in Abdominal Sepsis: A Controlled Clinical Study
Schein M, Gecelter G, Freinkel W, Gerding H, Becker PJ (Univ of the Witwatersrand, Johannesburg, South Africa)
Arch Surg 125:1132–1135, 1990 1–32

There is ongoing controversy regarding the value of intraoperative peritoneal lavage in the treatment of peritoneal contamination. However, evidence from well-constructed clinical trials does not support an improved outcome after intraoperative peritoneal lavage when compared with conventional surgical treatment plus perioperative broad-spectrum systemic antibiotic therapy.

During a 2-year study, 45 men and 42 women (mean age, 53 years)

Surgical and Medical Complications in Various Groups

	Group 1	Group 2	Group 3	Total
Wound infections, No. (%)				
Minor	4 (13)	3 (10)	3 (10)	**10** (11)
Major	2 (7)	2 (7)	2 (7)	**6** (7)
Total	**6** (20)	**5** (17)	**5** (17)	**16** (18)
Surgical complications, No. (%)	3 (10)	7 (24)	2 (7)	**12** (14)*
Medical complications, No. (%)	8 (24)	9 (31)	5 (17)	**22** (25)†

Note: group 1 received no introperative peritoneal lavage (IOPL), group 2 received IOPL with saline solution, and group 3 received IOPL to which chloramphenicol succinate had been added.
*P = .131 (chi-square test).
†P = .453 (chi-square test).
(Courtesy of Schein M, Gecelter G, Freinkel W, et al: *Arch Surg* 125:1132–1135, 1990.)

underwent emergency laparotomy for peritonitis. They were randomly allocated to receive no lavage, lavage with saline solution, or lavage with saline solution, to which 2 g of chloramphenicol succinate had been added. Systemic antibiotic therapy was started before operation and continued afterward for 24 hours or longer, depending on individual needs. The mean acute physiologic and chronic health evaluation (APACHE) II score was 9 in all 3 groups.

Fifteen of the 87 patients died: 6 (21%) had not received intraoperative peritoneal lavage, 6 (21%) had received lavage with saline only, and 3 (10%) had received lavage with saline plus antibiotics. The difference was not statistically significant. Mortality correlated well with the preoperative APACHE II scores.

There was no significant difference in the mean length of hospitalization among the 3 treatment groups. The incidence of surgical and medical complications and wound infections in the 3 treatment groups is shown in the table. Infections and other complications were significantly associated with APACHE II scores. The use of intraoperative peritoneal lavage with saline solution or antibiotics in patients undergoing emergency operation for peritonitis did not influence the outcome after laparotomy.

▶ This prospective randomized study suggests that intraoperative peritoneal lavage with saline or saline containing chloramphenicol succinate offers no advantage over no peritoneal lavage. There are problems with the study. Most important is the fact that the numbers are small and patients with severe forms of intra-abdominal sepsis likely to lead to infectious complications were deliberately excluded; thus the power of the study to detect a difference is low. Second, the use of chloramphenicol succinate is problematic, because the drug must be hydrolyzed to release antibacterially active chloramphenicol. I don't know at what rate this would occur in peritoneal fluid. Interestingly, the choices of antimicrobial agents for intraperitoneal application in other investigations of this matter have not been very relevant to our contemporary understanding of the organisms important in intra-abdominal infection. The choices have included cephalothin, cephaloridine, bacitracin with kanamycin, and tetracycline. I am not a fan of peritoneal lavage, at least in terms of the delivery of antimicrobial agents to the abdominal cavity, because systemic administration does this very well. Nevertheless, I don't think that the available literature on the subject allows one to draw reliable conclusions. In any event, this report, flawed as it may be, will serve as an update for those interested in the subject.—M.J. Barza, M.D.

The Efficacy of Palliative and Definitive Percutaneous Versus Surgical Drainage of Pancreatic Abscesses and Pseudocysts: A Prospective Study of 85 Patients

Lang EK, Paolini RM, Pottmeyer A (Louisiana State Univ)

South Med J 84:55–64, 1991 1–33

Delays in diagnosis and in the initiation of therapy contribute to the high mortality rates (40% to 80%) in pancreatic inflammatory disease. Prompt diagnosis had been aided by CT, and early percutaneous drainage of pancreatic abcesses and pseudocysts has helped to reduce morbidity and mortality significantly. Percutaneous drainage was compared to surgical drainage in a prospective study.

The 85 patients were assigned alternately to surgical (41) or percutaneous (44) management. In both groups the fluid was drained with either palliative or curative intent. In 18 patients with pancreatic abscesses, percutaneous drainage cured 3 patients and palliated 12 others who were cured subsequently by surgical ablation; 3 patients in this group died. Of 15 surgical patients with pancreatic abscesses, 4 were cured and 6 were palliated; 5 patients died. The 6 patients not cured by surgery alone were cured subsequently by percutaneous drainage and medical management or surgery (Table 1).

Eleven of 14 patients with infected pseudocysts were cured by percutaneous drainage. One of the other 3 was lost to follow-up, and 2 were cured subsequently by surgery. Surgical drainage cured 6 of 12 infected pseudocysts. Palliation and subsequent cure were achieved in the remaining 6 patients by further surgery or secondary percutaneous drainage (Table 2). There was a high rate of cure in the noninfected pseudocysts, either by percutaneous aspiration (9 of 12) or surgical drainage (13 of 14).

Aspirates from pancreatic abscesses and pseudocysts yielded valuable information on the offending organism or organisms. In 29 patients these organisms were not identified from earlier blood cultures. There were 14 cases in which data obtained from aspirates mandated a change in or addition of antibiotics (Table 3).

TABLE 1.—Success Rate of Percutaneous Versus Surgical Drainage of Pancreatic Abscesses

	Percutaneous Drainage		*Surgical Drainage*	
Expanded Ranson's score	>9	5-8	>9	5-8
Palliative intent	(n = 7)	(n = 1)	(n = 3)	
Palliated	5	1	1	-
Cured by additional procedure*	5	1	1	-
Died	2	-	2	-
Curative intent	(n = 5)	(n = 5)	(n = 4)	(n = 8)
Cured	1	2	0	4
Palliated	3	3	2	3
Cured by additional procedure*	3	3	2	3
Died	1	-	2	1

*Additional surgical or percutaneous drainage.
(Courtesy of Lang EK, Paolini RM, Pottmeyer A: *South Med J* 84:55–64, 1991.)

TABLE 2—Success Rate of Percutaneous Versus Surgical Drainage of Infected Pancreatic Pseudocysts

	Percutaneous Drainage		*Surgical Drainage*	
	(n = 4)	*(n = 10)*	*(n = 3)*	*(n = 9)*
Expanded Ranson's scores	>9	5-8	>9	5-8
No. of patients	4	10	3	9
Cure	2	9	2	4
Palliation	2	1*	1	5
Cure by additional procedure†	2	0	1	5
Lost to follow-up	0	1*	0	0

*Same patient.
†Palliation and cure were often effected by an additional procedure in the same patient.
(Courtesy of Lang EK, Paolini RM, Pottmeyer A: *South Med J* 84:55–64, 1991.)

TABLE 3.—Changes in Antibiotic Therapy Resulting From Microorganisms Identifiable Only From Aspirate

	Pancreatic Abscess	*Infected Pancreatic Pseudocyst*
No. of patients	33	26
Pathogen diagnosed only from aspirate	12	17
Change in antibiotic therapy reflecting resistance of organisms identified from aspirate	5	9

(Courtesy of Lang EK, Paolini RM, Pottmeyer A: *South Med J* 84:55–64, 1991.)

Percutaneous drainage was as effective as surgical drainage for palliation and can be used in critically ill, clinically unstable patients. The immediate use of percutaneous drainage should reduce the high morbidity and mortality from pancreatic abscesses and pseudocysts. Surgical management can be used after the patient has stabilized.

▶ Infection in the pancreas itself, or developing in a pseudocyst, is among the most dreaded of intra-abdominal infections. This is no wonder, because the mortality rates are approximately 40% to 80%. In view of this high mortality rate, an aggressive surgical approach has been recommended traditionally. However, the data in this report clearly indicate that percutaneous drainage is a valuable palliative and/or curative procedure in this patient population. Even in those patients with pancreatic abscesses, up to 20% were cured with percutaneous drainage plus antibiotics alone. Infected pseudocysts were highly responsive to percutaneous drainage and infrequently required surgical therapy for cure. Even in those patients with noninfected pseudocysts, percutaneous drainage was an excellent palliative procedure and there were no deaths in this group. Overall, it is clearly justified to approach patients with infections in the pancreatic bed through an initial percutaneous approach with surgery reserved for those in whom the more conservative management strategy fails.—M.S. Klempner, M.D.

Staphylococcus aureus Nasal Carriage and Infection in Patients on Continuous Ambulatory Peritoneal Dialysis

Luzar MA, Coles GA, Faller B, Slingeneyer A, Dah Dah G, Briat C, Wone C, Knefati Y, Kessler M, Peluso F (Baxter R & D Europe, Nivelles, Belgium; Cardiff Royal Infirmary, Wales; Ctr Hosp Gén L Pasteur, Colmar; Hôp de la Durance, Avignon; Hôp Saint André, Bordeaux, France; et al)
N Engl J Med 322:505–509, 1990 1–34

To determine the association between nasal carriage of *Staphylococcus aureus* and subsequent catheter exit site infection or peritonitis, 140 consecutive patients beginning continuous ambulatory peritoneal dialysis (CAPD) at 7 European hospitals were studied. The patients' anterior nares were cultured for the presence of *S. aureus*. Carriers were not treated with antibiotics. All patients were monitored for a median follow-up of 10.4 months for signs of infection.

At the beginning of CAPD, 63 patients (45%) carried *S. aureus*. Of the 30 patients with diabetes, 23 (77%) were carriers, compared with 40 patients (36%) who did not have diabetes. Patients who were carriers of *S. aureus* had significantly higher rates of exit site infections than those who were not carriers (table). Both groups had equal frequencies of peritonitis. Among carriers, 85% of the exit site infections were caused by *S. aureus* compared with only 2 of 8 episodes of exit site infections caused by *S. aureus* among noncarriers. In 85% of the patients with infections, the strain cultured from the nares and the strain causing the infection were similar in phage type and antibiotic profile.

These findings provide evidence that nasal carriage of *S. aureus* among patients beginning CAPD is associated with increased risk of catheter exit site infection by the same *S. aureus* strain. No particular strain was associated with infection. Patients at high risk of morbidity can be identified by isolation of *S. aureus* from the nares before insertion of the catheter.

Rate of Exit-Site Infection and Peritonitis Among Carriers and Noncarriers of *S. aureus*

Group	Exit-Site Infection	Peritonitis
	episodes/patient-year	
Carrier (n= 63)	0.40	0.50
Noncarrier (n = 77)	0.10	0.52
P value	0.012	>0.50

(Courtesy of Luzar MA, Coles GA, Faller B, et al: *N Engl J Med* 322:505–509, 1990.)

▶ This study raises some questions: (1) Why was there no difference in the rate of peritonitis between the 2 groups despite a much higher rate of exit site infections among carriers of *S. aureus?* Interestingly, in the carrier group, *S. aureus* caused 85% of exit site infections but only 35% of episodes of peritonitis, suggesting a differential ability to cause infection in the 2 sites. (2) Given that *S. aureus* carriage was associated strongly with diabetes, can one separate the carrier state from the diabetes in fostering infection? Although the numbers of patients in the subgroups are small, the rate of infection in carriers with and without diabetes was similar, suggesting that the diabetes does not determine the risk of infection. (3) Should one consider attempting to eradicate the carriage of *S. aureus* from CAPD patients? The data do not allow one to draw a conclusion, but the authors suggest that studies to answer this question are underway.—M.J. Barza, M.D.

Norfloxacin Prevents Spontaneous Bacterial Peritonitis Recurrence in Cirrhosis: Results of a Double-Blind, Placebo-Controlled Trial

Ginés P, Rimola A, Planas R, Vargas V, Marco F, Almela M, Forné M, Miranda ML, Llach J, Salmerón JM, Esteve M, Marqués JM, Jiménez de Anta MT, Arroyo V, Rodés J (Hosp Clinic i Provincial of Barcelona; Hosp Germans Trias i Pujol of Badalona; Hosp de la Vall d'Hebró of Barcelona; Hosp Mútua of Teressa; Residencia Virgen del Roció of Sevilla, Spain)

Hepatology 12:716–724, 1990 1–35

Spontaneous bacterial peritonitis (SBP) is a frequent and severe complication of cirrhosis that is caused by the passage of intestinal bacteria, particularly aerobic (facultative) gram-negative bacilli, into the general circulation and then into the ascitic fluid. The effectiveness of selective intestinal decontamination (defined as the elimination of aerobic gram-negative bacilli from the intestinal flora) with the long-term administration of norfloxacin in preventing SBP recurrence in patients with cirrhosis was evaluated in a multicenter, double-blind, placebo-controlled trial. Eighty patients with cirrhosis who had recovered from an episode of SBP were given either long-term norfloxacin treatment, 400 mg/day, or placebo. The mean follow-up period was 6.4 months (range, 1–19 months).

At entry, both treatment groups were similar in clinical and laboratory data, ascitic fluid protein and polymorphonuclear concentrations, number of previous episodes of SBP, and causative organisms of the index SBP. The incidence of SBP recurrence was significantly less in the norfloxacin-treated group (12%) compared with the placebo-treated group (35%). Similarly, the incidence of SBP recurrence caused by gram-negative bacilli was significantly less in the norfloxacin group (1 of 5) than in the placebo-treated group (10 of 14). The probability of SBP recurrence was significantly less at 1 year in the norfloxacin group (20%) compared with the placebo group (68%), primarily because of the significantly lower rate of SBP recurrence caused by gram-negative bacilli in the norfloxacin group (3% vs. 60%) (Fig 1–9). Only 1 patient had side effects related to norfloxacin.

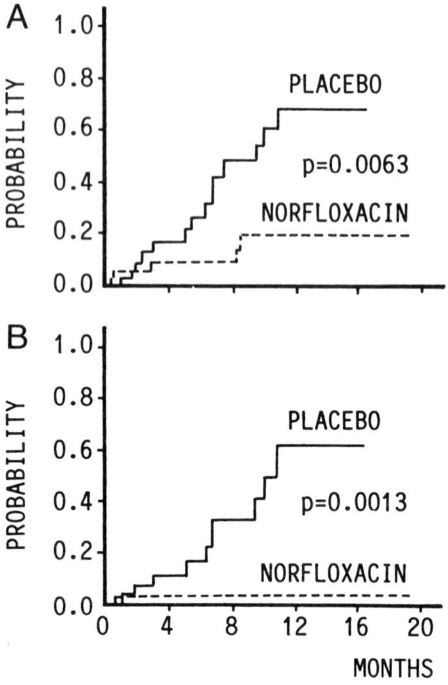

Fig 1–9.—A, cumulative probability of SBP recurrence in patients from both groups. B, cumulative probability of SBP recurrence caused by aerobic gram-negative bacilli in patients from both groups. (Courtesy of Ginés P, Rimola A, Planas R, et al: *Hepatology* 12:716–724, 1990.)

In a subgroup of 6 patients quantitative analysis of the fecal flora was performed. Norfloxacin administration resulted in selective intestinal decontamination, whereas no significant changes in the fecal concentration of aerobic gram-negative bacilli were observed in patients receiving placebo.

Patients with cirrhosis who recover from SBP are highly predisposed to experience new episodes during the course of their illness. Norfloxacin is highly effective and safe in preventing the recurrence of SBP caused by gram-negative bacilli in cirrhotic patients.

▶ This logically conceived, carefully done, and persuasive study may be influential in the management of patients who have had an episode of SBP. Norfloxacin was chosen because gram-negative bacilli are the usual culprits here. Although other fluoroquinolones are better absorbed and could therefore yield lower luminal concentrations, they might work just as well because the reductions in levels of gram-negative bacilli in the stool are similar to those produced by norfloxacin.—M.J. Barza, M.D.

Results of a Multicenter Trial Comparing Imipenem/Cilastatin to Tobramycin/Clindamycin for Intra-Abdominal Infections

Solomkin JS, Dellinger EP, Christou NV, Busuttil RW (Univ of Cincinnati; Har-

borview Med Ctr, Seattle; McGill Univ; Montreal, Quebec; Univ of California, Los Angeles)
Ann Surg 212:581–591, 1990 1–36

Studies of the clinical efficacy of antibiotic regimens for intra-abdominal infections have been hampered by several problems relating to study design. Using stricter enrollment criteria and the Acute Physiology and Chronic Health Evaluation (APACHE II) index of severity, 290 patients with established intra-abdominal infections were enrolled in a prospective, randomized, multicenter trial that compared the efficacy of tobramycin/clindamycin and imipenem/cilastatin in treatment of intra-abdominal infections.

Of the 162 evaluable patients, 81 received tobramycin/clindamycin and 81 received imipenem/cilastatin. Logistics regression analysis showed that the APACHE II score was a significant predictor of failure to control intra-abdominal infection and mortality (Fig 1–10). The treatment regimen was also a significant predictor of failure, favoring imipenem/cilastatin. The difference in outcome was attributed primarily to the higher failure rate in patients with gram-negative organisms treated with tobramycin/clindamycin. This was reflected in the significantly increased incidence of fasciitis requiring reoperation and prosthetic fascial replacement in the group given tobramycin/clindamycin (table). Among patients with gram-negative organisms treated with tobramycin/clindamycin, treatment failures and successes were achieved at similar peak levels at similar intervals into therapy.

Imipenem/cilastatin improves the outcome at the intra-abdominal site

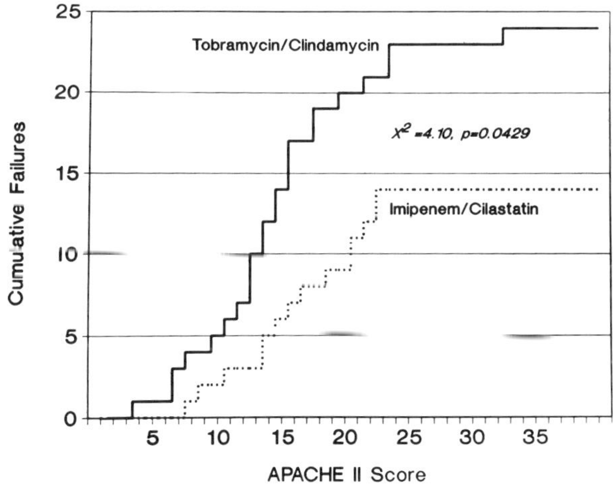

Fig 1–10.—The graph depicts failure as a function of the APACHE II score and antibiotic regimen for all evaluable patients. The APACHE II score was a significant predictor of failure ($\chi^2 = 10.11$, $P = .0015$). Treatment regimen was also a significant predictor for failure. There was a residual benefit of imipenem/cilastatin therapy for the entire study population with $\chi^2 = 4.10$, $P = .0429$. The model χ^2 was 14.46, $P = .0007$. (Courtesy of Solomkin JS, Dellinger EP, Christou NV, et al: *Ann Surg* 212:581–591, 1990.)

Anatomical and Other Bases for Failure

Basis for Failure	Tobramycin/ Clindamycin (n = 24)	Imipenem/ Cilastatin (n = 14)
Wound infection	2	3
Recurrent abscess	7†	6
Fasciitis	7	1*
Requiring prosthetic fascial substitute	6	0
Persisting peritonitis	—	2‡
Initially resistant gram-negative organisms	1	—
Expired with ongoing sepsis	5	3
Adverse reaction	3	1§

*$\chi^2 = 5.123$; $P < .05$.

†Treatment in 1 tobramycin/clindamycin-treated patient failed, with both abscess and fasciitis developing.

‡Treatment in 1 imipenem/cilastatin-treated patient failed, with both peritonitis and fasciitis developing.

§Treatment in 1 imipenem/cilastatin-treated patient failed, with both diarrhea and abscess developing.

(Courtesy of Solomkin JS, Dellinger EP, Christou NV, et al: *Ann Surg* 212:581–591, 1990.)

of infection compared to the results achieved by a conventional aminoglycoside-based regimen. The inclusion of severity scoring in the statistical analyses of outcome results is also supported.

▶ This is a well-done study. The antibiotic regimens and dosages were appropriate and serum concentrations of the aminoglycoside were adequate. The failure rate (postoperative infection despite adequate initial surgery) was significantly lower in patients treated with imipenem than in those treated with clindamycin and tobramycin. Imipenem was also superior in patients with gram-negative infections in the operative cultures, and this group accounted for most of the superiority of imipenem. Most failures were caused by infections by organisms that were initially susceptible to the antibiotic used for treatment. Several other studies comparing imipenem with combinations of clindamycin and aminoglycoside have shown a tendency to a superior outcome with imipenem, but none of them achieved statistical significance, as this one did. Based on those other studies, I have favored imipenem for intra-abdominal infections in patients who had a moderate or high risk of having resistant gram-negative bacilli in their flora, e.g., those who had received broad-spectrum antibiotics or had been hospitalized recently. This study suggests that imipenem should be considered as initial treatment in all patients with established intra-abdominal infection. The suggestion is difficult to refute.—M.J. Barza, M.D.

Antimicrobial Prophylaxis

Addition of Parenteral Cefoxitin to Regimen of Oral Antibiotics for Elective Colorectal Operations: A Randomized Prospective Study

Schoetz DJ Jr, Roberts PL, Murray JJ, Coller JA, Veidenheimer MC (Lahey Clinic Med Ctr, Burlington, Mass)
Ann Surg 212:209–212, 1990 1–37

Patients undergoing elective colorectal operations are prepared with mechanical cleansing combined with orally administered antimicrobial agents to reduce the incidence of septic complications. The value of adding perioperative parenteral antibiotics to this standard regimen has been questioned. The rates of wound infection and intra-abdominal infections were compared in 2 groups of patients, 1 of which received perioperative

Operation and Specific Septic Complications

Complication	Control (No Cefoxitin)		Treatment (Cefoxitin)	
	Total	Taking Steroids	Total	Taking Steroids
Wound infection	14	6	5	2
Anastomotic leakage	4	1	3	1
Intra-abdominal abscess/cellulitis	3	2	2	0

(Courtesy of Schoetz DJ Jr, Roberts PL, Murray JJ, et al: *Ann Surg* 212:209–212, 1990.)

cefoxitin in addition to mechanical preparation and orally administered antibiotics.

The series included 126 men and 71 women undergoing elective colorectal operations, most for carcinoma; 197 patients completed the study. The control group (96 patients) did not receive cefoxitin. Those in the treatment group (101 patients) were given cefoxitin in 3 doses of 2 g each, within 1 hour before incision, in the recovery room at 6 hours, and 6 hours thereafter.

The rate of wound infection differed significantly between the control group (14.6%) and the treatment group (5%). This difference remained significant after controlling for steroid use. The rates of intra-abdominal sepsis and pelvic abscesses were low and did not differ significantly in the 2 groups (table). Although recent studies have found parenteral antibiotics to be unnecessary in most patients, these results support the addition of perioperative parenteral cefoxitin to the regimen of mechanical cleansing and orally administered antibiotics during elective colorectal surgery.

▶ This study may be an influential one. Orally administered antimicrobial agents (mainly erythromycin and neomycin in the United States), together with mechanical cleansing of the bowel, are highly effective in preventing postoperative infection in elective colorectal surgery. Despite some controversy, the general consensus has been that there is no substantial benefit to adding a parenterally administered agent to the regimen. This study found a significant reduction in the incidence of wound infection (5% vs. 14.6%) after the addition of cefoxitin. A criticism I have of this study is that the rate of wound infection seems unusually high for elective surgery. There was no reduction in the incidence of intra-abdominal sepsis, but the authors suggest that this may be because the rate of intra-abdominal infection was too low to allow detection of a difference.—M.J. Barza, M.D.

Prevention of Nosocomial Lung Infection in Ventilated Patients: Use of an Antimicrobial Pharyngeal Nonabsorbable Paste

Rodríguez-Roldán JM, Altuna-Cuesta A, López A, Carrillo A, Garcia J, León J, Martínez-Pellús AJ (Gen Hosp; Virgen de la Arrixaca Hosp, Murcia, Spain)

Crit Care Med 18:1239–1242, 1990 1–38

Within the first week of mechanical ventilation, the oropharynx and/or digestive tract are colonized by hospital-acquired bacteria in 70% to 90% of patients. Reports of the beneficial effects of topically applied, nonabsorbable antibiotics against nosocomial infections in mechanically ventilated patients prompted a prospective, randomized, controlled study involving 28 patients who were mechanically ventilated because of respiratory failure of noninfectious origin. The incidence of infection in the lower airway was compared among 13 patients treated with nonabsorbable paste containing 2% tobramycin, 2% amphotericin B, and 2% polymyxin E administered locally to decontaminate the oropharynx and 15 controls who received topically applied paste without antibiotics.

Cultures of pharyngeal and tracheal aspirates showed no growth of potentially pathogenic organisms in 10 of 13 patients treated with the antimicrobial nonabsorbable paste, compared with 1 of 15 controls. Tracheobronchitis occurred in only 3, and pneumonia in none, of the patients treated with nonabsorbable antibiotics, compared with tracheobronchitis in 3 and pneumonia in 11 controls. The differences were highly significant. In addition, sepsis of pulmonary origin developed in 2 controls, but in none of the treated patients. The overall mortality was similar in both groups, but there was a clear relationship between pulmonary infection and mortality in 2 of 5 deaths in the control group. There were no alterations in the resistance patterns of bacteria to the antibiotics used. No serious side effects were noted.

These data indicate that local application of nonabsorbable antibiotics to the oropharynx can significantly reduce the incidence of nosocomial pneumonia in critically ill patients receiving mechanical ventilation. Further investigations are warranted to confirm these findings.

▶ There is a growing bandwagon of enthusiasts for prophylaxis of infection in intensive care unit (ICU) patients by application of broad-spectrum topical (oropharyngeal) and, in some studies, intravenous antibiotics. In this study, topical treatment alone was used. It is noteworthy to me that, although the incidence of colonization and of infection was reduced by the intervention, there was no effect on mortality. Length of stay in the hospital was not commented on. Interestingly, in the few other full-length papers (not abstracts) on the same topic, there has been no demonstrable effect of the prophylactic intervention on mortality or length of stay (see Abstract 1–39). Although these studies have not shown that the administration of prophylactic antibiotics to patients in the ICU fosters the development of antimicrobial resistance, past experience has amply illustrated this phenomenon. I would be very relucant to advise the approach suggested in this article until evidence accrues regarding improved survival or length of stay in the hospital. Even then, the issue of antimicrobial resistance will remain a major concern.—M.J. Barza, M.D.

Pilot Trial of Selective Decontamination for Prevention of Bacterial Infection in an Intensive Care Unit

Flaherty J, Nathan C, Kabins SA, Weinstein RA (Michael Reese Hosp and Med Ctr, Chicago; Univ of Chicago)

J Infect Dis 162:1393–1397, 1990 1–30

Selective decontamination of the oropharynx and gastrointestinal tract with nonabsorbable antimicrobials was compared with sucralfate, a cytoprotective antiulcer medicine, in patients in the cardiac intensive care unit (ICU). The 51 patients in the selective decontamination group received polymyxin, gentamicin, and nystatin orally as a paste and a solution. Sucralfate was given orally or by nasogastric tube to 56 patients.

Significantly less colonization of the oropharynx and stomach by gram-negative bacilli (12% vs. 55%), significantly fewer infections caused by

Colonization and Infection Rates of Patients Treated With Sucralfate or Selective Decontamination to Prevent Pneumonia

Patient status	Study regimen: Sucralfate (n = 56)	Study regimen: Selective decontamination (n = 51)	P
Oropharyngeal or gastric colonization by gram-negative bacilli			
On admission, no. (%)	22 (39)	19 (37)	NS
During study, no. (%)	31 (55)	6 (12)	<.001
P	.06	.003	
Infection			
No. infected (%)	15 (27)	6 (12)	.04
No. episodes	19*	7†	
Pneumonia	5‡	1‡	
Urinary tract infection	6	3	
Wound infection	6	2	
Bacteremia	3	1	

Abbreviation: NS, not significant.

* *Escherichia coli, Staphylococcus aureus,* and *Enterobacter, Proteus,* and *Klebsiella* species (3 each) and *Pseudomonas aeruginosa, Streptococcus pyogenes, Staphylococcus epidermidis,* and *Serrati, Hafnia,* and *Citrobacter* species (1 each) were cultured from 18 episodes; 1 episode was culture-negative.

†*Pseudomonas aerugniosa* (2) and *Pseudomonas fluorescens, E. coli,* and *S. epidermidis* (1 each were cultured from 5 episodes; 2 episodes were culture-negative.

‡Gram-negative bacilli were responsible for 3 and 0 episodes of pneumonia, respectively.

(Courtesy of Flaherty J, Nathan C, Kabins SA, et al: *J Infect Dis* 162:1393–1397, 1990.)

gram-negative bacilli (6% vs. 20%), and fewer infections overall (12% vs. 27%) occurred in the patients receiving selective decontamination. One episode of pneumonia occurred in the selective decontamination group and 5 in the sucralfate group (table). Of 8 wound infections, 2 involved deep sternal sites, and both occurred in patients treated with sucralfate.

This is the first known use of selective decontamination in an ICU in the United States. This mode of prophylaxis dramatically reduced both extrapulmonary and pulmonary infections. Patients receiving selective decontamination had less than one third as many days of systemic antibiotic therapy compared with those given sucralfate.

▶ As was suggested in the preceding comment (see Abstract 1–38), the prophylactic administration of antibiotics to prevent infections in patients in the ICU poses a risk of the development of antimicrobial resistance. In my opinion, prophylaxis is justified only if the data clearly indicate a clinically important benefit. In this study there was no difference in the mortality rate (only 1 death in the study patients) or length of postoperative hospital stay between the groups, which appears to me to be an argument against any "bottom line" benefit of prophylaxis.—M.J. Barza, M.D.

Antimicrobial Therapy

Emergence of Ciprofloxacin Resistance in Nosocomial Methicillin-Resistant *Staphylococcus aureus* Isolates: Resistance During Ciprofloxacin Plus Rifampin Therapy for Methicillin-Resistant *S. aureus* Colonization

Peterson LR, Quick JN, Jensen B, Homann S, Johnson S, Tenquist J, Shanholtzer C, Petzel RA, Sinn L, Gerding DN (VA Med Ctr, Minneapolis)

Arch Intern Med 150:2151–2155, 1990 1–40

There has been an increasing incidence of methicillin-resistant *Staphylococcus aureus* (MSRA) infection and colonization. The fluoroquinolone, ciprofloxacin, has in vitro activity against MRSA, and ciprofloxacin in combination with other agents has been suggested for possible use in the treatment of MRSA infections. The effectiveness of ciprofloxacin plus rifampin was compared with sulfamethoxazole and trimethoprim plus rifampin in the eradication of MRSA colonization in a randomized, single-blind, prospective study.

Of the 21 patients with MRSA infection who were treated for 2 weeks, 11 received ciprofloxacin plus rifampin; 10 received sulfamethoxazole and trimethoprim plus rifampin. The study was terminated early when ciprofloxacin resistance developed in 10 of 21 new MRSA isolates during

Eradication of MRSA Colonization After Therapy for MRSA Colonization

	No. (%) of Patients With Negative Cultures for MRSA			
Regimen	**1 wk** *	**2-3 wk**	**3 mo**	**6mo**
All patients				
Sulfamethoxazole and trimethoprim plus rifampin (n = 10)	6 (60)	5 (50)	5 (50)	4 (40)†
Ciprofloxacin plus rifampin (n = 11)	7 (64)	4 (37)	3 (27)	3 (27)†
Patients with isolates susceptible to all study agents				
Sulfamethoxazole and trimethoprim plus rifampin (n = 9)	6 (67)	5 (56)	5 (56)	4 (44)†
Ciprofloxacin plus rifampin (n = 8)	6 (75)	3 (38)	2 (25)	2 (25)†

*Time after completion of 2 weeks of therapy for MRSA colonization.

†Difference between eradication rates at any of the time points is not significant at $P < .1$.

(Courtesy of Peterson LR, Quick JN, Jensen B, et al: *Arch Intern Med* 150:2151–2155, 1990.)

the last 2 months of the study. Of the 10 patients with ciprofloxacin-resistant MRSA isolates, 5 had never received ciprofloxacin. At the 6-month follow-up period, only 27% of the patients given ciprofloxacin plus rifampin and 40% of those given sulfamethoxazole and trimethoprim plus rifampin remained free of MRSA; the difference was not significant (table).

The use of ciprofloxacin plus rifampin appeared to be associated with increased toxicity compared with what was previously reported when ciprofloxacin was used as a single agent. Except for a shift in plasmid bands in the ciprofloxacin-resistant isolates, no other changes were noted in whole-cell DNA restriction endonuclease analysis and the plasmid-profile pattern. All isolates appeared to be of single genomic type and highly resistant to most antimicrobials. These data indicate that ciprofloxacin plus rifampin is not effective in eradication of MRSA. Its use may risk the development of ciprofloxacin resistance in MRSA within the hospital environment.

Methicillin-Resistant Staphylococcal Colonization and Infection in a Long-Term Care Facility

Muder RR, Brennen C, Wagener MM, Vickers RM, Rihs JD, Hancock GA, Yee YC, Miller JM, Yu VL (Pittsburgh Veterans Affairs Med Ctr; Univ of Pittsburgh; Ctrs for Disease Control, Atlanta)

Ann Intern Med 114:107–112, 1991 1–41

Recent studies have shown the occurrence of endemic methicillin-resistant *Staphylococcus aureus* (MRSA) colonization and infection in long-term care facilities, but none has shown the effect of MRSA on patient

Comparison of Persistent Staphylococci Carriers (MRSA and MSSA) With Noncarriers

Variable	MRSA Carriers (*n* = 32)	MSSA Carriers (*n* = 44)	Non-carriers (*n* = 88)
Demographics			
Mean age (± SD), *y*	67.6 ± 16	67.4 ± 14	67.1 ± 14
Median duration of hospitalization (range), *d*	172 (4-3507)	130 (5-3953)	153 (4-5789)
Mean duration of follow-up, *d*	241	164	197
Residence on intermediate unit, %	78	44	46 *
Underlying conditions, %			
Chronic obstructive lung disease	22	23	19
Liver disease	6	4.5	6
Malignancy	28	20	26
Diabetes	13	13	20
Renal disease	25	33	21
Dialysis	14	9	12
Outcomes† %			
Staphylococcal infection	25	4.5	4 ‡
Death during study	53	29	34 ‡

* $P < .05$.
†risk ratio for staphylococcal infection for MRSA carriers compared with others is 3.6; risk ratio for death during study for MRSA carriers compared with others is 2.
‡ $P < .01$.
(Courtesy of Muder RR, Brennen C, Wagener MM, et al: *Ann Inter Med* 114:107–112, 1991.)

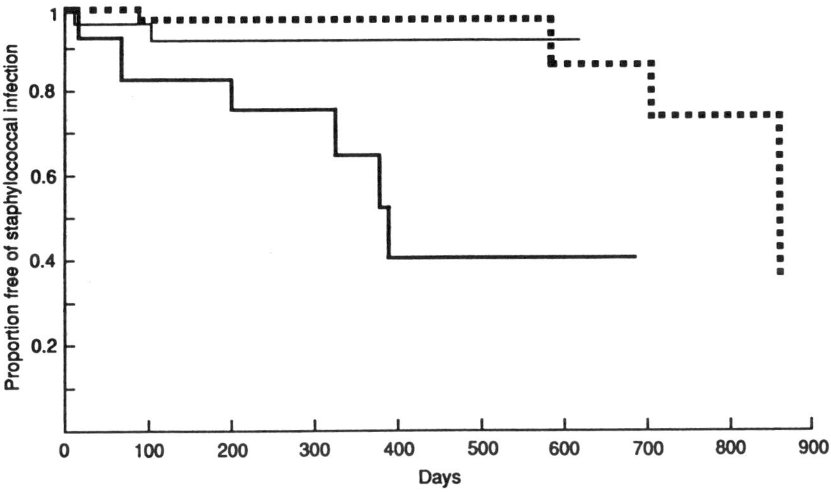

Fig 1–11.—Kaplan-Meier plot of rate of development of staphylococcal infection over time for MRSA carriers *(heavy solid line)*, MSSA carriers *(light solid line)*, and noncarriers *(dashed line)*. There was a significantly higher rate of infection among MRSA carriers over time than in the other 2 groups. (Mantel-Cox log-rank test). Only 2 noncarriers were followed beyond 800 days. (Courtesy of Muder RR, Brennen C, Wagener MM, et al: *Ann Intern Med* 114:107–112, 1991.)

morbidity and mortality. In a 3-year prospective study, 197 patients residing in 2 units of a Veterans Administration Affairs long-term care facility were followed with regular surveillance cultures of the anterior nares to determine the natural history of colonization by MRSA in these facilities, particularly the development of staphylococcal infection. Patients had been hospitalized in the facility for 4 days to 17 years.

Thirty-two patients were persistent carriers of MRSA and 44 were persistent carriers of methicillin-sensitive *S. aureus*. Staphylococcal infection occurred in 25% of MRSA carriers; the incidence was 4.5% in methicillin-sensitive *S. aureus* carriers and 4% in 88 noncarriers (table). The relative risk for staphylococcal infection in the MRSA carriers was 3.6 (confidence interval, 2–6.4), compared with the other 2 groups. Life-table analysis showed that the risk for staphylococcal infection was 15% for every 100 days of MRSA carriage (Fig 1–11).

Multiple logistics regression analysis showed that persistent MRSA carriage was the most significant predictor of infection. The finding of persistent colonization of the nares predicted 73% of all MRSA infections. Phage typing and plasmid analysis of MRSA isolates in 7 patients showed the same phage type in the colonizing and infecting strains in all patients and the same pattern of plasmid *Eco*RI restriction endonuclease fragments in 5 patients. Only 1 death occurred during a staphylococcal infection. Carriage of MRSA is widespread and prolonged in a long-term care facility, and the risk for staphylococcal infection in MRSA-colonized patients is substantial.

▶ This study shows persuasively that carriage of MRSA is associated with a substantially increased risk of the development of staphylococcal infection compared to the risk in patients carrying methicillin-sensitive *S. aureus* or not carrying *S. aureus*. What to do about the problem is less clear. In short-term facilities (e.g., acute care hospitals) isolation is routine. In long-term facilities, isolation of all patients with MRSA has not proven beneficial and may be traumatizing to patients. Efforts to eradicate MRSA by the use of antibiotics have been disappointing, with high rates of failure, recolonization, and the emergence of resistant strains after treatment. Nevertheless, this study may provide further impetus to efforts at eradication.—M.J. Barza, M.D.

Complement and Immunoglobulin Studies in 15 Cases of Chronic Meningococcemia: Properdin Deficiency and Hypoimmunoglobulinemia

Nielsen HE, Koch C, Mansa B, Magnussen P, Bergmann OJ (Statens Seruminst; Rigshospitalet, Copenhagen; Marselisborg Hosp, Århus, Denmark)

Scand J Infect Dis 22:31–36, 1990 1–42

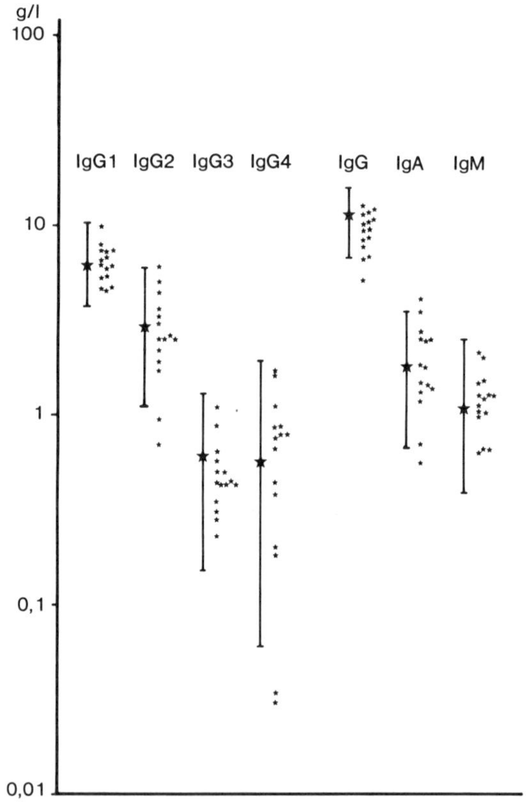

Fig 1–12.—Plasma Ig classes and IgG subclasses in plasma of 15 patients who previously had chronic meningococcemia *(stars)*. The 2.5–97.5 percentiles of the normal distributions are indicated by *bars*, 50 percentiles by *asterisks*. (Courtesy of Nielsen HE, Koch C, Mansa B, et al: *Scand J Infect Dis* 22:31–36, 1990.)

Chronic or prolonged meningococcemia is a rare form of meningococcal disease in which a prolonged, usually relapsing, fever is accompanied by the presence of meningococci in the bloodstream for up to several months. It has been suspected that the unusually long duration of this meningococcal disease is because of host factors, rather than variations of bacterial virulence. To determine whether the abnormal course of this infection is caused by a deficiency of complement or immunoglobulins, blood samples obtained from 15 patients who had recovered from chronic meningococcemia that occurred as early as 1948 were studied. The samples were assayed for the components of the classic and alternative complement pathways, and for the levels of IgA, IgG, IgM, and IgG subclasses.

The mean plasma IgG concentration in the 15 patients was significantly less than the mean in the normal group (Fig 1–12). The mean concentrations of IgA, IgM, and the IgG subclasses of the patient group were normal. Two patients had levels of IgG_2 and IgG_4 less than reference levels, and 1 of these patients also had reduced levels of total IgG and IgA. Only 1 patient had any complement system defects; this patient had a complete lack of properdin.

These data suggest that properdin deficiency and reduced plasma IgG levels may predispose to chronic meningococcal disease. However, most of these patients seem to have normal humoral immune systems.

▶ Studies of patients with acute meningococcal infection have shown appreciable incidences of unsuspected deficiencies of various components of the complement system. This study looks at the humoral limb of resistance in a much rarer form of meningococcal infection, chronic meningococcemia. With 1 exception, the complement levels were normal. In most of the patients, immunoglobulin studies also were normal. The bottom line is that the reason why the infection cannot be eradicated from patients with chronic meningococcemia is not known.—M.J. Barza, M.D.

Serologic Evidence of *Yersinia* Infection in Patients With Anterior Uveitis

Wakefield D, Stahlberg TH, Toivanen A, Granfors K, Tennant C (Univ of New South Wales, Sydney, Australia; Turku Univ, Finland)

Arch Ophthalmol 108.219–221, 1990 1–43

Anterior uveitis, an acute inflammation of the iris or ciliary body, or both, is associated with the HLA-B27 antigen, which is linked to a group of rheumatic diseases frequently seen in patients with anterior uveitis. It has also been noted that anterior uveitis often follows infection with a variety of gram-negative bacteria, and a number of recent studies have found anterior uveitis in patients who had *Yersinia* infection.

To examine the possible role of *Yersinia* infection in the pathogenesis of anterior uveitis, as well as the relationship between the HLA-B27 phenotype and associated rheumatic diseases, 28 consecutive patients with anterior uveitis and 28 matched, healthy controls were studied. Because

15 patients were HLA-B27 positive, the control group chosen contained a similarly high proportion of subjects with HLA-B27 antigen.

Serologic evidence of *Yersinia* infection was detected in 12 of the patients but in none of the controls (table). Eight patients with a significantly increased *Yersinia* antibody titer were HLA-B27 positive. Eight of the 15 patients who were HLA-B27 positive had seronegative arthritis. Five of those with arthritis were positive for *Yersinia* and 4 had elevated levels of IgM, which suggested recent infection.

In this series, patients with anterior uveitis, whether HLA-B27 positive or HLA-B27 negative, had an increased incidence of positive *Yersinia* se-

Yersinia Serologic Findings in Different Subject Groups

Subject Group	HLA	SNA*	No.	No. With Positive Serologic Findings	Yersinia Antibodies IgM	IgG	IgA
Uveitis	B27+	...	15	8†‡	6	3	2
		+*	8	5	4	2	1
		−*	7	3	2	1	1
	B27−	...	13	4§	2	2	2
		+	4	0	0	0	0
		−	9	4	2	2	3
	All patients	...	28	12‖	8	5	5
Controls							
	B27+	...	13	0	0	0	0
	B27−	...	15	0	0	0	0
	All subjects	...	28	0	0	0	0

*SNA indicates seronegative arthritis; +, present; −, absent.
†$P < .01$; statistical significance between HLA-B27–positive patients and controls.
‡Difference between HLA-B27–positive and HLA-B27–negative patients not statistically significant.
§$P < .05$; statistical significance between HLA-B27–negative patients and controls.
‖$P < .001$; statistical significance between patients with uveitis and control subjects.
(Courtesy of Wakefield D, Stahlberg TH, Toivanen A, et al: *Arch Ophthalmol* 108:219–221, 1990.)

rologic findings. A recent study detected *Yersinia* antigen in the joint fluid of patients with reactive arthritis, a disease that is also associated with HLA-B27. Taken together, the results suggest the need for a closer examination of the role of *Yersinia* as a trigger in the development of anterior uveitis.

▶ This report of a high prevalence of antibody to *Yersinia* species (the antibody recognizes antigens of *Yersinia enterocolitica* and *Yersinia pseudotuberculosis*) among patients with anterior uveitis, especially those positive for HLA-B27, is confirmatory of other studies. Indeed, almost half of the patients, but none of the controls, had such antibody. There has been considerable interest lately in the use of antibody detection systems for *Yersinia* infection, and it is not clear that the system described here is the most sensitive one. Nevertheless, the results of the various studies suggest that *Yersinia* infection may trigger a reaction of anterior uveitis, particularly but not exclusively in subjects who are positive for the HLA-B27 antigen.—M.J. Barza, M.D.

The Role of Skin Testing for Penicillin Allergy
Redelmeier DA, Sox HC Jr (Stanford Univ; Palo Alto VA Med Ctr, Calif)
Arch Intern Med 150:1939–1946, 1990 1–44

Decision analysis was used to determine when the penicillin allergy skin test should be performed. The threshold model of decision making (Fig 1–13) assumes that skin testing should be performed only if the results could change therapy. This model makes use of the treatment threshold concept, defined as the probability of a severe allergic reaction at which penicillin therapy is abandoned and an alternative antibiotic is selected. Skin testing is useful when the pretest probability of a severe allergic reaction lies between P1 and P2. Below P1, penicillin is always preferred, regardless of skin test results. Similarly, above P2 always indicates use of an alternative antibiotic.

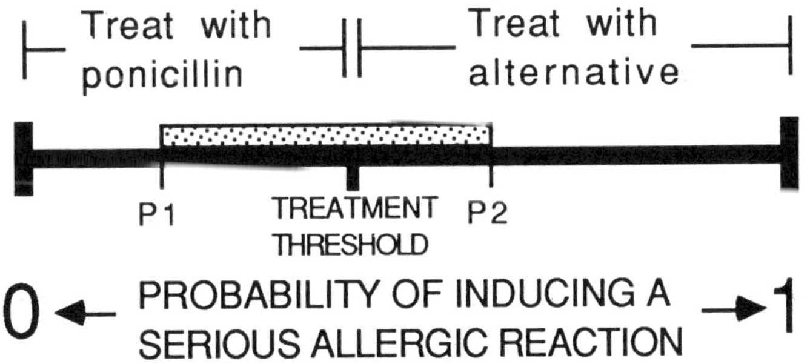

Fig 1–13.—Threshold model of decision making for dealing with diagnostic uncertainty. Penicillin can be used whenever the probability of inducing a serious allergic reaction is sufficiently low. The threshold represents the highest acceptable probability; above this point, penicillin should be abandoned and alternative antibiotics should be selected. If an imperfect diagnostic test is available, P1 and P2 define the range (shown by *stippling*) where test results are useful in guiding therapy. (Courtesy of Redelmeier DA, Sox HC Jr: *Arch Intern Med* 150:1939–1946, 1990.)

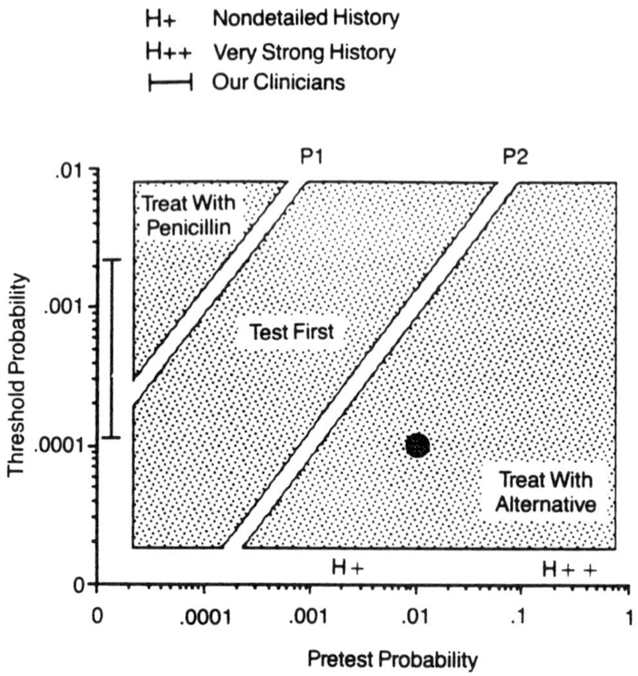

Fig 1–14.—Two-way sensitivity analysis: a guide for determining when to use the penicillin allergy skin test. The position on the *abscissa* is determined by the risk of a severe allergic reaction based on the clinical setting. The position on the *ordinate* is determined by the threshold probability at which a clinician would switch from penicillin to an alternative antibiotic based on the clinical situation. Representative pretest probabilities are plotted for a patient who has an extremely strong history of penicillin allergy (H++) or a history of penicillin allergy for which no details are available (H+). Representative threshold probabilities are plotted for *Streptococcus viridans* endocarditis, as perceived by clinicians. Patients located in the *middle stippled area* should have therapy guided by the results of penicillin allergy skin testing, whereas those located in the *lateral strippled areas* should proceed directly to treatment. The *large gray cross-hatched dot* demarcates the location of the patient described in the text of the original article. (Courtesy of Redelmeier DA, Sox HC Jr: *Arch Intern Med* 150:1939–1946, 1990.)

The attitudes of 12 physicians toward the outcomes of treatment with penicillin or vancomycin for *Streptococcus viridans* endocarditis in patients with a history of penicillin allergy were assessed. In this situation, calculating the treatment threshold requires identifying both the probability and the value of the clinical outcomes with the 2 agents. A negative skin test result in this setting is worthwhile in a patient with a weak history of allergy.

Skin test results are negative in approximately 5% of patients who would have a severe allergic reaction. Thus if the patient's history of a reaction to penicillin is convincing, there should be no skin test and no penicillin therapy. With a less certain history of penicillin allergy, the decision to perform the skin test must be individualized (Fig 1–14).

▶ It is striking that even after more than 50 years of penicillin usage there is still controversy over when an allergic history should preclude its use. There are at least 2 fundamental problems that make this a controversial issue. The first is that a negative skin test does not exclude an anaphylactic reaction. The authors of this paper reviewed this literature extensively and found that about 5% of patients with a strong history of penicillin allergy will have an anaphylactic reaction despite a negative skin test. Because of the unreliability of the predictive value of the skin test, it is my opinion that no patient with a history of acute allergic reactions (e.g., angioedema, urticaria, or previous anaphylaxis) should either be skin tested or receive penicillin. The second major difficulty muddies the waters even more. Patients' histories of allergic reactions to penicillin are not entirely reliable. When one combines these 2 problems, the very limited utility of penicillin skin testing becomes apparent. With each passing year that alternative antibiotics prove their effectiveness, the need to ever skin test should further diminish.—M.S. Klempner, M.D.

Childhood Brucellosis: A Study of 102 Cases

Al-Eissa YA, Kambal AM, Al-Nasser MN, Al-Habib SA, Al-Fawaz IM, Al-Zamil FA (King Khalid Univ Hosp, Riyadh; King Saud Univ, Riyadh, Saudi Arabia)

Pediatr Infect Dis J 9:74–79, 1990 1–45

Brucellosis appears to be common and widespread in Saudi Arabia. The epidemiologic, clinical, and laboratory features and outcome of antimicrobial therapy were reviewed in 102 children treated for brucellosis in a 4-year period. The source of infection was unpasteurized goat's milk in 80% of patients. The disease was prevalent throughout the year, with the highest incidence in late winter and early summer. The predominant symptoms and signs were fever, arthralgia, malaise, weight loss, arthritis, hepatosplenomegaly, and lymphadenopathy (Table 1).

Most joint involvement was monarticular, involving the hips and knees. The severity of the disease did not correlate with the duration of illness before diagnosis. Diverse nonspecific hematological and biochemical abnormalities were found. *Brucella melitensis* was isolated in 75% of 87 patients, and only 4 were resistant to trimethoprim-sulfamethoxazole (TMP-SMX); all other isolates were susceptible to other drugs.

Treatment consisted of various durations and combinations of TMP-SMX or tetracycline plus streptomycin or rifampin. Of the 85 patients evaluable after an average follow-up period of 14 months (range, 9–36 months), 17 (20%) had relapses. Relapse occurred significantly more often among those given 2-drug combination therapy for 3 weeks (85.7%) than among patients treated for at least 6 weeks (8%) (Table 2). No relapses occurred among the 9 patients treated with a combination of TMX-SMX and rifampin for 8–12 weeks. All 17 of 85 patients (20%) who relapsed were treated successfully with a 6-week course of antibiotics other than the initial regimen.

Brucellosis appears to be common in endemic areas and its treatment remains a problem. However, these data suggest that a longer duration of treatment with combination antibiotic therapy may improve the outcome and prevent relapse.

▶ There has been interest in the use of fluoroquinolones for brucellosis recently, with mixed results in small series. However, these agents would not be

TABLE 1.—Distribution of Clinical manifestations in 102 Children With Brucellosis

Symptom or Sign	Males (n=52) No.	Females (n=50) No.	Total (n=102) No (%)
Fever	48	45	93 (91)*
Arthralgia	34	40	74 (73)
Malaise	28	33	61 (60)
Weight loss	25	24	49 (48)
Anorexia	19	22	41 (40)
Chills	10	10	20 (20)
Sweating	11	8	19 (19)
Backache	5	11	16 (16)
Headache	2	9	11 (11)
Abdominal pain	3	8	11 (11)
Nausea/Vomiting	4	6	10 (10)
Arthritis	15	23	38 (37)
Splenomegaly	15	21	36 (35)
Hepatomegaly	12	17	29 (28)
Lymphadenopathy	11	5	16 (16)
Osteomyelitis	-	2	2 (2)
Myocarditis	2	-	2 (2)

*Numbers in parentheses indicate percent.
(Courtesy of Al-Eissa YA, Kambal AM, Al-Nasser MN, et al: *Pediatr Infect Dis J* 9:74–79, 1990.)

an attractive choice for the treatment of infections in children.—M.J. Barza, M.D.

The Incidence of Aminoglycoside Antibiotic-Induced Hearing Loss

Brummett RE, Morrison RB (Oregon Health Sciences Univ, Portland)

Arch Otolaryngol Head Neck Surg 116:406–410, 1990 1–46

TABLE 2.—Antibiotic Regimens and Outcome of Treatment in 85 Children With Brucellosis

Antibiotic regimen*	No. of patients treated / No. of patients relapsed	
	Short duration*	Long duration †
TMP-SMZ + Stm	4/4	40/2
Tet + Stm	5/3	10/2
TMP-SMZ + Rif	4/4	9/1
Tet + Rif	1/1	3/0
TMP-SMZ+Rif+Stm	-	9/0
TOTAL	14/12	71/5

Abbreviations: Stm, streptomycin; *Tet,* tetracycline; *Rif,* rifampin.
*TMP-SMX, Tet and Rif were given for 3 weeks and Stm for the first 2 weeks.
†TMP-SMX, Tet and Rif were given for at least 6 weeks and Stm for the first 3 weeks.
(Courtesy of Al-Eissa YA, Kambal AM, Al-Nasser MN, et al: *Pediatr Infect Dis J* 9:74–79, 1990.)

Studies in both humans and animals have shown that ototoxicity can result from aminoglycoside antibiotics. The true incidence of hearing loss that results from such drugs has not, however, been determined. One cause for the discrepancy between studies is the definition of ototoxicity in terms of auditory threshold changes: an increase in pure-tone threshold from a baseline audiogram ≥15 dB at 2 or more frequencies, or ≥20 dB at 1 or more frequencies. However, pure-tone threshold changes of at least 15 dB occur in normal humans. Furthermore, most studies have not included control or comparison groups in addition to the aminoglycoside-treated group. The 2 criteria for ototoxicity were applied to 20 normal volunteers not using any known ototoxic drugs.

All of the subjects had measurable hearing at all test frequencies. Three pure-tone air conduction audiograms were obtained for each volunteer. These audiograms simulated a baseline before aminoglycoside antibiotic therapy, at the end of 1 week of therapy, and 1 week after therapy.

Most threshold changes were ≤10 dB, indicating no meaningful change. Yet, differences >10 dB were observed. Using the 2 accepted criteria for aminoglycoside antibiotic-induced ototoxicity, the incidence of "ototoxicity" in these subjects ranged from 20% to 33%. Because the subjects were not taking ototoxic agents, the changes observed may have resulted from the many variables that can affect auditory threshold measurements. The auditory changes may also represent the normal test-retest variability of pure-tone audiometry.

Pure-tone thresholds can be variable enough to be interpreted erroneously as drug-induced ototoxicity, thus exaggerating the reported incidence of hearing loss from aminoglycoside antibiotics. High-frequency hearing tests are recommended to minimize the risk of error.

▶ This is a seminal study in many ways, looking at the measurement variability in pure-tone air conduction audiograms over time in normal volunteers, 25–63 years old, using no ototoxic drugs. The results are rather surprising in that 20% to 33% satisfied the 2 criteria for ototoxicity. The authors conclude that the incidence of aminoglycoside-induced ototoxicity may be exaggerated. Exaggerated, perhaps, but probably not "never." I have seen profound hearing loss develop in patients, particularly in the old days when kanamycin was commonly used, and I didn't need an audiogram to measure the change. High-frequency loss is the common effect of aminoglycosides, and the authors suggest using only high-frequency testing as a more reliable method to specifically detect aminoglycoside-induced changes. However, as they point out, such tests are difficult to do in those very sick patients most likely to be receiving the drugs. They are trying to develop such a method, and when they do and apply it to the problem, I hope they include controls and attempt to follow patients with a high probability of repeat courses of aminoglycosides, because aminoglycoside toxicity is probably cumulative over the lifetime of exposure to these drugs.—G.T. Keusch, M.D.

2 Lyme Borreliosis

Lyme Disease in Childhood: Clinical and Epidemiologic Features of Ninety Cases

Williams CL, Strobino B, Lee A, Curran A, Benach JL, Inamdar S, Cristofaro R (New York Med College, Valhalla; Westchester County Health Dept, White Plains, NY; New York State Dept of Health, Stony Brook)

Pediatr Infect Dis J 9:10–14, 1990 2–1

Ninety patients aged 19 years and younger who had Lyme disease in 1982–1983 were studied. They represented 43% of all cases reported in Westchester County during this time. The mean patient age was 10 years. Nearly three fourths of the patients had onset of symptoms in the summer months. Half of them reported a tick bite before symptom onset.

Two thirds of the patients had a skin rash consistent with erythema chronicum migrans, and the same proportion reported flulike symptoms (Fig 2–1). Joint involvement tended to occur in older children, and in most cases multiple joints were affected. The knee was the most commonly involved joint (Fig 2–2), and seventh nerve palsy was the most frequent neurologic symptom.

Antibiotics, most often orally administered penicillin, were prescribed for 79% of the children. Only 10% of them received more than 1 course. Compared with adults seen in the same period, the pediatric patients were more likely to have fever and joint complaints and less likely to have erythema chronicum migrans (table).

Careful examination of the skin in a febrile child seen during the summer in an endemic region may reveal annular skin lesions with central clearing. Facial nerve paralysis was the most common neurologic presentation in this series. Tetracycline is effective in adults, but penicillin gen-

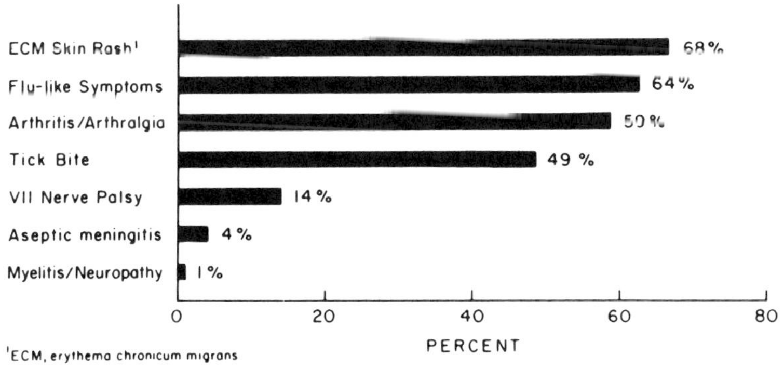

Fig 2–1.—Clinical characteristics of 90 children with Lyme disease. (Courtesy of Williams CL, Strobino B, Lee A, et al: *Pediatr Infect Dis J* 9:10–14, 1990.)

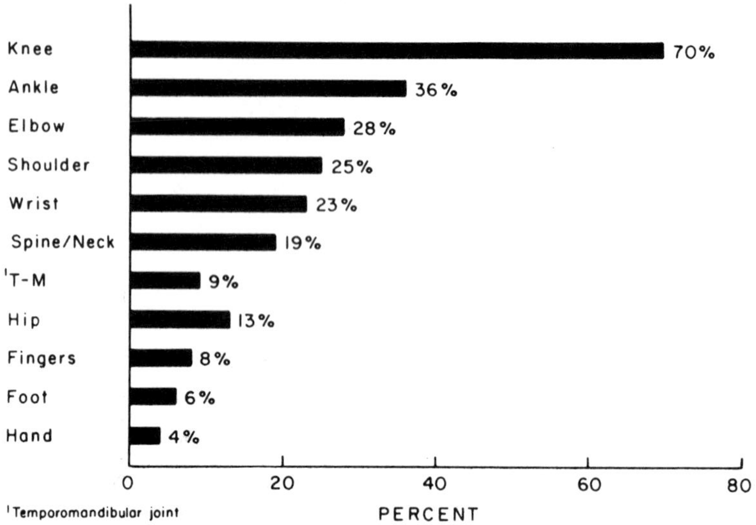

Fig 2–2.—Frequence of specific joint involvement in 53 children with Lyme disease. (Courtesy of Williams CL, Strobino B, Lee A, et al: *Pediatr Infect Dis J* 9:10–14, 1990.)

erally is prescribed for young children. Erythromycin appears to be less effective than either penicillin or tetracycline.

▶ There is a major need to define whether the spectrum of Lyme disease, both acutely and chronically, is different in the pediatric and adult populations. This report of 90 patients ranging in age from 1 to 19 years points out how similar the presentation of Lyme disease is in pediatric and adult cases. Although fever was more common and erythema chronicum migrans (ECM) less

Comparison of Pediatric Vs. Adult Cases of Lyme Disease: Frequency of Reported Characteristics With Odds Ratio

	Pediatric Cases (n = 90)		Adult Cases (n = 119)		Odds Ratios*
	n	%	n	%	
Tick bite	44	49	43	36	1.69 (0.97, 2.95)†
Fever	57	63	48	40	2.55 (1.45, 4.49) ‡
ECM	60	67	96	81	0.48 (0.25, 0.90) ‡
Joint complaints §	53	59	52	44	1.85 (1.06, 3.21) ‡
Joint pain only	19	21	28	24	0.48 (0.22, 1.05)
Joint swelling	34	38	24	20	2.09 (0.95, 4.57)
Neurologic symptoms	14	16	23	19	0.77 (0.31, 1.59)
Seventh nerve palsy	12	13	11	9	

*Odds ratios compare the presence of each characteristic in pediatric cases with that in adults.
†Numbers in parentheses, 95% confidence limits.
‡$P < .05$.
§Pain, swelling, or both.
(Courtesy of Williams CL, Strobino B, Lee A, et al: *Pediatric Infect Dis J* 9:10–14, 1990.)

common in pediatric patients, these differences are not helpful diagnostically. It is important to recall that only 50% of patients with ECM alone have a positive serology initially, again pointing out the need for better diagnostic tests, especially in early disease. The long-term follow-up studies of both pediatric and adult patients with Lyme disease are now appearing, and it is becoming more clear that there is reason for concern for both late neurologic and musculoskeletal problems.—M.S. Klempner, M.D.

Chronic Neurologic Manifestations of Lyme Disease

Logigian EL, Kaplan RF, Steere AC (Tufts Univ; New England Med Ctr, Boston)
N Engl J Med 323:1438–1444, 1990 2–2

Lyme disease is associated with a wide range of neurologic abnormalities, both acute and chronic. The chronic abnormalities were investigated in a series of 27 patients with neurologic symptoms after an episode of Lyme disease. All had current evidence of immunity to *Borrelia burgdorferi*, and the patients lacked evidence of other causes for their symptoms. Eight patients were followed prospectively for 8–12 years after onset of infection.

Signs and Symptoms of Chronic Neurologic Abnormalities

Signs and Symptoms	No. of Patients (%)
Encephalopathy	24 (89)
Memory loss	22 (81)
Depression	10 (37)
Sleep disturbance	8 (30)
Irritability	7 (26)
Difficulty finding words	5 (19)
Polyneuropathy	19 (70)
Spinal or radicular pain	11 (41)
Distal paresthesia	7 (26)
Sensory loss	12 (44)
Lower-motor-neuron weakness	2 (7)
Ankle hyporeflexia	2 (7)
Leukoencephalitis	1 (4)
Upper-motor-neuron weakness	1 (4)
Hyperreflexia	1 (4)
Increased muscle tone	1 (4)
Other symptoms	27 (100)
Fatigue	20 (74)
Headache	13 (48)
Hearing loss	4 (15)
Tinnitus	2 (7)
Fibromyalgia	4 (15)

(Courtesy of Logigian EL, Kaplan RF, Steere AC: *N Engl J Med* 323:1438–1444, 1990.)

About 40% of patients had severe headache, mild neck stiffness, or spinal pain during the acute illness. Symptoms of chronic peripheral neurologic disorder were seen a median of 16 months after onset of infection, and CNS involvement began after a median of 26 months. Twenty-four patients had a mild encephalopathy, usually manifested by difficulty in remembering things and compensatory list-making (table). Nineteen patients had polyneuropathy, which nearly always included sensory symptoms. One patient had evidence of leukoencephalitis 6 years after the onset of Lyme disease.

Improvement often did not begin until several months after completion of intravenous ceftriaxone therapy. Nerve conduction and neuropsychological function tended to improve, but serum and CSF antibody responses often were unchanged. Five patients with abnormal cerebral MR images improved clinically despite a lack of change in the lesions. Seventeen of the 27 patients were improved when last seen; 6 others improved but later relapsed; 4 were no better.

The response to antibiotic therapy supports a role for spirochetal infection in the pathogenesis of chronic neurologic syndromes. The results, however, were not as good as those in previous reports. Some nonresponders may have irreversible damage to the nervous system.

▶ I suspect that many of the editors and readers of this YEAR BOOK will acknowledge, on careful examination, difficulty in remembering things and compensatory list-making. Nevertheless, the population studied here did not simply have nonspecific CNS abnormalities and a positive antibody titer to *B. burgdorferi.* Rather, 85% of the patients had had erythema migrans days to weeks before onset of neurologic symptoms (their memory for that feature seems to be quite good!) and the rest had arthritis preceding the neurologic symptoms. One third of the patients had CNS involvement early on, including facial palsy, meningitis, or thoracic radiculoneuritis. Within a median of 6 months after onset of disease, 70% of the patients had episodes of arthritis. In terms of the chronic neurologic abnormalities, aside from memory loss and other central phenomena, 70% had polyneuropathy and 1 patient had leukoencephalitis. The analogy to syphilis is striking. That the results of treatment were variable with more than one third of the patients having no improvement or relapse after 6 months is also reminiscent of the findings with CNS syphilis. Whether patients with unexplained neurologic symptoms whose only evidence of *B. burgdorferi* infection is a positive antibody titer should be treated cannot be answered by the available evidence.—M.J. Barza, M.D.

Randomized Comparison of Ceftriaxone and Cefotaxime in Lyme Neuroborreliosis

Pfister H-W, Preac-Mursic V, Wilske B, Schielke E, Sörgel F, Einhäupl KM (Univ of Munich; Ludwig Maximilians Univ, Munich; Inst for Biomedical and Pharmaceutical Research, Nürnberg-Heroldsberg, Germany)
J Infect Dis 163:311–318, 1991 2–3

TABLE 1.—Clinical Data of 30 Patients With Lyme Neuroborreliosis at the Onset of Antibiotic Therapy

					Cerebrospinal fluid (CSF)				Antibody titers‡		
Patient, sex, age, years	AB*	EM*	Neurologic symptoms and signs	Disease duration, days†	WBC/μl	Protein, g/l	CSF-to-serum albumin ratio, $\times 10^{-3}$	Oligoclonal IgG bands	Serum IgG	Serum IgM	CSF/serum index
Ceftriaxone											
1, M, 68	+	–	Pareses of anterior tibialis and gastrocnemius muscles, R&L; pain and hypesthesia at L5/S1, R&L	304	18	0.75	15.2	–	1:128	Neg	Neg
2, M, 49	–	+	Facial palsy, L; cervical pain	8	23	0.46	4.6	–	Neg	1:64	Neg
3, M, 53	+	–	Facial palsy, L; paresis of arm, R; of supra- and infraspinatus, deltoid, brachioradialis, and biceps muscles, L; radicular pain at C7, R&L	30	37	0.90	9.9	+	1:512	1:64	Neg
4, F, 26	+	–	Radicular pain at S1, L&R; headache	9	451	0.77	10.7	–	Neg	Neg	Neg

(Continued)

TABLE 1. (continued)

				Cerebrospinal fluid (CSF)							
5, F, 84	+	+	Paresis of interossei muscles, L; radicular pain and hypesthesia at C7, R&L, and C8, R	60	26	0.69	7.2	+	1:1024	Neg	2.9
6, F, 33	+	+	Lumbar pain; pain at S1, R&L	4	6	0.34	5.8	–	Neg	Neg	Neg
7, M, 79	–	–	Radicular pain at C7, R&L; hypesthesia of both hands	19	89	0.75	ND	+	1:512	Neg	27.0
8, M, 72	–	–	Facial palsy, L; paravertebral pain; paresthesia at C7, R	36	50	1.12	16.5	+	1:1024	Neg	4.5
9, M, 58	+	+	Radicular pain at C7, R&L	18	82	0.75	9.6	+	Neg	1:128	2.3
10, F, 66	+	+	Pareses of iliopsoas and quadriceps muscles, R; radicular pain at L3/L4, R	27	109	0.72	10.0	+	1:64	Neg	6.0
11, M, 66	+	–	Abducent paresis, R; pareses of both arms; cervical pain; hypesthesia of both hands	38	288	1.91	34.3	+	1:64	1:128	38.9
12, M, 25	–	+	Radicular pain and hypesthesia at C7/C8, R&L, and S1, L	46	21	0.32	5.2	+	Neg	1:32	Neg
13, M, 61	–	–	Pareses of both legs, dysesthesia and pain at S1, R&L	184	5	0.24	5.0	+	1:512	Neg	Neg
14, F, 82	+	+	Pareses of interossei muscles, R; dysesthesia at C7/C8, L	120	5	0.46	5.0	–	1:128	Neg	Neg

Patient, sex, age, years	AB*	EM*	Neurologic symptoms and signs	Disease duration, days†	WBC/μl	Protein, g/l	CSF-to-serum albumin ratio, $\times 10^{-3}$	Oligoclonal IgG bands	Antibody titers‡ Serum IgG	Serum IgM	CSF/serum index
Cefotaxime											
15, F, 62	+	–	Facial palsy, R; headache	35	26	0.75	11.7	+	1:128	1:64	Neg
16, F, 63	–	+	Paresis of anterior tibialis muscle, R; radicular pain and hypesthesia at L5, R	83	16	0.47	8.1	+	1:64	Neg	Neg
17, M, 12	–	–	Facial palsy, L	21	15	0.32	4.5	–	1:64	1:128	Neg
18, F, 57	+	+	Radicular pain and dysesthesia at C7, R&L; radicular pain at T10, R&L	29	71	0.53	9.0	+	1:64	1:64	13.4
19, M, 52	+	+	Facial palsy, R; radicular pain and paresthesia at C7/C8, R&L	40	155	0.97	16.9	+	1:256	Neg	14.0
20, F, 69	–	–	Facial palsy, L	62	5	0.27	3.7	–	1:128	Neg	Neg
21, M, 28	–	–	Facial palsy, R; vertebral pain	32	1207	1.92	34.9	+	Neg	Neg	27.8
22, F, 71	–	–	Pareses of both legs; hypesthesia at T7, R&L; radicular pain at L4, R&L	77	367	1.46	31.3	+	1:32	Neg	1:32§

(Continued)

TABLE 1. (continued)

23, M, 59	–	+	Facial palsy, R&L; radicular pain at S1, R&L	32	44	1.47	ND	ND	1:32	Neg	100.1
24, F, 78	+	–	Paravertebral and cervical pain	29	31	0.99	ND	ND	1:32	Neg	4.1
25, M, 48	+	–	Pareses of anterior tibialis and gastrocnemius muscles, R; hypesthesia at L5, R, and both hands; pain at S1, R&L	71	52	0.83	13.7	+	1:128	Neg	21.2
26, M, 63	+	+	Radicular pain and dysesthesia at T12/L1, R&L, and S1, L	17	62	0.38	6.7	–	1:64	Neg	Neg
27, F, 61	+	+	Radicular pain and hypesthesia at L4/S1, L	10	17	0.37	5.8	–	1:128	Neg	Neg
28, F, 39	+	+	Facial palsy, L; vertebral pain and dysesthesia at T10/T11, R&L	11	34	0.96	8.2	+	Neg	Neg	7.3
29, F, 43	+	+	Radicular pain at L3/L4, R	47	13	0.37	4.6	+	Neg	Neg	Neg
30, M, 54	–	+	Facial palsy, L; radicular pain at C7, S1, R&L	22	50	0.60	16.3	+	1:32	Neg	Neg

*Arthropod bite (AB) or erythema migrans (EM) within 3 months before onset of neurologic disease.
†From onset of neurologic symptoms to therapy.
‡Titers to *Borrelia burgdorferi.*
§Cerebrospinal fluid/serum index could not be determined in this patient.
‖*Abbreviations: WBC,* white blood cells; *M,* male; *F,* female; *R,* right; *L,* left; *ND,* not done; *Neg,* no detectable antibodies.
(Courtesy of Pfister H-W, Preac-Mursic V, Wilske B, et al: *J Infect Dis* 163:311–318, 1991.)

The most frequent neurologic manifestations of Lyme borreliosis are meningitis, cranial neuritis, and painful radiculoneuritis. Although high-dose penicillin administered intravenously has been used to treat the neurologic complications of Lyme disease, recent studies have shown third-generation cephalosporins to be more effective. Two of these drugs, ceftriaxone and cefotaxime, were compared in a randomized open clinical study.

Thirty-three patients with Lyme neuroborreliosis were randomly assigned to either ceftriaxone (2 g every 24 hours) or cefotaxime (2 g every 8 hours), both given intravenously for 10 days. Lumbar punctures were performed to determine CSF antibiotic concentrations and antibodies to *Borrelia burgdorferi.*

Twenty-seven of the 30 patients eligible for efficacy analysis (Table 1) were reexamined at a mean of 8.1 months after antibiotic therapy. Seventeen were clinically asymptomatic at follow-up. Two patients in each group did not improve or even deteriorated during treatment. Lumbar puncture was performed in 23 patients. In nearly all cases, the CSF antibiotic concentrations were above the minimal inhibitory concentration 90 level for *B. burgdorferi* (Table 2). In 1 patient, however, *B. burgdorferi* was isolated from the CSF 7.5 months after treatment.

TABLE 2.—Clinical Findings on Follow-Up Examination

	Ceftriaxone (n = 12)	Cefotaxime (n = 15)
Follow-up period, months, mean ± SD	7.4 ± 2.1	8.6 ± 1.8
Neurologic findings		
Normal, no complaints	8	9
Clinically symptomatic	4	6
Mild residual symptoms	3	5
Facial pareses	0	2
Pareses of extremities	2	3
Sensory disturbances	2	3
Episodes of radicular pain, headache, arthralgias, fever	1*	0
Recurrent radicular pain	0	1†
Repeated lumbar puncture	10	13
Cerebrospinal fluid		
Lymphocytic pleocytosis	0	2‡
Protein elevation	0	0
Oligoclonal IgG bands	5	7
Isolation of *B. burgdorferi*	1	0

**Borrelia burgdorferi* was isolated from the CSF of this patient 7.5 months after antibiotic therapy.

†Lymphocytic pleocytosis in CSF 9 months after antibiotic therapy.

‡Eight and 6 cells/μL at follow-up periods of 7 months and 9 months, respectively.

(Courtesy of Pfister H-W, Preac-Mursic V, Wilske B, et al: *J Infect Dis* 163:311–318, 1991.)

Both drugs were generally well tolerated. Most patients showed clinical improvement on days 3–5 of therapy. There were no clinical differences between the 2 antibiotics, either during the 10-day treatment period or at follow-up. A longer period of antibiotic therapy might have improved the outcome in the 10 patients who remained symptomatic at follow-up.

▶ Optimal treatment for Lyme disease involving the CNS has not been defined. With an appreciation of possible long-term neurologic effects of Lyme disease, the importance of answering this question looms larger. This study showed no differences between a 10-day treatment course with ceftriaxone (2 g every 24 hours) and cefotaxime (2 g every 8 hours). It was striking to me, however, that at least a third of the patients in both groups remained symptomatic at follow-up more than 6 months after treatment. Residual symptoms included facial paralysis, paralysis of an extremity, sensory disturbances, and radicular pain. Perhaps of even greater concern was the isolation of *B. burgdorferi* from the spinal fluid of a patient treated with ceftriaxone 7½ months later. Most experts now believe that a 10-day course of parenteral antibiotics for patients with Lyme disease involving the CNS is inadequate. A minimum duration of 14–21 days of parenteral therapy with ceftriaxone or penicillin seems prudent. There is an excellent review by Rahn and Malawista in the *Annals of Internal Medicine* (1).—M.S. Klempner, M.D.

Reference

1. Rahn DW, Malawista SE: *Ann Intern Med* 114:472, 1991.

Association of Chronic Lyme Arthritis With HLA-DR4 and HLA-DR2 Alleles

Steere AC, Dwyer E, Winchester R (New England Med Ctr, Boston; Tufts Univ; New York Univ)

N Engl J Med 323:219–223, 1990 2–4

Joint involvement occurs in about 80% of patients with Lyme disease, and arthritic episodes may become longer-lasting as the disease continues. Chronic joint involvement may have an immunogenic basis. Immunogenetic profiles were determined in 130 patients who had various manifestations of Lyme disease, including 80 with arthritis.

Among the 80 patients with arthritis, 57% of those affected for longer than 1 year had the HLA-DR4 specificity compared with 23% of patients who had arthritis for 6–11 months and 9% of those with involvement for 1–5 months. Excluding HLA-DR4-positive patients, HLA-DR2 occurred in 75% of those with chronic arthritis, 50% of patients with arthritis of moderate duration, and 20% of those affected for less than 6 months. The disease in patients with HLA-DR4 tended to resist antibiotic therapy.

These findings support a role for immunogenetic factors in chronic Lyme arthritis. Class II molecules of the HLA-DR4 or DR2 haplotype may combine with an arthritogenic epitope of *Borrelia burgdorferi* that mimics a host component at the molecular level. The interaction of T helper cells with this complex could produce an ongoing autoimmune response. Alternatively, affected patients may, during thymic maturation, delete T cell clones that are required to eliminate the spirochete.

▶ As Alan Steere's office is directly below mine, I would have to be tactful if I felt too critical of his study. But there is no need for tact, because this is a very nice, sufficiently large (80 patients) study clearly showing the association between both HLA DR types 2 and 4 with chronic arthritis in patients with Lyme disease. The challenge to my neighbor and colleague is to discover why these patients are at risk and to apply this information to therapeutic interventions. If he, and his coworkers, can accomplish this, they may also provide clues to the pathogenesis and therapy of other microbially induced reactive arthritis states. As a devotee of *Shigella,* I eagerly await the results. So, no long lunches, Alan, I'm watching.—G.T. Keusch, M.D.

3 Viral Infections

Herpesviruses

Predictors of Morbidity and Mortality in Neonates With Herpes Simplex Virus Infections

Whitley R, Arvin A, Prober C, Corey L, Burchett S, Plotkin S, Starr S, Jacobs R, Powell D, Nahmias A, Sumaya C, Edwards K, Alford C, Caddell G, Soong S-J, and the Natl Inst of Allergy and Infectious Diseases Collaborative Antiviral Study Group (Univ of Alabama, Birmingham; Stanford Univ; Univ of Washington; Joseph Stokes Jr Research Inst, Philadelphia; Univ of Arkansas; et al)

N Engl J Med 324:450–454, 1991 3–1

In other investigations the study group found no detectable differences in mortality and morbidity after vidarabine and acyclovir therapy for neonatal herpes simplex virus (HSV) infection. Based on this finding, the clinical, laboratory, and outcome factors that influence the prognosis of neonatal HSV infection were studied in a controlled trial of 202 infants.

Disease in the 202 infants was classified in 3 categories based on extent of involvement at entry into the trial: infection confined to skin, eyes, or

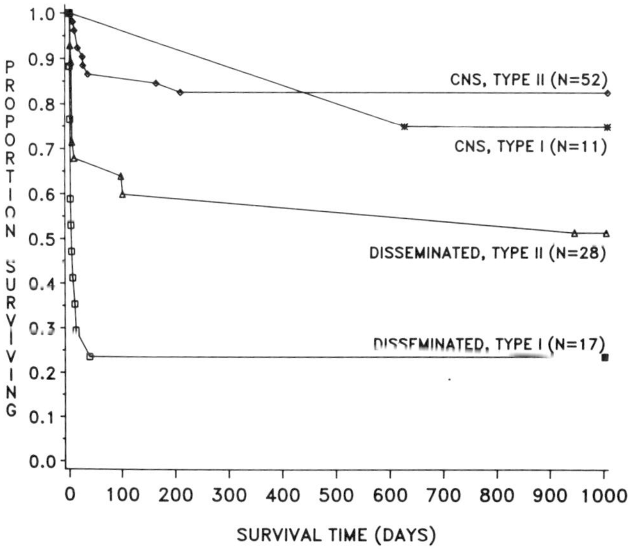

Fig 3–1.—Survival of infants with neonatal HSV infection with CNS involvement or disseminated disease. In group with disseminated disease infants with HSV type 1 had significantly poorer survival than those with type 2. (Courtesy of Whitley R, Arvin A, Prober C, et al: *N Engl J Med* 324:450–454, 1991.)

Prognostic Factors Identified by Multivariate Analyses for Neonates with HSV Infection

Dominant Factors	Relative Risk	
	Mortality	Morbidity
Total group (n = 202)		
Extent of disease		
Skin, eyes, or mouth	1	1
CNS *	5.8†	4.4†
Disseminated	33†	2.1†
Level of consciousness		
Alert or lethargic	1	NS
Semicomatose or comatose	5.2†	NS
Disseminated intravascular coagulopathy	3.8†	NS
Prematurity	3.7†	NS
Virus type		
1	2.3‡	1
2	1	4.9†
Seizures	NS	3.0†
Infants with disseminated disease (n = 46)		
Disseminated intravascular coagulopathy	3.5†	NS
Level of consciousness		
Alert or lethargic	1	1
Semicomatose or comatose	3.9†	4.0†
Pneumonia	3.6†	NS
Infants with CNS involvement (n = 71)		
Level of consciousness		
Alert or lethargic	1	NS
Semicomatose or comatose	6.1†	NS
Prematurity	5.2†	NS
Seizures	NS	3.4†
Infants with infection of the skin, eyes, or mouth (n = 85)		
No. of skin-vesicle recurrences		
<3	NA	1
≥3	NA	21†
Virus type		
1	NA	1
2	NA	14‡§

Abbreviations: NS, not statistically significant; *NA,* not applicable (no infant with disease confined to skin, eyes, or mouth died).

*Central nervous system.

†$P < .01$.

‡$P < .05$.

§Because of correlation between virus type and skin-vesicle recurrence, virus type was not significant in multivariate model; however, it was significant as single factor.

(Courtesy of Whitley R, Arvin A, Prober C, et al: *N Engl J Med* 324:450–454, 1991.)

mouth; encephalitis; or disseminated infection. The highest mortality rate was 57% in the 46 neonates with disseminated infection, compared to 15% in the 71 infants with encephalitis and no deaths in neonates with localized infections. The mortality risk was increased in neonates in or near coma at entry, neonates with disseminated intravascular coagulopathy, or premature neonates. In infants with disseminated disease, HSV pneumonitis was also associated with increased mortality. As shown in Figure 3–1, infants with HSV type 1 disseminated infection had poorer outcomes than those with HSV type 2 infection. Three or more recurrences of vesicles limited to the skin, eyes, or mouth were also associated with an increased risk of neurologic impairment (table).

Morbidity and mortality from neonatal HSV infection were closely related to extent of the disease. Prognostic factors for neonatal HSV infection include level of consciousness, development of disseminated intravascular coagulopathy or pneumonia, gestational age, and type of virus. Treatment before development of CNS disease, disseminated disease, or a depressed consciousness significantly improves outcome.

▶ This study will be the classic one cited regarding the natural history of neonatal HSV infection. Surprisingly, morbidity with HSV type 1 infection of the CNS appears to have a better prognosis than type 2. The lower sensitivity for HSV type 2 isolates to acyclovir provides a rational basis for the increased dosing regimen.

As the authors note, in individuals with HSV limited to the skin, eyes, or mouth, 3 or more skin recurrences in 6 months correlated with long-term neurologic sequelae. Therefore, oral therapy with acyclovir as long-term suppression will be studied to prevent the potential development of silent viremia.—D.R. Snydman, M.D.

Primary and Recurrent Herpes Simplex Virus Type 2-Induced Meningitis

Bergström T, Vahlne A, Alestig K, Jeansson S, Forsgren M, Lycke E (Univ of Göteborg; Stockholm County Council, Sweden)

J Infect Dis 162:322–330, 1990 3–2

Herpes simplex virus type 2 (HSV-2) may cause fatal encephalitis in neonates and immunocompromised patients, but severe postnatal CNS infections are rare. Nevertheless, HSV-2 might induce nonfatal meningeal infection. Data were reviewed concerning 27 patients after a first episode of confirmed HSV-2-induced meningitis. Seven other patients had recurrent meningitis possibly caused by HSV-2.

Herpes simplex virus type 2 was isolated from the CSF in the first episode of meningitis in 21 patients and typed as HSV-2; in 6 others the diagnosis was based on seroconversion against HSV-2. Five patients had recurrence of meningitis. Genital lesions preceded meningitis by a mean of about 1 week. All patients had severe headaches and a stiff neck. The most frequent complications of HSV-2 meningitis were urinary retention, dysesthesias/paresthesias, neuralgias, and motor weakness/paraparesis.

In contrast to the initial episode of HSV-2 meningitis, viral isolation and HSV antigen detection are not helpful in diagnosing recurrences. The immunoblotting method may be used to detect intrathecally produced IgG antibody to the HSV-2 type-specific protein gG-2 during recurrent episodes.

▶ Several years ago I saw a patient with recurrent HSV-2 meningitis and had a difficult time finding much of value in the literature. Thus I welcome this report.—S.M. Wolff, M.D.

▶ ↓ Physicians should be aware that even with relatively early therapy of *Herpes simplex* encephalitis and a clinical response, long-term neuropsychological residual deficits are likely. Families and patients need to be counseled in this regard.—D.R. Snydman, M.D.

Long-Term Cognitive Sequelae of Acyclovir-Treated Herpes Simplex Encephalitis

Gordon B, Selnes OA, Hart J Jr, Hanley DF, Whitley RJ (Johns Hopkins Univ; Univ of Alabama, Birmingham)

Arch Neurol 47:646–647, 1990 3–3

Survival from untreated herpes simplex type 1 encephalitis (HSE-1) is associated with severe cognitive and behavioral sequelae. Early diagnosis and prompt antiviral therapy may significantly reduce the mortality and morbidity of this illness. To investigate further, the long-term cognitive changes of 4 patients who received acyclovir during the early stages of biopsy-proven HSE-1 were studied. Patients received their first acyclovir treatment an average of 9.75 days (range, 5–20 days) after the onset of fever and headache. Their Glasgow Coma Scale scores were between 9 and 15. Neuropsychological tests were performed 1–3 years after onset of illness.

Although 3 of 4 patients had normal performance on a standard clinical mental status test, all 4 showed significant residua, most commonly dysnomia and impaired new learning for both verbal and visual material. These deficits were consistent with the temporal lobe localization of HSE-1. None of 4 patients was able to return to his/her pre-illness life and work.

Despite early acyclovir treatment of HSE-1, long-lasting or permanent residua are likely. Furthermore, these deficits may not be evident on clinical screening.

Varicella With Delayed Hemiplegia

Ichiyama T, Houdou S, Kisa T, Ohno K, Takeshita K (Tottori Univ, Yonago, Japan; Shimane Prefectural Central Hosp, Izumo, Japan)

Pediatr Neurol 6:279–281, 1990 3–4

Contralateral hemiplegia that occurs from several days to 6 months after herpes zoster ophthalmicus is a distinct CNS syndrome caused by the varicella zoster virus (VZV). Two boys and 2 girls aged 1–7 years had acute hemiplegia 7 weeks to 4 months after varicella infection. Computed tomography scans demonstrated low-density lesions in the left basal ganglia (Fig

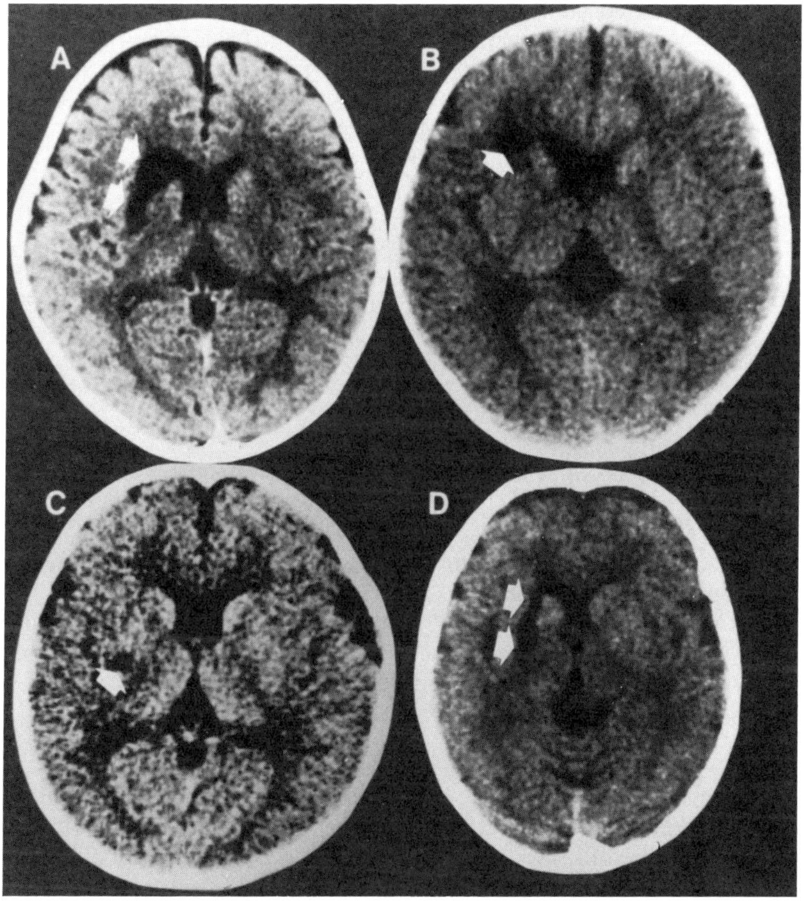

Fig 3–2.—Computed tomography scans of 4 patients show low-density lesions in left basal ganglia *(arrows)*. **A,** boy aged 4 years; **B,** girl aged 1 year; **C,** boy aged 7 years; and **D,** girl aged 2 years. (Courtesy of Ichiyama T, Houdou S, Kisa T, et al: *Pediatr Neurol* 6:279–281, 1990.)

3–2). Carotid angiography revealed segmental narrowing and occlusion of the middle cerebral artery in 2 patients. Within 1–8 months of the onset of hemiplegia 2 children were asymptomatic and 2 had residual weakness.

Because varicella and herpes zoster are different clinical manifestations of the same causative agent, VZV, the appearance of acute hemiparesis with antecedent varicella strongly suggests a causal relationship. Hemiplegia after varicella appears to result from vasculitis caused by VZV infection. The 4 cases reported here occurred during a period in which there were 26,001 cases of varicella; thus the frequency of delayed hemiparesis was approximately 1/6,500 varicella patients.

▶ Hemiplegia following ophthalmic zoster is a rare entity, with only a few dozen patients reported in the literature. Hemiplegia following the primary infection, varicella, apparently is rarer still. It was first described in 1983, and there have been only a couple of patients reported. The pathogenesis is presumed to be the same in hemiplegia following varicella as in that following zoster, namely, a cerebral vasculitis caused by infection of middle and anterior cerebral arteries producing low-density CT lesions, presumably infarcts, of the basal ganglia, internal capsule, and thalamus.—M.J. Barza, M.D.

Hepatitis

▶ ↓ Last year I reviewed a surveillance study implying that occasional transmission of hepatitis C may occur by sexual contact (1). However, this study did not rely on anti-HCV antibody testing. The 2 studies cited below both confirm that sexual transmission, either by heterosexual or homosexual contact, is much less common than that occurring with hepatitis B.—D.R. Snydman, M.D.

Reference

1. 1991 Year Book of Infectious Diseases, pp 112–113.

Sexual Transmission of Hepatitis C Virus: Cohort Study (1981–9) Among European Homosexual Men

Melbye M, Biggar RJ, Wantzin P, Krogsgaard K, Ebbesen P, Becker NG (Rigshospitalet and Inst of Cancer Epidemiology, Copenhagen; Natl Cancer Inst, Bethesda, Md; Hvidore Hosp, Copenhagen; Danish Cancer Society, Aarhus; La Tnobe Univ, Bundoora, Vic, Australia)

Br Med J 301:210–212, 1990 3–5

Transmission of hepatitis C virus (HCV) by exposure to blood has been described in drug addicts and in patients with hemophilia, but little has been reported on the frequency of sexual transmission of this virus. The prevalence, incidence, and persistence of positivity for antibodies to HCV (anti-HCV) and the potential for sexual transmission of the virus were investigated. The cohort analysis of 259 male members of a Danish homosexual organization used data from 1981 to 1989. Comparison of anti-HCV data was made with data on hepatitis B core antigen (anti-HBc) and antibodies to HIV (anti-HIV).

Four men were positive for anti-HCV in 1981 and another 3 seroconverted between 1981 and 1984. One man seroconverted between 1981 and 1989. Three of these men lost reactivity to HCV within 3–5 years later. None of the 8 anti-HCV positive men had ever had a transfusion, and only 1 had a history of intravenous drug abuse. None of the sexual life-style variables correlated with the presence of anti-HCV.

The estimated cumulative incidence of positivity for anti-HCV was 1.6% in 1981, 4.1% in 1984, and 4.1% in 1989. The corresponding values for anti-HBc were 44%, 52.7%, and 58.8%, and those for anti-HIV were 8.8%, 24%, and 30.1%. Seroconversion rates for anti-HCV were 2.5% between 1981 and 1984 and 0% between 1984 and 1989. Corresponding rates for anti-HBc were 15.5% and 12.9%, and those for anti-HIV were 16.7% and 8%. Sexual transmission of HCV is rare compared to that of hepatitis B virus, and individuals with antibodies to HCV may lose them after several years.

Risk for Non-A, Non-B (Type C) Hepatitis Through Sexual or Household Contact With Chronic Carriers

Everhart JE, Di Bisceglie AM, Murray LM, Alter HJ, Melpoder JJ, Kuo G, Hoofnagle JH (Natl Insts of Health, Bethesda, Md; Chiron Corp, Emeryville, Calif)

Ann Intern Med 112:544–545, 1990 3–6

Antibody to hepatitis C virus (HCV) appears late in the course of infection and persists in high titer when chronic infection is present. Testing for anti-HCV should make it easier to assess risk factors for transmission of non-A, non-B hepatitis.

Forty-four patients with chronic non-A, non-B hepatitis were studied. Most had received blood transfusions, but several patients were intravenous drug abusers. Sixty-two contacts of the index patients also were studied; a majority were sexual partners.

Five contacts, all sexual partners, had increased alanine aminotransferase (ALT) activity (table). All 5 had normal physical findings and normal hepatobiliary sonographic studies. One patient who underwent liver biopsy had mild nonspecific hepatitis. Anti-HCV was found in 40 of the 44 index patients but not in any of the contacts.

This study failed to yield conclusive evidence of transmission of hepa-

Demographic Characteristics, Unexplained Elevation, of Alanine Aminotransferase, and Antibody to Hepatitis C Virus of Contacts of Patients With Chronic Non-A, Non-B Hepatitis

Contacts of Patients with Chronic Non-A, Non-B Hepatitis	Type of Contact: Sexual	Household	Total
Number	42	20	62
Mean age, *y*	44.8	16.3	35.6
Mean exposure, *y*	4.2	3.1	3.8
Female, %	76.2	60.0	71.0
Elevated ALT activity			
Number, *n(%)*	3 (7.1)	0 (0)	3 (4.8)
95% CI, *% to %*	1.5 to 19.5	0 to 16.8	1.0 to 13.5
Antibody to HCV			
Number, *n(%)*	0 (0)	0 (0)	0 (0)
95% CI, *% to %*	0 to 8.4	0 to 16.8	0 to 5.8

Abbreviations: ALT, alanine aminotransferase; *HCV,* hepatitis C Virus; *CI,* confidence interval.

(Courtesy of Everhart JE, Di Bisceglie AM, Murray LM, et al: *Ann Intern Med* 112:544–545, 1990.)

titis to sexual contacts or relatives of adults having chronic non-A, non-B hepatitis. Even if the index patients are not representative of patients in general with this disease, the risk of infection via personal contact is not high.

Miscellaneous

A Randomized, Controlled Trial of Vitamin A in Children With Severe Measles

Hussey GD, Klein M (Univ of Cape Town, South Africa)
N Engl J Med 323:160–164, 1990 3–7

It has been suggested that vitamin A may be beneficial in measles. This appears to be biologically plausible, because hyporetinemia occurs almost invariably in children with severe measles, and the reduction in the serum level of retinol is associated with increasing mortality.

In a randomized, double-blind placebo-controlled trial, 189 children with acute measles who were hospitalized because of associated complications (e.g., pneumonia, diarrhea, and croup) received either 400,000 IU of retinyl palmitate or placebo orally beginning within 5 days of onset of rash. The outcome variables were death and severity of illness.

Mortality and Morbidity in 189 Children With Measles, According to Treatment Group

Characteristic	Placebo (N = 97)	Vitamin A (N = 92)	Relative Risk (95% CI) *	P Value
Death	10	2	0.21 (0.05–0.94)	0.046
Age at death (mo)				
<6	1	0		
6–12	7	1		
13–23	1	1		
≥24	1	0		
Pneumonia (days)				
Duration	*12.37 (5, 8, 17)*	*6.53 (3, 5, 8.5)*		<0.001
≥10	29	12	0.44 (0.24–0.80)	0.008
Diarrhea (days)				
Duration	*8.45 (5, 7, 10)*	*5.61 (3, 5, 7)*		<0.001
≥10	21	8	0.40 (0.19–0.86)	0.023
Postmeasles croup	27	13	0.51 (0.28–0.92)	0.033
With airway intervention	9	3	0.35 (0.10–1.26)	0.16
Herpes stomatitis	9	2	0.23 (0.05–1.06)	0.08
Intensive care	11	4	0.38 (0.13–1.16)	0.13
Adverse outcome †	52	25	0.51 (0.35–0.74)	<0.001
Hospital stay (days) ‡	*15.24 (8, 11, 19)*	*10.52 (7, 9, 13)*		0.004

Abbreviation: CI, confidence interval.

Note: In columns representing treatment groups values in italics are means, followed in parentheses by 25th percentiles, medians, and 75th percentiles. All other values are numbers of patients.

*Relative risk denotes ratio of incidence of event in vitamin A group to incidence of event in placebo group.

†Defined as death, pneumonia of at least 10 days' duration, diarrhea of at least 10 days' duration, postmeasles croup, or transfer for intensive care.

‡Refers to children who survived.

(Courtesy of Hussey GD, Klein M: *N Engl J Med* 323:160–164, 1990.)

Baseline characteristics were similar in both the treatment and placebo groups. Although vitamin A deficiency was uncommon in this patient population, serum levels of retinol, retinol-binding protein, and albumin were markedly low. Serum levels of retinol were below .7 μmol/L in 92% of the children, which is indicative of hyporetinemia, and 46% had levels below .35 μmol/L, which placed them at risk for xerophthalmia.

Children who received vitamin A had markedly diminished morbidity and mortality, compared with the placebo group (table). Vitamin A reduced the duration of pneumonia by about half and the duration of diarrhea and hospitalization by about a third. Vitamin A also reduced the incidence of postmeasles croup, herpes stomatitis, and the need for intensive care. Overall, the risk for an adverse outcome in children treated with vitamin A was half that in the placebo group, particularly in a child aged 2 years or older, compared to younger children. No adverse effects to vitamin A were noted. It is recommended that all children with severe measles should receive vitamin A supplements at a dose of 400,000 IU.

▶ After reading this paper, I couldn't help but recall my days working in a small rural hospital in Nigeria and the helpless feeling watching so many children die of measles. I often thought that I could have done more good with a few vials of measles vaccine than any other medical remedy. Treatment with 400,000 IU of vitamin A dramatically reduced the mortality and complications of measles in this and a previous study. This practice should be rapidly incorporated into the therapy of patients with serious measles infections even when vitamin A levels are not measured routinely. There is also probably an important basic mechanism to this effect that deserves further study. I commend this paper to you because it references a number of other papers on the relationship of vitamin A and infections, a literature with which I was not familiar.—M.S. Klempner, M.D.

Unexplained Rabies in Three Immigrants in the United States: A Virologic Investigation

Smith JS, Fishbein DB, Rupprecht CE, Clark K (Ctrs for Disease Control, Atlanta; Wistar Inst of Anatomy and Biology, Philadelphia; Texas State Health Dept, Austin)

N Engl J Med 324:205–211, 1991 3–8

Although more than 90% of patients with rabies have had a definite or probable history of exposure to an animal, a progressively larger proportion of cases in the United States cannot be linked to contact with animals. Three such cases were reviewed, all involving patients who had immigrated to the United States from countries in which rabies is endemic.

The patients included a 12-year-old girl from Laos who was living in Houston, a 13-year-old boy from the Philippines who was living in San Francisco, and an 18-year-old man from Mexico who was working as an agricultural laborer in Oregon. All 3 died of rabies. The disease was not immediately suspected at the time of their hospitalization, and in 2 cases the diagnosis was made post mortem.

Brain tissue was collected from samples that had been submitted for immunofluorescent-antibody tests for rabies. Rabies viruses isolated from the 3 patients, from other patients with a known source of exposure, and from animals in the United States, Thailand (because no samples could be obtained from Laos), the Philippines, and Mexico underwent antigenic and genetic analysis. Identical variants of the 3 viral isolates were found in specimens from rabid animals obtained from or near the country in which each patient lived before immigrating to the United States. These variants were not found among isolates collected from rabid animals in the United States.

Several possible sources of rabies infection in these patients were considered. The most likely explanation was that they had been bitten by a rabid animal in their native countries. The disease appears to have remained latent for long periods of time (1–7 years). Although the patients' families and friends could not recall an episode leading to the infection, dog bites are common among children in developing countries. Thus rabies virus can persist for years without producing clinical signs.

▶ Rabies infections for which the incubation period is longer than 1 year occur in less than 3% of the total cases. Longer incubation periods have been reported only in patients who may have had a second exposure. This is an elegant use of molecular biological techniques to suggest an incubation period of 1–7 years in these 3 patients. I continue to marvel at the endless number of surprises in this wonderful subspecialty of infectious diseases.—M.S. Klempner, M.D.

Occurrence of Adverse Effects and High Amantadine Concentrations With Influenza Prophylaxis in the Nursing Home

Degelau J, Somani S, Cooper SL, Irvine PW (Ramsey Clinic, St Paul; St Paul-Ramsey Med Ctr; Hennepin County Med Ctr, Minneapolis)

J Am Geriatr Soc 38:428–432, 1990 3–9

Amantadine hydrochloride, 100 mg/day, is recommended for the prevention of influenza A in nursing home residents. Because most nursing home residents are older than age 75 years and are female, differences in renal function and volume distribution may alter the pharmacokinetics of amantadine in this population. An amantadine prophylaxis protocol was instituted in a 98-bed community nursing home. The mean age of the residents was 87.4 years, and 96% were female. Adverse effects and serum concentrations of creatinine and amantadine were monitored.

On confirmation of an influenza A outbreak, 55 residents received amantadine, 100 mg/day, for 14 days. No further influenza infections were diagnosed, but 22% of amantadine recipients experienced adverse events, e.g., weakness, fatigue, nausea, delirium, and falls. Amantadine was discontinued because of possible toxicity in 14.5% of recipients.

Those who had adverse effects received a significantly higher mean daily dose of amantadine than those who did not (2.24 vs. 1.76 mg/kg/day) (table). Adverse effects were also more frequent in residents who weighed

Adverse Events in Amantadine Recipients

	No Adverse Events	Adverse Events
n	43	12
Age (years)	87.4 ± 6.0	88.8 ± 6.3
Sex (% female)	93	100
% Walking	70	67
% Disoriented	33	8*
Level of care (% ICF)	72	75
Weight (kg)	59.1 ± 10.6	56.9 ± 18.0
Mean dose (mg/kg/day)	1.76 ± .35	2.24 ± .98†
Weight < 50 kg (%)	16	42‡

Note: walking, independent with or without a device; *disoriented,* at least partial disorientation observed by nursing staff; *ICF,* intermediate level of care.
*$P < .01$ (chi-square).
†$P < .01$ (t test).
‡$P < .06$ (chi-square).
(Courtesy of Degelau J, Somani S, Cooper SL, et al: *J Am Geriatr Soc* 38:428–432, 1990.)

less than 50 kg. Concentrations of amantadine in 32 recipients ranged from 128 ng/mL to 5,810 ng/mL, including 6 with amantadine concentrations of more than 1,000 ng/mL. High serum concentrations of amantadine strongly correlated with elevated serum levels of creatinine and high daily doses. On the basis of the estimated creatinine clearance, 78% of residents would have qualified for a further reduction in the amantadine dose.

Amantadine in a dose of 100 mg/day may be excessive for influenza prophylaxis in older nursing home residents. The cost, safety, and efficacy of lower doses should be evaluated and compared with other prophylactic agents.

▶ I'm not clear why these patients apparently were not immunized with influenza vaccine, but the study emphasizes once again the narrow therapeutic margin of amantadine. Whether lower doses would be effective remains to be seen.—M.J. Barza, M.D.

B Virus *(Herpesvirus simiae)* Infection in Humans: Epidemiologic Investigation of a Cluster

Holmes GP, Hilliard JK, Klontz KC, Rupert AH, Schindler CM, Parrish E, Griffin G, Ward GS, Bernstein ND, Bean TW, Ball MR Sr, Brady JA, Wilder MH, Kaplan JE (Ctrs for Disease Control, Atlanta; Southwest Found for Med Research, San Antonio; Florida Dept of Health and Rehabilitative Services, Tallahassee; Naval Hosp, Pensacola; Baptist Hosp, Pensacola)

Ann Intern Med 112:833–839, 1990 3–10

B virus *(Herpesvirus simiae)* is enzootic in Old World monkeys, particularly in macaques (genus *Macaca*). Several *Macaca* species, particularly rhesus and cynomolgus monkeys, are commonly used in biomedical research and thus have frequent contact with humans. An epidemiologic investigation was made of a cluster of symptomatic B virus infections that occurred in 4 humans.

In March 1987, 4 adults were hospitalized in Pensacola, Florida, with virologically confirmed acute B virus infection. Patients 1, 2, and 3 worked regularly with rhesus monkeys at a research facility, and patient 4 was the wife of 1 of the infected patients. Patients 1 and 2 apparently were bitten by 1 clinically ill monkey (monkey X). Patient 3 had handled a second, clinically healthy monkey (monkey Y). Patient 4 was evidently infected by autoinoculation through use of nonprescription skin cream used by her infected husband.

Restriction endonuclease digestion patterns of DNA from viral isolates from patients 1, 2, and 4 were identical to those of monkey X, and the isolate of patient 3 matched that of monkey Y. Contact tracing identified 159 persons who may have been exposed to B virus, including 21 who had been exposed to monkeys at the facility and 138 who had been exposed to 1 or more of the patients. No further cases were identified.

These 4 cases represent the first reported cluster of human B virus infection since its discovery and the first known person-to-person transmission of B virus infection. The risk of person-to-person transmission is very low and may be limited to direct contact with fresh drainage from active lesions that are shedding B virus. Human infection among monkey handlers could be avoided through use of mechanical or chemical restraints for monkeys before handling and use of protective gear.

▶ B virus *(Herpesvirus simiae)* is an often fatal illness, as illustrated by the 50% mortality in this series. More than 70% of the human cases reported have been fatal. One of the survivors received intravenous acyclovir, although the sensitivity of the isolate was not stated in the case report. The potential for person-to-person spread requires appropriate isolation of all suspected cases of this rare virus.—D.R. Snydman, M.D.

Syncytial Giant-Cell Hepatitis: Sporadic Hepatitis With Distinctive Pathological Features, a Severe Clinical Course, and Paramyxoviral Features

Phillips MJ, Blendis LM, Poucell S, Patterson J, Petric M, Roberts E, Levy GA, Superina RA, Greig PD, Cameron R, Langer B, Purcell RH (Hosp for Sick Children, Toronto; Univ of Toronto; Toronto Gen Hosp; Natl Insts of Health, Bethesda, Md)

N Engl J Med 324:455–460, 1991 3–11

A new form of giant cell hepatitis that causes acute or chronic hepatic necrosis was seen in 10 patients aged 5 months to 41 years. All were seen in a 6-year period. Five patients had liver transplantation and survived with no recurrence of disease; the other 5 patients died.

Woman, 32, the index patient, received a diagnosis of non-A, non-B hepatitis in November 1985. Jaundice resolved within several months and the patient returned to work. During the summer of 1986 she had fluctuating jaundice and a liver biopsy was performed. The specimen revealed syncytial giant cells and chronic hepatitis. Complement-fixing antibodies to the paramyxovirus groups of viruses were sought, and the results of tests for parainfluenza viruses 1 and 2, measles, and mumps were negative. By January 1987 the patient had increased anemia and jaundice, together with hepatosplenomegaly and ascites. The specimen from a second liver biopsy showed the formation of more syncytial giant cells, now in columns. While awaiting a liver transplant, the patient had a rash typical of measles for several days. She has had no recurrence of disease since the transplant in March 1987.

This condition is characterized by the presence of syncytial giant cells that replace the liver cell cords. The syncytial cells, which were easily recognized on light microscopy, were large and contained many nuclei within a single large cytoplasmic body. In 8 of the 10 cases structures that resembled the nucleocapsids of paramyxovirus were detected on electron microscopy.

When 2 chimpanzees were injected with a liver homogenate from the index patient, 1 had an increase in the titer of paramyxoviral antibodies, which suggested that a paramyxoviral antigen, but not a viable virus, was present in the liver homogenate. Molecular studies are needed for precise classification of the virus. The possibility of paramyxovirus should be considered in patients with severe sporadic hepatitis.

▶ The paramyxoviruses are generally pathogenic for animals, although some are human pathogens. The particles seen on electron microscopy had characteristics of 150 nm to 250 nm spheroids with nucleocapsids of 12–17 nm with surface projections. Presumably, the disease reported here is a variant of this family.—D.R. Snydman, M.D.

A School-Based Measles Outbreak: The Effect of a Selective Revaccination Policy and Risk Factors for Vaccine Failure

Hutchins SS, Markowitz LE, Mead P, Mixon D, Sheline J, Greenberg N, Preblud SR, Orenstein WA, Hull HF (Ctrs for Disease Control, Atlanta; Dartmouth-Hitchcook Med Ctr, Hanover, NH; New Mexico Health and Environment Dept, Santa Fe; Albuquerque Public Schools, NM)

Am J Epidemiol 132:157–168, 1990 3–12

Although significant progress has been made in the control of measles in the United States, the goal to eliminate the disease by October 1982 has not been realized. Outbreaks continue to occur, even in appropriately vaccinated children. Because persons who received measles vaccine between the ages of 12 and 14 months are at increased risk of measles compared with those vaccinated at age 15 months or older, the Public Health Service now recommends that those vaccinated between the ages of 12 and 14 months be revaccinated.

To assess the effectiveness of this strategy, during a 1987 school-based measles outbreak in Albuquerque, New Mexico, 88,486 students were

Measles Attack Rates (Per 1,000 Students) in Students Before and After Revaccination in 21 Affected Schools, by Age at Vaccination, Albuquerque, New Mexico, 1987

Age (months) at vaccination†	Total population	Before revaccination‡		After revaccination§		Attack rate decrease (%)‖	p
		No.	Attack Rate	No.	Attack Rate		
12–14	7,051	50	7.1	0	0.0	100	<0.001
≥15	15,641	44	2.8	26	1.7	41	<0.001
Total	22,692	94	4.1	26	1.1	73	<0.001

*Not limited to single-dose vaccinees.

†Age at most recent vaccination before revaccination in school clinics.

‡Before the effect of revaccination (interval between onset of rash in index case and 14 days after revaccination in school clinics). Before revaccination, 12- to 14-month vaccinees were at a significantly increased risk for measles (relative risk = 2.5, $P < .001$).

§After the effect of revaccination (interval > 14 days after revaccination in school clinics to the end of the outbreak). After revaccination, ≥ 15-month vaccines were at a significantly increased risk for measles (relative risk undefined, $P < .001$).

‖The difference between 100% and 41% (59%) is significant ($P < .001$).

(Courtesy of Hutchins SS, Markowitz LE, Mead P, et al: *Am J Epidemiol* 132:157–168, 1990.)

enrolled in the school district. A total of 16,150 students who had been vaccinated between the ages of 12 and 14 months underwent mandatory revaccination.

Before the expected effect of this revaccination campaign, the overall attack rate in persons vaccinated at age 12 months or older was 4.1 cases per 1,000 students (table). After the expected effect of revaccination, the overall attack rate was reduced by 73% to 1.1 per 1,000 students. There was a 100% decline in the attack rate among students targeted for revaccination as they had originally been vaccinated between 12 and 14 months of age compared with a 41% reduction in the attack rate among students not targeted for revaccination because they had originally been vaccinated at age 15 months or older.

In a retrospective cohort study of 1,389 students who had received only a single dose of measles vaccine before this measles outbreak, age at vaccination was not associated with risk of disease. However, students who had been vaccinated 10 years or more before the measles outbreak were at significantly increased risk of disease compared with students vaccinated less than 10 years earlier, independently of age at vaccination. During school-based measles outbreaks, a policy of mandatory selective revaccination of persons initially vaccinated between the ages of 12 and 14 months may prevent intraschool transmission of measles.

▶ Immunization policies and recommendations are regularly reviewed as new vaccines become available and problems associated with previous vaccines become apparent. Nowhere is this more needed than for measles. School outbreaks have shown that those immunized before 15 months of age are at greater risk of measles infection compared to those immunized after 15 months, and that revaccination during an outbreak reduces the risk in the former to a greater extent than it does in the latter. However, as more and more children receive routine reimmunization, and as the use of higher titer or more immunogenic vaccines becomes widespread, the characteristics of the high-risk group may change.

In addition, a current controversy relates to data suggesting that use of the Edmonston-Zagreb (EZ) vaccine, which is more immunogenic than the current measles vaccine, in young children in developing countries is associated with late deaths. This has led a WHO consultative group to evaluate the data, and although it was concluded that there is little merit in the suggestion that the finding is real or that EZ is responsible, the group did call for further study. This is now going on. The issue is at present of little concern for medicine in the United States because EZ vaccine is not used here, but it is of public health policy importance in developing countries where earlier immunization could prevent measles deaths during the interval between the waning of maternally derived immunity and later vaccination. Perhaps next year we will at least be able to resolve the EZ controversy.—G.T. Keusch, M.D.

Hantavirus Infection in the United States: Epizootiology and Epidemiology

Yanagihara R (Natl Inst of Neurological Disorders and Stroke, Bethesda, Md)
Rev Infect Dis 12:449–457, 1990 3–13

The causative agent of hemorrhagic fever with renal syndrome (HFRS) was identified in 1976 as a virus of the *Hantavirus* genus. Multiple species of murid and arvicolid rodents serve as the reservoir hosts of hantaviruses.

About half of the approximately 200,000 cases of HFRS each year are found in the People's Republic of China. Mortality from the disease ranges from 2% to 10%. Epidemic outbreaks usually appear after invasion of rodent habitats or eruptions of reservoir rodent populations. Viral transmission to human beings can occur via the respiratory droplet or airborne route, by direct contamination of food or household articles with excreta from infected rodents, or by an animal bite.

Strains of Seoul virus have been isolated from Norway rats captured in New Orleans, Houston, Philadelphia, and Baltimore. *Hantavirus*-infected rats have also been trapped in New York City, San Francisco, and Columbus, Ohio. Another *Hantavirus*, known as the Leakey virus, was isolated recently from a house mouse captured in Leakey, Texas. This virus is antigenically distinct from the 4 known serotypes of *Hanta virus*.

Fluorescent antibodies against *Hantavirus* have been found in cats in Maryland, particularly those living in alleys inhabited by seropositive rats and other small predatory mammals. A report from India suggests that birds may also be involved in the maintenance and transmission of hantaviruses.

Although antibodies to *Hantavirus* have been reported in a number of different groups in the United States, including longshoremen, zoo and granary employees, renal biopsy patients, and persons attending clinics for sexually transmitted diseases, seropositivity could not be verified in most cases.

In the United States the absence of *Apodemus*-derived hantaviruses, which are associated with the severe form of HFRS, would seem to preclude serious disease. The overall risk of *Hantavirus* infection appears to be low in this country, but precautions should be taken in major port facilities and research laboratories.

▶ Bunyaviruses such as the Hantaviruses are causes of hemorrhagic fever with renal syndrome (HFRS), in which acute interstitial nephropathy with renal failure, hemorrhage, and shock are the major manifestations and mortality is reported to range between 2% and 10%. Other related viruses can cause less severe illness. Classic HFRS is most prevalent in China, but as the causative virus is carried by rodents, it represents a potential epizootic threat to other nations entering via the ports where ships carrying infected rodents from China may dock. In fact, large numbers of port rats in the United States are infected with a virus that is serologically indistinguishable from the virus in China, but severe HFRS is not seen. The author speculates that subclinical infection may predominate in the United States, or that the presentation is of hepatitis (this is readily testable), or that late sequelae such as chronic renal disease and hypertension follow subclinical infection. For the moment, American infectious disease clinicians need only be aware of the presence of a virus related to HFRS viruses from the Orient and consider it in patients with hemorrhagic fever or hepatitis associated with thrombocytopenia and proteinuria. There are no therapeutic options.—G.T. Keusch, M.D.

Parvovirus

Management and Outcomes of Pregnancies Complicated by Human B19 Parvovirus Infection: A Prospective Study

Rodis JF, Quinn DL, Gary GW Jr, Anderson LF, Rosengren S, Cartter ML, Campbell WA, Vintzileos AM (Univ of Connecticut, Farmington; Connecticut Dept of Health Services, Hartford; Ctrs for Disease Control, Atlanta)
Am J Obstet Gynecol 163:1168–1171, 1990 3–14

Although intrauterine infection with human B19 parvovirus has been associated with fetal hydrops and death, most pregnancy outcomes have been normal. During a 1988 outbreak of erythema infectiosum (fifth disease) in Connecticut, 1,000 pregnant women were tested for the presence of IgG and IgM parvovirus-specific antibodies.

Of 1,000 pregnant women tested, 39 were positive for B19 IgM antibody, indicating recent B19 parvovirus infection. Targeted fetal ultrasonography to detect signs of fetal hydrops was performed at intervals for 6–8 weeks after maternal exposure or a positive blood test result. Of the 39 seropositive women, 37 had healthy infants; the fetal loss rate was 5% (2 miscarriages).

A management protocol involves identifying women at risk, serologic testing, and targeted fetal ultrasonograms for 6–8 weeks from time of infection. It may be necessary to follow a normal ultrasonogram with repeated ultrasonograms. If fetal anemia is detected on sonographic examination, fetal blood sampling and intrauterine fetal transfusion or immune globulin therapy may be considered.

Prospective Study of Human Parvovirus (B19) Infection in Pregnancy
Hall SM, for the Public Health Lab Service Working Party on Fifth Disease (PHLS Communicable Disease Surveillance Ctr, London)
Br Med J 300:1166–1170, 1990 3–15

Case reports and retrospective studies have suggested that human parvovirus (B19) infection in pregnancy may result in an adverse outcome. A prospective study of 190 pregnant women with serologically confirmed B19 infection in pregnancy was conducted to determine the risk of adverse fetal outcome, transplacental transmission rate, and neonatal and longer term outcome associated with B19 infection in pregnancy.

Of the 186 who elected to go to term, 156 (84%) delivered a normal infant. Follow-up of 114 of these infants up to age 1 year showed no congenital or serious neurodevelopmental anomalies, although 27 had serologic evidence of intrauterine infection, i.e., persistent B19 IgG. Thirty fetuses (16%) were lost, and the rate of fetal loss tended to be substantially higher among women infected before 20 weeks' gestation (table). Based on virologic findings in the aborted fetuses, the risk of fetal death caused by B19 was estimated to be 9%. The transplacental transmission rate was estimated to be 33%.

Most women with B19 infection during pregnancy have a satisfactory outcome, but the infection is associated with a substantial excess risk of fetal loss during the second trimester. Because of the absence of adverse effects in infants who survive maternal infection, therapeutic termination of pregnancy is not indicated.

▶ The study reviewed in Abstract 3–12, which was carried out in Connecticut, and that in Abstract 3–13, which was conducted in the United Kingdom, are reports of cohorts of pregnant women followed prospectively after recent parvovirus B19 infection. In the series described in Abstract 3–12, 37 of 39 infected women delivered healthy babies; the other 2 women had miscarriages. Abstract 3–13 reports that 30 of 186 fetuses were lost, the loss rate being highest among women infected in the first 20 weeks of gestation. By examination of the products of conception in a subset of fetuses, it is estimated that only 9% of the fetuses died of the infection. These results are in contrast to those of retrospective studies in which much higher rates of hydrops and fetal loss were reported.

The authors whose work is reported in Abstract 3–13 conclude that for pregnant women working in schools or nurseries, the decision to excuse them from work during an epidemic or erythema infectiosum must be made on an individual basis. Most women in that study did not know the source of infection, or

Outcome of Maternal Infection With B19 in Relation to Stage of Pregnancy

Weeks of gestation maternal B19 infection occurred*	No of cases	No of live births	Weeks of gestation spontaneous abortion or fetal death occurred					
			1-12	13-20	21-27	28-40	Not known	Total
1-12	117†	96	7	14	–	–	–	21
13-20	49	42	–	6	1	–	–	7
21-27	10	10	–	–	–	–	–	0
28-40	7	6	–	–	–	1	–	1
Not known	3	2	–	–	–	–	1	1
Total	186†	156	7	20	1	1	1	30

*Occurrence defined as onset of symptoms or first positive blood test result if asymptomatic.
†Includes 4 terminations of pregnancy.
(Courtesy of Public Health Laboratory Service Working Party on Fifth Disease: *Br Med J* 300:1166–1170, 1990.)

inferred that it was contracted from their own children. The authors further conclude that there is no role for routine antenatal screening for antibody to B19, and that infection is not an indication for termination of pregnancy. Finally, they also express skepticism about the utility of ultrasound examinations and α-fetoprotein measurements to detect fetal hydrops and to correct it by intrauterine transfusion.—M.J. Barza, M.D.

Genital Human Papillomavirus Infection in Female University Students as Determined by a PCR-Based Method

Bauer HM, Ting Y, Greer CE, Chambers JC, Tashiro CJ, Chimera J, Reingold A, Manos MM (Cetus Corp, Emeryville, Calif; Univ of California, Berkeley; Roche Biomed Lab, Research Triangle Park, NC)

JAMA 265:472–477, 1991 3–16

Many methods used to detect human papillomavirus (HPV) are limited to the HPV types to which they are applicable and exclude some known and all unidentified HPV types. A polymerase chain reaction (PCR) DNA amplification method was developed that uses degenerate consensus primers to target the highly conserved late region 1, which encodes a viral capsid protein.

The prevalence of cervical and vulvar HPV infection was studied in a cross-sectional survey by using the Food and Drug Administration-approved ViraPap tests and the PCR DNA amplification method. A total of 467 women attending a university health service for routine annual gynecologic examination were studied. Most were young (mean age, 22.9 years), white, and sexually active.

Infection with HPV was evident at 1 or both genital sites in 46% of women when the PCR method was used and in 11% of women when the ViraPap test was used. Both cervical and vulvar infection was present in 69% of women when the PCR method was used, compared to infection found in only 45% of women when the ViraPap test was used. When the PCR method was used, HPV-type analysis showed that 33% of women were infected with types 6, 11, 16, 18, 31, 33, 35, 39, 45, 51, 52, or other previously isolated types, and 13% were infected with other HPVs of yet unidentified types. For the 12 women with condylomatous atypia or dysplasia on Papanicolaou smears, 11 tested HPV positive by the PCR method, although 1 tested positive on the vulvar site alone. In contrast, only 2 women tested HPV positive with the ViraPap test.

The improved generic HPV probe used in this study was significantly more effective in detecting amplified types than the generic oligonucleotide probe mixture previously described. The PCR DNA amplification technique is a highly sensitive and useful method in detecting a broad spectrum of HPV types, compared with the ViraPap test.

▶ This paper demonstrates the superiority of PCR detection of HPV compared to the ViraPap test. The 46% positivity rate with PCR in healthy, sexually active, female university students is, in and of itself, remarkable. Clearly, PCR techniques will be the method of choice for doing the necessary epidermiologic studies to continue to define the natural history of this widespread infection.—M.S. Klempner, M.D.

Persistent B19 Parvovirus Infection in Patients Infected With Human Immunodeficiency Virus Type I (HIV-1): A Treatable Cause of Anemia in AIDS

Frickhofen N, Abkowitz JL, Safford M, Berry JM, Antunez-de-Mayolo J, Astrow A, Cohen R, Halperin I, King L, Mintzer D, Cohen B, Young NS (Natl Heart, Lung, and Blood Inst, Bethesda, Md; Univ of Washington; Miriam Hosp, Providence, RI; Pacific Presbyterian Med Ctr, San Francisco; Univ of Miami; et al)
Ann Intern Med 113:926–933, 1990 3–17

To determine the role of B19 parvovirus in red blood cell aplasia of patients with HIV-1, 7 patients with a syndrome identical to pure red cell aplasia (PRCA) and serologic evidence of infection with HIV-1 were studied in an uncontrolled clinical trial (table). Serum, peripheral blood cells, and bone marrow samples were tested for the presence of parvovirus using DNA hybridization and immunocytochemistry techniques and for the presence of antivirus antibodies using immunoassays.

All patients had giant pronormoblasts in their bone marrow. Patients had anemia for 2–9 months before diagnosis of B19 infection. High levels of viremia, $1-8 \times 10^{11}$/mL, were found in all patients. Virus was detected in serum, often at constant levels for periods of months, and in the saliva of 1 patient and the bone marrow of 3. No patient had detectable levels of antibodies against B19 proteins, or any symptoms of fifth disease (which are known to be mediated by immune complexes). All 6 patients treated with commercial immunoglobulin infusions of .4 g/kg/day for 5 or 10 days recovered, with a rapid reduction in the serum virus concentration and full recovery of erythropoiesis. After treatment, some patients had symptoms suggestive of fifth disease. Only the 2 patients with CD4+ cell counts greater than $.3 \times 10^9$/L had remissions longer than 6 months. All patients with relapses were treated successfully with a repeat course of immunoglobulin.

These findings provide evidence that B19 parvovirus is responsible for severe chronic anemia in some HIV-infected patients. This infection is easily treated with immunoglobulin therapy. A positive diagnosis requires DNA hybridization studies, but the clinical picture, especially the bone marrow morphology, suggests infection and the need for these studies.

▶ The development of a routine clinical assay has been difficult because parvovirus B19 cannot be grown in any conventional cell culture system. Although antibody assays are on the horizon, the patients reported here lacked detectable antibody. Therefore, diagnosis will require a high index of suspicion based on bone marrow morphology, DNA hybridization studies, or perhaps a therapeutic trial of intravenous immunoglobulin.—D.R. Snydman, M.D.

Clinical Data for 7 Patients Infected With HIV-1 and With Persistent B19 Parvovirus

Patient	Sex,	Age	Risk Group	HIV Status*		Location	Initial Presentation		Interval between Diagnosis and Treatment	Transfusions
				Walter Reed (WR) Classification	CD4+ Count		Diagnosis	Hemoglobin		
		y			*×10⁹/L*			*g/L*		*units*
1	M,	24	Homosexual	WR 5	NA	Philadelphia	PRCA	39	7 wk	14
2	M,	27	Drug abuser	WR 3	0.03	Miami	Staphylococcal arthritis	40	No treatment	>8
3	M,	26	Homosexual	WR 3	0.08	Seattle	PRCA	48	11 mo	35
4	M,	37	Homosexual	WR 6	0.08	New York	PRCA	26	4 wk	6
5	M,	40	Homosexual	WR 3	0.36	New York	PRCA	30	4 mo	20
6	M,	39	Homosexual	WR 5	0.33	San Francisco	PRCA	44	7 wk	11
7	M,	26	Homosexual	WR 5	0.06	Providence	PRCA	38	8 wk	9

Abbreviations: NA, not available; *PRCA,* pure red cell aplasia.
*Human immunodeficiency virus status at the time of diagnosis.
(Courtesy of Frickhofen N, Abkowitz JL, Safford M, et al: *Ann Intern Med* 113:926–933, 1990.)

Occupational Risk of Human Parvovirus B19 Infection for School and Day-Care Personnel During an Outbreak of Erythema Infectiosum

Gillespie SM, Cartter ML, Asch S, Rokos JB, Gary GW, Tsou CJ, Hall DB, Anderson LJ, Hurwitz ES (Ctrs for Disease Control, Atlanta; Connecticut State Dept of Health Services, Hartford; Torrington Area Health District, Torrington, Conn)

JAMA 263:2061–2065, 1990 3–18

Infection with human parvovirus B19, the cause of erythema infectiosum, has been associated with adverse fetal outcomes including death. The risk of acquiring B19 infection was examined in the course of a large outbreak of erythema infectiosum that occurred in northwestern Connecticut in 1988. Most (571) of 634 school and day-care personnel were surveyed. An enzyme-linked immunosorbent assay was used to detect serologic evidence of infection.

Fifty-eight percent of the personnel evaluated had evidence of past B19 infection. The minimum rate of infection in susceptible personnel during the outbreak was 19%. Teachers and day-care providers who had contact with younger children and with greater numbers of ill children were especially at risk. Most infected adults reported no symptoms in the 4 months before serum collection. All 6 pregnant subjects, 1 of whom was infected in the outbreak and 3 of whom had evidence of past infection, delivered healthy infants. These findings suggest that infection by human parvovirus B19 is an occupational risk for school and day-care personnel.

▶ Pregnancy raises an incredible variety of issues, from the abortion crisis now becoming the focus of politics, through the safety of drugs used in pregnant women and the medicolegal implications of manufacturing or prescribing medications, to the occupational risks of exposure of pregnant women to infectious agents with possible teratogenic effects, and much much more. In this study, a clear risk of transmission of parvovirus B19 to adult teachers or day-care attendants from children with fifth disease was shown. Given the nature of the world, some of these teachers or caretakers will be pregnant women, and their exposure to the virus will result in a potential risk to their fetus. We can't always know what that risk is (magnitude or severity), and what to do with these women in the workplace remains a question with unsolved medical, social, and legal ramifications. But, having raised the issue, it had better be openly discussed with personnel "at risk" and a clear, if not satisfactory, policy established in advance.—G.T. Keusch, M.D.

Antiviral Therapy

Acyclovir Treatment of Varicella in Otherwise Healthy Children

Balfour HH Jr, Kelly JM, Suarez CS, Heussner RC, Englund JA, Crane DD, McGuirt PV, Clemmer AF, Aeppli DM (Univ of Minnesota; Burroughs Wellcome Co, Research Triangle Park, NC)

J Pediatr 116:633–639, 1990 3–19

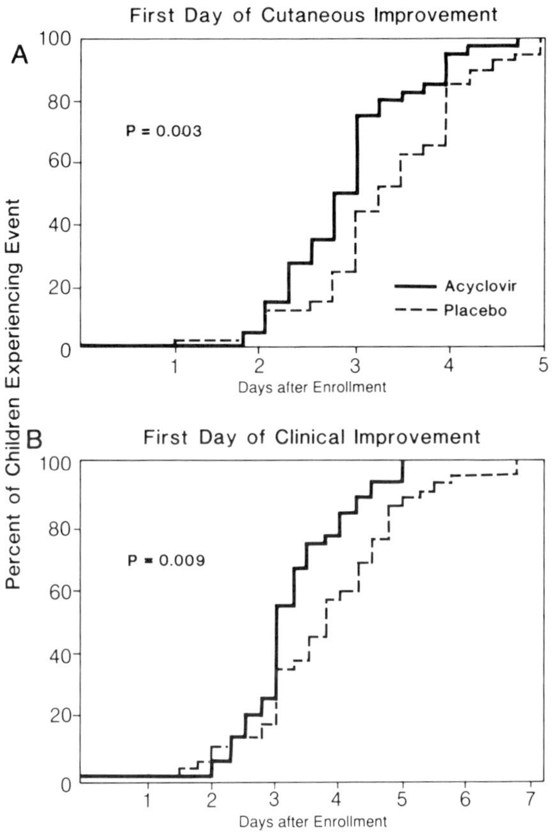

Fig 3–3.—Kaplan-Meier plots showing effect of acyclovir on time required to experience cutaneous improvement (**A**) and clinical improvement (**B**), (*P* values by Breslow test). (Courtesy of Balfour HH Jr, Kelly JM, Suarez CS, et al: *J Pediatr* 116:633–639, 1990.)

Previous studies have shown that intravenously administered acyclovir prevents visceral dissemination of varicella in immunocompromised children and provides a modest clinical benefit in immunocompetent adults. To determine whether orally administered acyclovir moderates the duration and severity of varicella in otherwise normal children, studies were made in 102 children aged 5–16 years with laboratory-confirmed varicella. They were randomly assigned to receive acyclovir orally 4 times daily for 5–7 days, or placebo. The dose for children aged 5–7 years was 20 mg/kg; the dose for those aged 7–12 years was 15 mg/kg; and the dose for those aged 12–16 years was 10 mg/kg.

Acyclovir significantly accelerated the rates of cutaneous and clinical improvement (Fig 3–3), shortened the time required to achieve a decrease in the number of lesions, and reduced the total number of lesions (table). Furthermore, acyclovir-treated children defervesced significantly sooner and had quantitatively less fever than placebo-treated children. The complication rates from varicella were 13.5% in placebo recipients

Effect of Acyclovir on Fever and Cutaneous Events in 102 Children With Varicella

	Treatment group		
Clinical observation	Placebo (n = 52)	Acyclovir (n = 50)	p*
Maximum No. of lesions	500 (290- > 500)	336 (263- > 500)	0.02
Area under time-temperature curve†	2.4 (1.0-2.4)	1.6 (1.0-1.6)	0.035
Median days from enrollment			
Defervescence†	2 (1-3)	1 (0-1)	0.001
No new lesions	3 (3-5)	3 (3-4)	0.2
Maximum number of lesions	2 (1-3)	1 (1-2)	0.02
Decrease in number of lesions	4 (3-7)	3 (2-4)	0.001
Cessation of itching	3 (2-4)	3 (2-4)	0.4

Note: Data shown are medians, with interquartile ranges in parentheses.
*Wilcoxon test.
†Placebo recipients, number = 42; acyclovir recipients, number = 37.
(Courtesy of Balfour HH Jr, Kelly JM, Suarez CS, et al: *J Pediatr* 116:633–639, 1990.)

and 10% in acyclovir recipients. Thus acyclovir did not significantly affect the frequency of complications from varicella. There were no adverse drug effects.

Acyclovir did not alter the transmission rate of varicella to susceptible household members. At 4 weeks after onset of chickenpox, acyclovir recipients had lower geometric mean serum antibody titers to varicella zoster virus than did placebo-treated children. However, antibody titers in both groups were similar 1 year later. Because of the substantial overall economic impact of chickenpox on school and workdays lost, and because of the safety and efficacy of orally administered acyclovir, this practical and specific treatment can be recommended for use in otherwise healthy children with chickenpox.

▶ The use of acyclovir for therapy of chickenpox in healthy children is very controversial, not because it was not shown to be effective in this study but, rather, because of the economic impact such broad use would have on the cost of health care. Is 1 day less of fever a clinically significant and economically significant effect? Is the reduction by 1 day of decreased vesicle formation a clinically significant effect? I don't know, but a cost-benefit analysis is needed.

Data suggesting more rapid cutaneous healing in the group receiving the 20 mg/kg dose has resulted in the use of this dose in a large, multicenter, controlled trial. Although I have no doubt that these results will be reproducible in the next study, a careful economic analysis will of necessity be required to support the use of this drug in normal hosts.

The long-term consequences of acyclovir use in children have not been defined. The widespread use of acyclovir may encourage resistance in a virus that is already less susceptible than herpes simplex and may affect acyclovir sensitivity in others of the herpes family.—D.R. Snydman, M.D.

Early Treatment With Acyclovir for Varicella Pneumonia in Otherwise Healthy Adults: Retrospective Controlled Study and Review

Haake DA, Zakowski PC, Haake DL, Bryson YJ (Univ of California, Los Angeles; Cedars-Sinai Med Ctr, Los Angeles)

Rev Infect Dis 12:788–798, 1990 3–20

Acyclovir is effective and safe when used to treat disseminated varicella in immunocompromised children or herpes zoster in immunocompromised and immunocompetent patients. The efficacy of early acyclovir therapy was assessed in previously healthy adults, all immunocompetent, who had a clinical diagnosis of primary varicella, a chest x-ray study consistent with varicella pneumonia, and significant arterial hypoxia.

Eleven of 38 adult patients received a course of acyclovir intravenously starting within 36 hours of hospitalization; the mean interval was 10 hours. The other 27 patients served as a control group. Early treatment began with a dose of 9–10 mg/kg every 8 hours in most instances. Six patients subsequently received oral acyclovir therapy.

Patients given early acyclovir treatment had lower temperatures and respiratory rates after 5–6 days in the hospital. Oxygenation improved significantly starting on day 6; control patients improved relatively slowly. Patients treated early approached 80% of normal oxygenation by the end of the first week in hospital.

The early intravenous administration of acyclovir can enhance clinical recovery and promote oxygenation in adults with varicella pneumonia. Acyclovir is much less likely to be helpful if treatment is delayed until pulmonary injury has developed.

▶ Retrospective analyses are often difficult and inconclusive. This analysis was probably difficult, but the results support the authors' (and others') contention that early institution of acyclovir therapy in varicella pneumonia is of value.—S.M. Wolff, M.D.

A Controlled Trial Comparing Vidarabine With Acyclovir in Neonatal Herpes Simplex Virus Infection

Whitley R, Arvin A, Probor C, Burchett S, Corey L, Powell D, Plotkin S, Starr S, Alford C, Connor J, Jacobs R, Nahmias A, Soong S-J, and the Natl Inst of Allergy and Infectious Diseases Collaborative Antiviral Study Group (Univ of Alabama, Birmingham; Stanford Univ; Univ of Washington; Ohio State Univ, Univ of Pennsylvania; et al)

N Engl J Med 324:444–449, 1991 3–21

Ongoing therapeutic trials have tested the efficacy of intravenous vidarabine therapy in the treatment of neonatal herpes simplex virus (HSV) infection. In a comparative study of vidarabine and acyclovir therapy, 202 infants younger than age 1 month with confirmed HSV infection were randomly and blindly assigned to receive vidarabine (95 infants) or acyclovir therapy (107 infants). Actuarial rates of morbidity and mortality after 1 year were compared according to the extent of disease at the time of entry into the trial (infection limited to the skin, eyes, or mouth; encephalitis; or disseminated disease).

None of the 85 infants with disease confined to the skin, eyes, or mouth died, and 90% of these infants were developing normally at follow-up (table). Mortality was lower in infants with brain infection than in those with disseminated disease, but the proportion of children who functioned normally in these 2 disease categories was similar.

Acyclovir and vidarabine therapy appear to be equally effective in the management of neonatal HSV infection. Acyclovir, 30 mg/kg, for 10 days is recommended for its ease of administration. The outcome varied significantly according to the extent of disease, but no comparison of treatments within disease categories was statistically significant (Fig 3–4). Increased knowledge of HSV natural history, mortality, and morbidity will aid future therapeutic strategies, but future efforts should also emphasize disease prevention.

▶ The power of this study was insufficient to detect a difference between vidarabine and acyclovir. In fact, with disseminated disease there is a suggestion that vidarabine is superior. However, overall, no difference could be detected; acyclovir was associated with more rapid cessation of viral shedding, and vidarabine was more likely to be associated with thrombocytopenia. Because acyclovir is much easier to administer, it is the drug of choice.—D.R. Snydman, M.D.

▶ ↓ There are very limited data on the frequency of acyclovir-resistant *H. simplex.* The large study reported in Abstract 3–22 demonstrates a surprisingly

Assessment of Morbidity After 12 Months in Infants With Neonatal HSV Infection Treated With Vidarabine or Acyclovir

Extent of Disease	Morbidity after 12 Mo					Alive after 12 Mo, Morbidity Unknown	Dead within 12 Mo	Total
	normal	mild	moderate	severe	subtotal			
	number of infants							
Skin, eye, or mouth infection								
Vidarabine	22	1	1	1	25	6	0	31
Acyclovir	45	0	1	0	46	8	0	54
Central nervous system infection								
Vidarabine	13	1	5	11	30	1	5	36
Acyclovir	8	5	6	9	28	2	5	35
Disseminated disease								
Vidarabine	7	1	0	4	12	2	14	28
Acyclovir	3	1	0	1	5	2	11	18
Total	98	9	13	26	146	21	35	202

(Courtesy of Whitley R, Arvin A, Prober C, et al: *N Engl J Med* 324:444–449, 1991.)

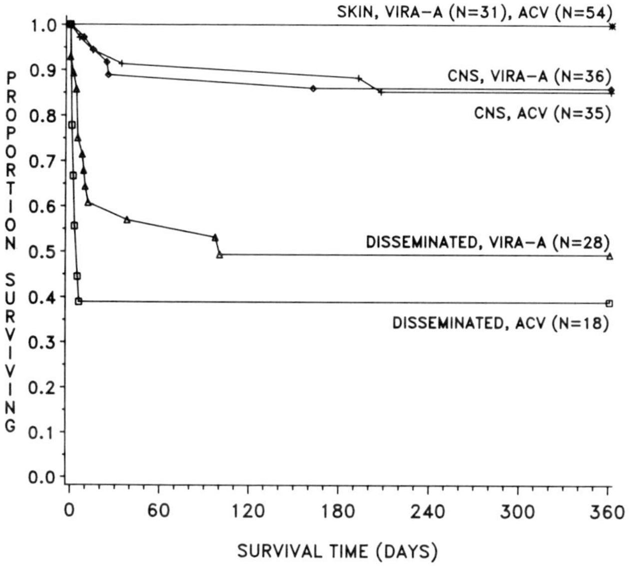

Fig 3–4.—Survival of infants with neonatal HSV infection, according to treatment and extent of disease. Infection was classified as confined to skin, eyes, or mouth; affecting the CNS; or producing disseminated disease. After adjustment for extent of disease with use of stratified analysis, overall difference between vidarabine and acyclovir was not statistically significant by a log-rank test. No comparison of treatment within disease categories was statistically significant. (Courtesy of Whitley R, Arvin A, Prober C, et al: *N Engl J Med* 324:444–449, 1991.)

high rate of acyclovir resistance, all in immunocompromised patients receiving acyclovir therapy.

As Abstract 3–23 illustrates, the optimal management of such patients is not known. Generally, acyclovir should be discontinued and alternatives such as foscarnet considered. However, as these cases demonstrate, very high-dose, continuous infusions of acyclovir may control the infection. Alternatively, stopping acyclovir may allow the wild type to preferentially grow in relation to the thymidine-kinase deficient mutants, thereby allowing reinstitution of acyclovir therapy.

In any event, viral surveillance, especially of chronic acyclovir recipients by a laboratory that can detect such mutants, is necessary. In high dose, continuous infusion therapy, monitoring acyclovir levels may be necessary; however, I am not aware of the ready availability of such determinations.—D.R. Snydman, M.D.

Herpes Simplex Virus Resistant to Acyclovir: A Study in a Tertiary Care Center

Englund JA, Zimmerman ME, Swierkosz EM, Goodman JL, Scholl DR, Balfour HH Jr (Univ of Minnesota; St Louis Univ; Diagnostic Hybrids, Inc, Athens, Oh)
Ann Intern Med 112:416–422, 1990 3–22

Acyclovir-resistant herpes simplex virus infections have been reported in patients with AIDS. In a retrospective study all herpes simplex virus isolates cultured in a 1-year period from 207 patients in a tertiary care center were evaluated to determine the sensitivity of these isolates to acyclovir and the pathogenicity of resistant isolates. A rapid nucleic acid hybridization method was used to assess susceptibility to acyclovir.

Herpes simplex viruses with an in vitro ED_{50} of more than 90 μM of acyclovir were recovered from 7 patients (3%). Acyclovir-resistant isolates were recovered only from immunocompromised patients who received prolonged acyclovir therapy (median duration, 46 days). Six of these patients were transplant recipients and 1 had AIDS. In contrast, none of the 59 immunocompetent patients harbored acyclovir-resistant isolates. Clinical disease was present in all 7 patients with acyclovir-resistant isolates and was more severe in pediatric patients. Plaque autoradiography showed absent or altered thymidine kinase activity in all acyclovir-resistant isolates tested.

Herpes simplex viruses resistant to acyclovir are relatively frequent in immunocompromised patients and may cause serious disease. Prolonged exposure to acyclovir and severe immunosuppression appear to be the "2-edged sword" in the development of resistance. The discriminatory use of acyclovir in immunocompromised patients should be encouraged. Antiviral susceptibility testing should also be encouraged to monitor viral resistance, particularly in tertiary care settings.

Treatment of Resistant Herpes Simplex Virus With Continuous-Infusion Acyclovir

Engel JP, Englund JA, Fletcher CV, Hill EL (Univ of Minnesota; Burroughs Wellcome Co, Research Triangle Park, NC)
JAMA 263:1662–1664, 1990 3–23

Herpes simplex virus (HSV) infection can often be controlled by acyclovir, but acyclovir resistance can develop after long treatment courses. Data were reviewed on 2 patients with severe ulcerative proctitis caused by HSV type 2 (HSV-2) that was resistant to acyclovir.

Both patients had AIDS and severe HSV-2-induced ulcerative proctitis. Viruses cultured from the lesions were resistant to acyclovir in vitro. Both patients were treated successfully with 6 weeks of high-dose, continuous-infusion acyclovir sodium, 1.5–2 mg/kg/hr, in an outpatient setting. This response occurred despite previous failure with prolonged oral and intravenous acyclovir treatment given in traditional divided doses and plasma levels of acyclovir that were well below the median infective dose of the resistant isolate. Plaque autoradiography showed deficient thymidine-kinase activity (TK) from the first patient's isolate and an altered substrate specificity of the TK from the second patient's isolate. Serum creatinine levels were normal in both patients.

High-dose, continuous-infusion acyclovir is a safe and effective therapeutic alternative for clinical significant acyclovir-resistant HSV-induced mucocutaneous disease. The infusions are administered through Hickman catheters in the outpatient setting with weekly visits and monitoring of creatinine and acyclovir levels.

Randomized, Double-Blind, Placebo-Controlled, Patient-Initiated Study of Topical High- and Low-Dose Interferon-α With Nonoxynol-9 in the Treatment of Recurrent Genital Herpes

Sacks SL, Varner TL, Davies KS, Rekart ML, Stiver HG, DeLong ER, Sellers PW (Univ of British Columbia Herpes Clinic; University Hosp-UBC Site; British Columbia Ctr for Disease Control, Vancouver; Quintiles Inc, Chapel Hill, NC; Exovir Inc, Great Neck, NY)

J Infect Dis 161:692–698, 1990 3–24

The effectiveness of systemic interferon-α (IFN-α) for the treatment of genital herpes simplex virus (HSV) infection has been variable, and significant adverse effects have been reported. Systemic toxicity can be avoided by applying IFN-α topically. A single-center, randomized, double-blind, patient-initiated trial evaluated a topical gel containing placebo or natural IFN-α in 1 or 2 doses.

Of the 105 patients with prodromal symptoms who began the study, 34 patients using low-dose and 35 using high-dose therapy were assessable at the time the study ended. Patients applied IFN-α within several hours of prodrome onset. More than 90% had lesional episodes. Times to complete healing in men and in patients applying the medication before the appearance of a genital lesion were somewhat longer in placebo recipients than in high-dose therapy recipients. The duration of virus shedding was reduced by high-dose therapy overall and in the early treatment group. The duration of lesion symptoms was decreased in high-dose treatment recipients. Four patients receiving high-dose therapy had adverse effects.

Topical high-dose IFN-α with 1% nonoxynol-9 in 3.5% methylcellulose gel appears to be effective and safe. This treatment may be an effective alternative to oral acyclovir for recurrences in patients whose rate of recurrence does not necessitate long-term acyclovir suppression. When used at the first sign of recurrence, IFN-α can relieve the symptoms of genital herpes faster than placebo.

▶ For most comparisons in this study, the effect of the high-dose IFN was significant but clinically unimpressive. The median shortening of time before cultures became negative and complete reepithelialization occurred was about a day less in those treated with high-dose IFN than in those given placebo. The role of nonoxynol-9 in this study is difficult to ascertain; in vitro it has some synergistic effect with IFN. The placebo group was not given nonoxynol-9 because that agent alone appears to delay the healing of genital herpetic lesions. The authors explain the poorer results in earlier trials of IFN by the delay in application of the drug (most of the studies were clinic initiated rather than patient initiated) and by differences in the vehicle that might have impaired delivery of the IFN. The authors conclude that topical IFN may be useful in patients whose recurrent attacks are not so frequent as to merit the use of chronic suppressive treatment with oral acyclovir.—M.J. Barza, M.D.

Cytomegalovirus Esophagitis in Patients With AIDS: A Clinical, Endoscopic, and Pathologic Correlation

Wilcox CM, Diehl DL, Cello JP, Margaretten W, Jacobson MA (Univ of California, San Francisco, San Francisco Gen Hosp)

Ann Intern Med 113:589–593, 1990 3–25

Cytomegalovirus esophagitis is a recognized, although uncommon, complication in patients with AIDS. However, the natural history of this infection has not been well described. To examine the clinical presentation, endoscopic features, laboratory diagnosis, and outcome of cytomegalovirus esophagitis in patients with AIDS, the records of 16 patients seen by gastroenterology consultants at 1 center were reviewed retrospectively. All had undergone endoscopy, with multiple mucosal biopsies and viral culture of all esophageal mucosal lesions.

Cytomegalovirus disease was verified through immunohistochemical antibody staining of mucosal biopsy specimens. The most prominent esophageal symptom was odynophagia, which was seen in 14 patients. Ulcerations of the esophagus, which typically appeared as large, solitary, shallow lesions, were found in all but 1 patient. Routine hematoxylin-eosin staining of esophageal mucosal and submucosal specimens demonstrated intranuclear inclusions in all patients. By contrast, cytomegalovirus cultures were positive in only 8 of 14 patients. Patients with cytomegalovirus esophagitis had a poor long-term prognosis.

Cytomegalovirus esophagitis in patients with AIDS is a well-defined entity with characteristic clinical symptoms, endoscopic findings, and histopathologic features. Patients with AIDS who have dysphagia alone should receive an initial empirical trial of antifungal treatment, even in the absence of thrush. If odynophagia is the major symptom, however, or if dysphagia is not ameliorated within 7–10 days while the patient is receiving effective antifungal therapy, upper endoscopy should be done with esophageal biopsy of any endoscopic mucosal anomalies.

▶ Despite using appropriate antiviral therapy with ganciclovir, these authors caution that cytomegalovirus esophagitis in AIDS patients may not be very responsive. Certainly, results here are consistent with the evidence of lack of effect of ganciclovir on cytomegalovirus enteritis in marrow transplant recipients.

▶ ↓ As Abstract 3–23 illustrates, controlled trials are sorely needed to document ganciclovir efficacy for cytomegalovirus disease in a variety of settings. Early therapy to prevent the pathogenic events triggered by early viral replication may be the way in which ganciclovir will ultimately be used (1).—D.R. Snydman, M.D.

Reference

1. Schmidt GM, et al: *N Engl J Med* 324:1005, 1991.

Ganciclovir for the Treatment of Cytomegalovirus Gastroenteritis in Bone Marrow Transplant Patients: A Randomized, Placebo-Controlled Trial

Reed EC, Wolford JL, Kopecky KJ, Lilleby KE, Dandliker PS, Todaro JL, McDonald GB, Meyers JD (Fred Hutchinson Cancer Research Ctr, Seattle; Univ of Washington)

Ann Intern Med 112:505–510, 1990 3–26

Ganciclovir has exhibited both in vitro and in vivo activity against cytomegalovirus. Ganciclovir, in a dose of 2.5 mg/kg every 8 hours for 2 weeks, was evaluated in patients seen consecutively with biopsy-proved cytomegalovirus infection of the gastrointestinal tract. Eighteen patients received active drug and 19 were given placebo. The esophagus was the most frequent site of cytomegalovirus infection.

Oropharyngeal and urinary excretion of virus ceased in the patients given ganciclovir, and repeated esophageal cultures were negative more often than in placebo recipients. There were no differences in symptoms or endoscopic findings between the actively treated patients and those given placebo (table). Four patients given ganciclovir and 6 placebo re-

Severity of Disease of Esophagus, Stomach, and Duodenum as Determined by Upper Endoscopy

Variable	Mean Endoscopic Score*	
	Ganciclovir Group	Placebo Group
All patients before treatment†	4.1 (0.5)‡	3.9 (0.5)‡
Patients with paired examinations§		
Before treatment	3.8 (0.6)	3.8 (0.6)
After treatment	4.1 (0.6) ‖	3.6 (0.4) ‖

*Data are expressed as mean ± 1 SE of the sum of the endoscopic scores from esophagus, stomach, and duodenum. Results of sigmoidoscopy are not included.

†Based on 18 ganciclovir recipients and 17 placebo recipients who had a complete upper endoscopic examination before treatment. One placebo recipient who did not have a duodenal examination before treatment is not included; 1 other placebo recipient had only a sigmoidoscopic examination before treatment.

‡$P = .40$ by 1-tailed Wilcoxon test.

§Results from the 14 patients in each group who had complete upper endoscopic examinations before and after treatment.

‖The change in endoscopy scores within the ganciclovir and placebo groups was analyzed using 1-tailed P values based on the signed rank test of the differences between pre- and posttreatment scores. The P values were .31 and .43 for the ganciclovir and placebo groups, respectively. The change in endoscopy scores between the ganciclovir and placebo groups was analyzed by 1-tailed Wilcoxon test. The P value was .35.

(Courtesy of Reed EC, Wolford JL, Kopecky KJ, et al: *Ann Intern Med* 112:505–510, 1990.)

cipients had cytomegalovirus pneumonia. One ganciclovir recipient and 4 placebo recipients were withdrawn from the study because of neutropenia.

Ganciclovir suppresses the proliferation of cytomegalovirus, but its use for 2 weeks did not promote clinical or endoscopic improvement in patients with gastroenteritis. Whether the addition of immunoglobulin would improve the results remains speculative.

Cytomegalovirus Retinitis in AIDS: Treatment With Intravitreal Injections of Ganciclovir

Cochereau-Massin I, Le Hoang P, Lautier-Frau M, Zazoun L, Marcel P, Robinet M, Besingue A, Rousselie F (Hôp la Pitié-Salpêtrière, Paris)
Presse Med 19:1313–1316, 1990 3–27

Cytomegalovirus retinitis is the most common ocular infection and the principal cause of blindness among patients with AIDS. Systemic ganciclovir therapy has proven effective in the treatment of AIDS-associated cytomegalovirus, but it is often poorly tolerated. In these cases, local intravitreal ganciclovir injection offers a useful therapeutic alternative. The results of a prospective, open study to evaluate the efficacy of intravitreally injected ganciclovir in patients with AIDS who had cytomegalovirus retinitis were assessed.

The study was done in 17 patients with AIDS aged 25–62 years with clinically confirmed cytomegalovirus retinitis in 25 eyes. Nine patients had unilateral and 8 had bilateral involvement. Fifteen patients had been treated previously with systemic antiviral agents for a mean of 2.3 induction courses. The mean duration of AIDS was 16.4 months and the mean duration of retinitis, 4.9 months. Intravitreal injections at a dose of 400 μg of ganciclovir were given twice weekly during the acute phase and once a week thereafter for maintenance therapy. Because of death or treatment intolerance, 10 of the 25 eyes were treated only once by the intravitreal route.

Twenty-three induction courses in 13 patients were assessable, showing cure after an average of 6 intravitreal ganciclovir injections over an

Evaluation of Maintenance Therapy in 11 Patients

Results	Regular maintenance	Irregular maintenance	Discontinued reg. maintenance	Number
Relapse	4 (29 days)	1 (45 days)	2 (26 days)	7
No relapse	10 (48 days)	0	0	10
Total no.	14	1	2	17

(Courtesy of Cochereau-Massin I, Le Hoang P, Lautier-Frau M, et al: *Presse Méd* 19:1313–1316, 1990.)

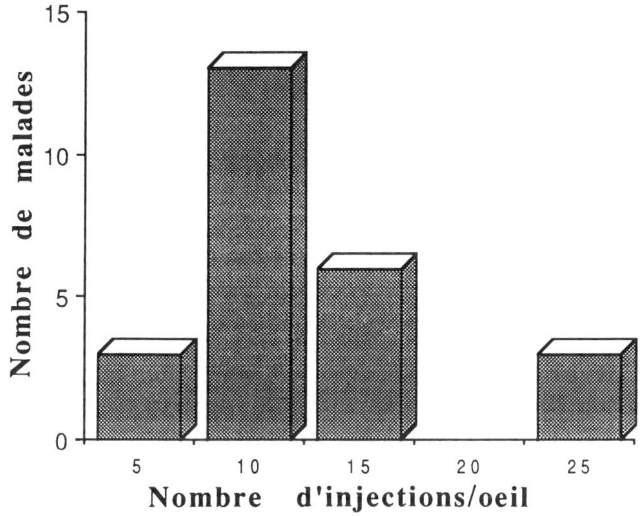

Fig 3–5.—Distribution of the patients according to the number of injections per eye. Average number of injections per eye: 9.4 (4–25). (Courtesy of Cochereau-Massin I, Le Hoang P, Lautier-Frau M, et al: *Presse Med* 19:1313–1316, 1990.)

average treatment period of 18 days. Ophthalmologic follow-up ranged from 21 days to 67 days (mean, 43 days). Seventeen maintenance courses in 11 patients were assessable. The mean number of maintenance injections per eye was 5.2, and the range was 2–8 injections per eye. At 48 days after treatment for cure, 10 of 14 eyes had not relapsed with maintenance therapy. The other 4 eyes relapsed after a mean interval of 29 days (table). The overall number of injections given in the study was 231, and the average number of injections per eye was 9.4 (Fig 3–5). Eleven patients considered the injection painful. Pain lasted for several minutes and increased with the number of injections given. None of the patients had cataracts or endophthalmia. Intravitreal ganciclovir injection in the treatment of cytomegalovirus retinitis in patients with AIDS appears to be an effective alternative for those who do not tolerate systemic antiviral therapy.

▶ There are several reports of the use of intravitreal injections of ganciclovir for the maintenance of patients with infection clinically limited to the eye who cannot tolerate the drug systemically. This is among the larger collections of patients treated in this way. The estimated half-life of the drug in the vitreous humor is 13.5 hours, and it has been estimated that inhibitory concentrations remain in the vitreous humor for 60 hours after injection of 200 μg. The authors used double this dosage to achieve a longer effect. A mean of 6 injections, given in 3 weeks was needed to achieve scarring (inactivity) of the lesions; the authors note that this is the same duration as the course of drug usually given intravenously for this purpose. Interestingly, only 1 of 17 patients in this study contracted extraocular cytomegalovirus infection during the period of observation.—M.J. Barza, M.D.

A Randomized Controlled Trial of Interferon Alfa-2b Alone and After Prednisone Withdrawal for the Treatment of Chronic Hepatitis B

Perrillo RP, Schiff ER, Davis GL, Bodenheimer HC Jr, Lindsay K, Payne J, Dienstag JL, O'Brien C, Tamburro C, Jacobson IM, Sampliner R, Feit D, Lefkowitch J, Kuhns M, Meschievitz C, Sanghvi B, Albrecht J, Gibas A, and the Hepatitis Interventional Therapy Group (Washington Univ; Univ of Miami; Brown Univ; Univ of California, Los Angeles; Rush-Presbyterian-St Luke's Hosp, Chicago; et al)

N Engl J Med 323:295–301, 1990 3–28

The value of recombinant interferon alfa-2b in the treatment of chronic hepatitis B virus (HBV) infection was assessed in a randomized study. The patients were assigned randomly to an untreated control group (43), prednisone in decreasing daily doses for 6 weeks followed by 16 weeks of recombinant interferon alfa-2b at a dose of 5 million units daily (44), placebo followed by 5 million units of interferon daily for 16 weeks (41), or placebo followed by 1 million units of interferon daily for 16 weeks (41).

Seroconversion of HBeAg and a sustained loss of HBV DNA occurred

TABLE 1.—Responses to Treatment in the Multicenter Trial of Patients With Chronic Hepatitis B

Characteristic	Prednisone plus Interferon	Interferon Alone 5 million U	Interferon Alone 1 million U	Untreated Controls
No. of patients	44	41	41	43
		number (percent)		
Loss of HBV DNA and HBeAg	16 (36)†	15 (37) *	7 (17) †	3 (7)
Indeterminate response at 24-week follow-up	4 (9)	3 (7)	4 (10)	2 (5)
Loss of HBsAg	5 (11)	5 (12)‡	1 (2)	0
ALT, AST normal at last follow-up	19 (43)	18 (44)	11 (27)	8 (19)
Reactivation of HBeAg or HBV DNA during follow-up	1 (2)	0	1 (2)	0

Abbreviations: ALT, alanine aminotransferase; *AST,* aspartate aminotransferase.
$^*P < .001$ for the comparison with controls by Fisher's exact test.
†*P* not significant for the comparison with controls.
‡$P = .024$ for the comparison with controls by Fisher's exact test.
(Courtesy of Perrillo RP, Schiff ER, Davis GL, et al: *N Engl J Med* 323:295–301, 1990.)

TABLE 2.—Association Between Serum Levels of HBV DNA and Alanine Aminotransferase Before Treatment and Response to Treatment

Variable	Prednisone plus Interferon	Interferon Alone		Untreated Controls
		5 million U	1 million U	
No. of patients	44	41	41	43
		no. with response/total (%)		
HBV DNA (pg/ml)*				
2–99	11/23 (48)	10/19 (53)	6/14 (43)	2/23 (9)
100–200	4/13 (31)	5/15 (33)	0/13 (0)	0/12 (0)
>200	1/8 (13)	0/7 (0)	1/14 (7)	1/8 (13)
Alanine aminotransferase (U/liter)				
<100	8/18 (44)	2/12 (17)	1/12 (8)	1/16 (6)
100–200	4/16 (25)	6/15 (40)	3/18 (17)	1/16 (6)
>200	4/10 (40)	7/14 (50)	3/11 (27)	1/11 (9)

*$P < .0001$ by Cox regression analysis.
(Courtesy of Perrillo RP, Schiff ER, Davis GL, et al: *N Engl J Med* 323:295–301, 1990.)

in 36% of the patients treated with prednisone plus interferon and in 37% of those treated with 5 million units of interferon alone (Table 1). In contrast, only 7% of untreated controls had clearance. Those receiving 1 million units of interferon did not fare significantly (17%) better than controls. In about 10% of the treated patients, hepatitis B surface antigen disappeared from serum.

The most important predictor of response was the HBV DNA level before treatment. Fewer than 7% of patients with circulating HBV DNA in excess of 200 pg/mL responded to the 5-million-unit dose compared to a 50% response in those given 100 pg/mL. A dose-response effect could be demonstrated in alanine aminotransferase levels as well (Table 2). Patients who had a sustained loss of viral replication, including those who continued to have detectable HBcAg, had both a clinical and a histologic response. Yet many patients, particularly those with high levels of viral replication, had no response to interferon either alone or with a short course of corticosteroids.

▶ The results from several small clinical trials for therapy of the hepatitis B carrier have suggested that a short course of corticosteroids may be synergistic when combined with interferon alfa-2b or vidarabine (1,2). This is the first comparative trial of such an approach.

These results, although not dramatic, show some loss of viral markers of replication in a proportion of patients who received the larger dose of interferon alfa-2b. Loss of hepatitis B surface antigen was more likely to occur in patients who had a shorter duration of the carrier state. The potential benefit of prednisolone therapy was small and limited to a subset of patients with lower alanine aminotransferase levels.

Although these results are encouraging, a large number of patients did not respond, particularly those with high levels of viremia. Therefore, other management regimens clearly are needed.—D.R. Snydman, M.D.

References

1. Perrillo RP, et al: *Ann Intern Med* 109:95, 1988.
2. Alexander GJ, et al: *J Med Virol* 21:81, 1987.

Treatment of Condyloma Acuminatum With Three Different Interferon-α Preparations Administered Parenterally: A Double-Blind, Placebo-Controlled Trial

Reichman RC, Oakes D, Bonnez W, Brown D, Mattison HR, Bailey-Farchione A, Stoler MH, Demeter LM, Tyring SK, Miller L, Whitley R, Carveth H, Weidner M, Krueger G, Choi A (Univ of Rochester, New York; Univ of Alabama, Birmingham; Univ of Utah)

J Infect Dis 162:1270–1276, 1990 3–29

Condyloma acuminatum, or anogenital warts, is an increasingly prevalent sexually transmitted disease caused by human papillomaviruses (HPV). There is evidence that parenterally administered interferon preparations can be an effective treatment. A randomized, placebo-controlled multicenter study compared different preparations of subcutaneously injected interferon with placebo in 175 adult patients in good general health who had anogenital warts.

Complete and incomplete resolution of lesions was greater in interferon-treated patients than in placebo-treated recipients. Women were more likely to respond than men. The outcome could not be related to virologic measurements in paired lesion biopsy specimens. Toxicity from interferon was frequent but did not necessitate withdrawal from the trial or even dose reductions.

Subcutaneous interferon-α can reduce lesion size and numbers in patients who have anogenital warts; toxicity is acceptable. Women appear to respond more readily than men to interferon treatment.

▶ The use of interferon to treat condylomata has been suggested by a variety of studies, including its intralesional use. This carefully done, double-blind trial demonstrates that interferon-α given subcutaneously is of value in the treatment of this common condition.—S.M. Wolff, M.D.

4 Fungal Infections

Fungal Burn Wound Infection: A 10-Year Experience

Becker WK, Cioffi WG Jr, McManus AT, Kim SH, McManus WF, Mason AD, Pruitt BA Jr (US Army Inst of Surgical Research, Fort Sam Houston, San Antonio)

Arch Surg 126:44–48, 1991 4–1

In recent years, burn wound infections caused by yeast and fungi have been increasing despite the decline in bacterial burn wound infections. A 10-year experience with fungal burn wound infections was reviewed and compared with experience with bacteria from wound infections in the same period.

Burn wound infections were diagnosed by biopsy specimen and histopathologic examination (Table 1). For bacterial burn wound infections treatment consisted of systemic antibiotics, subeschar cylsis of a semisynthetic penicillin, and topical chemotherapy with mafenide acetate and/or silver sulfadiazine. Fungal wound infections were treated primarily with wide surgical excision of all infected tissues. Antifungal topical chemotherapeutic agents (e.g., 1% clotrimazole cream) were used in some patients and systemic amphotericin B was given only to patients with disseminated fungal infection or to patients with microvascular (stage 2c) invasion.

From 1979 to 1989, a total of 2,114 patients with thermal injury were seen and 209 (9.9%) contracted proved burn wound infection. There were 141 fungal burn wound infections and 68 bacterial infections. The annual incidence of fungal burn wound infections remained relatively stable during the study period, but there was a marked reduction in the incidence of bacterial wound infections (Table 2).

Patients with either fungal or bacterial burn wound infection had massive injury, with burn sizes averaging more than 50% of the total body

TABLE 1.—Classification of Microbial Status of Wounds

Stage 1: Wound colonization	
	1a: Superficial colonization
	1b: Microorganisms in nonviable tissue
	1c: Microorganisms at the interface of viable tissue
Stage 2: Invasive infection	
	2a: Microinvasion of viable tissue
	2b: Deep or generalized invasion of viable tissue
	2c: Microvascular invasion

(Courtesy of Becker WK, Cioffi WG Jr, McManus AT, et al: *Arch Surg* 126:44–48, 1991.)

TABLE 2.—Annual Incidence of Burn Wound Infections

Year	No. of Admissions	Bacterial Burn Wound Infection	Fungal Burn Wound Infection
1979 (0.5 year)	140	9 (6.4)	7 (5)
1980	225	20 (8.9)	23 (10.2)
1981	229	12 (5.3)	6 (2.6)
1982	209	12 (5.7)	19 (9.1)
1983	188	3 (1.6)	15 (8)
1984	186	2 (1.1)	19 (10.2)
1985	197	2 (1)	10 (5.1)
1986	206	1 (0.5)	13 (6.3)
1987	221	3 (1.4)	11 (5)
1988	223	3 (1.3)	9 (4)
1989 (0.5 year)	90	1 (1.1)	9 (10)

Note: Values are number (percent of total admissions).
(Courtesy of Becker WK, Cioffi WG Jr, McManus AT, et al: *Arch Surg* 126:44–48, 1991.)

surface area. Factors that appeared to have markedly reduced bacterial wound infection (e.g., patient isolation, topical chemotherapeutic agents, and burn wound excision) did not have a similar effect on fungal wound infection. During the early part of the study 3 patients underwent amputation to control progressive fungal infection. However, with the early diagnosis of fungal infection from biopsy specimens followed by topical therapy and wound débridement, only 2 patients had disseminated fungal infection and none required amputation.

The incidence of fungal burn wound infection has remained relatively stable despite the marked decline in bacterial burn wound infection. Early biopsy and diagnosis of fungal burn wound infection, followed by surgical débridement of the infected area, appears to have limited some of the adverse consequences of this infection, such as the need for amputation and the development of disseminated fungal infection.

▶ Because we don't have a burn unit at our hospital, we rarely come across these patients. I was struck to read in this article that fungal burn infection is the most common complication seen at this very experienced burn wound center. It occurs in approximately 7.5% of their admissions. The most common organisms were *Aspergillus* followed distantly by *Candida, Mucor* and *Rhizopus, Microspora,* and *Alterneria* species. Aggressive early biopsy diagnosis and surgical débridement have markedly reduced the complication of disseminated fungal infections in these patients.—M.S. Klempner, M.D.

Fluconazole Compared With Amphotericin B Plus Flucytosine for Cryptococcal Meningitis in AIDS: A Randomized Trial

Larsen RA, Leal MAE, Chan LS (Los Angeles County Hosp; Univ of Southern California)
Ann Intern Med 113:183–187, 1990 4–2

Cryptococcal meningitis is an opportunistic infection that is devastating to patients with AIDS. Nearly 60% of AIDS patients who contract the infection die of it. Amphotericin B, alone or in combination with flucytosine, may prevent death, but causes significant morbidity. Alternative treatments would be desirable. Fluconazole, a triazole antifungal agents, appears to be effective against infections caused by *Cryptococcus neoformans*.

Twenty male patients with AIDS and evidence of cryptococcal meningitis were randomly assigned to receive treatment with either fluconazole or amphotericin B and flucytosine. There were 14 patients in the fluconazole trial and 6 in the amphotericin trial. Patients received fluconazole orally at a dosage of 400 mg/day for 10 weeks and thereafter at 200 mg/day. Fluconazole doses were increased to 400 mg/day when warranted by positive urine cultures. Patients given amphotericin B received .7 mg/kg daily, administered intravenously, for the first 7 days. The dose was then reduced to 3 times weekly for the next 9 weeks. Patients assigned to amphotericin B treatment also received flucytosine, 150 mg/kg/day in 4 orally administered, divided doses during the initial 10-week treatment period. Patients were followed for 62 weeks or until death, treatment failure, or withdrawal from the study.

Fluconazole treatment failed in 8 of 14 subjects, whereas amphotericin B plus flucytosine treatment failed in none of 6. Cerebrospinal fluid cultures remained positive for a mean of 40.6 days in patients receiving fluconazole and for 15.6 days in patients receiving amphotericin B plus flucytosine. Four patients assigned to fluconazole died. There were no deaths of patients receiving amphotericin.

Treatment with amphotericin B plus flucytosine is apparently superior to treatment with fluconazole in AIDS patients with cryptococcal meningitis. Both clinical and mycologic failure was significantly more common in patients treated with fluconazole. Although less toxic alternatives to amphotericin B would be highly desirable, fluconazole does not appear to be an effective treatment.

▶ Fluconazole has become the mainstay of maintenance treatment among patients with AIDS and cryptococcal infection that is in remission, but the role of the drug in the treatment of active cryptococcal infection remains unclear. This trial argues against a role for fluconazole in initiation of treatment in AIDS patients but, as the authors point out, the study was a small one and, by chance, the CD4 counts were lower among the fluconazole-treated patients than in those given amphotericin B (44/mm^3 vs. 97/mm^3; P = .055). The authors speculate that the better results with fluconazole in previous series may relate to the fact that most of the patients had received some amphotericin B before the fluconazole. Despite the present report, some authorities continue to regard fluconazole as a reasonable initial treatment for patients with mild cryptococcal meningitis. The authors do not believe that their study militates against the continued use of fluconazole for maintenance treatment.—M.J. Barza, M.D.

Treatment of Systemic Sporotrichosis With Ketoconazole

Calhoun DL, Waskin H, White MP, Bonner JR, Mulholland JH, Rumans LW, Stevens DA, Galgiani JN (VA Med Ctr, Tucson; Univ of Arizona; VA Med Ctr, Albuquerque; Med Service, Fort Huachucha, Ariz; Univ of Alabama, Birmingham; et al)

Rev Infect Dis 13:47–51, 1991 4–3

Deep soft tissue infection with the dimorphic fungus *Sporothrix schenckii* is uncommon. Patients with such infection often require toxic drugs. Ketoconazole is a well-tolerated, orally absorbed antifungal agent. Ketoconazole was used in the treatment of deep-seated sporotrichosis in 11 patients. Eight infections involved at least 1 joint, and 3 involved thoracic, cervical, and widespread cutaneous sites, respectively.

All signs of infection resolved during treatment in 8 patients. Six patients had sustained remissions lasting for 6 months to 5 years after all treatment was discontinued. These encouraging findings suggest that ketoconazole may be a viable alternative to amphotericin B in some patients with serious *S. schenckii* infections.

▶ The results of this study are modestly supportive of a role for ketoconazole in the treatment of systemic sporotrichosis. As the authors point out in their review, previous reports have been less sanguine. Only 7 of 18 patients reported previously had an appreciable response to treatment without relapse. One hopes that other oral antifungal agents (e.g., itraconazole) will be more effective.—M.J. Barza, M.D.

Candidemia in Children With Central Venous Catheters: Role of Catheter Removal and Amphotericin B Therapy

Dato VM, Dajani AS (Wayne State Univ; Children's Hosp of Michigan, Detroit)

Pediatr Infect Dis J 9:309–314, 1990 4–4

To determine the optimal therapy of catheter-related *Candida* infection, data were reviewed on 31 children with candidemia who had central venous catheters. Follow-up ranged from 20 days to 5 years (median, 6½ months).

The catheter-related infection rate remained relatively constant at 3% to 4%, despite a marked increase in the number of central catheters inserted (Table 1). The infection rate was significantly higher in toddlers

TABLE 1.—Annual Rates of Candidemia

Year	No. of Infections/ No. of Catheters Inserted	Rate (%)
1981	0/30	0
1982	0/34	0
1983	2/68	2.9
1984	3/97	3.1
1985	7/179	3.9
1986	8/215	3.7
Total	20/623	3.2

(Courtesy of Dato VM, Dajani AS: *Pediatr Infect Dis J* 9:309–314, 1990.)

aged 1–5 years compared with other age groups (8.4% vs. 2.2%). Serious complications developed in 11 patients (35%) at a mean of 16 days (range, 3–52 days) after the first positive blood culture. Five patients died; *Candida* endocarditis occurred in 2 others, as well as renal abscesses, meningitis, arthritis, and osteomyelitis in 1 patient each. Complications were significantly more common in infants younger than 1 year compared with older children (56% vs. 13%). There were no complications among the 6 patients in whom the catheters were removed within 1 day of having a positive blood culture. In contrast, in 4 of the 5 children who died, catheters were left in place for a significantly greater number of days.

Another 43 patients with catheter-related candidemia in 11 studies were identified in a literature survey, for an average *Candida* infection rate of 2.7%. Analysis of data from this survey and the present study indicated that patients treated with catheter removal within 4 days of a first positive blood culture plus amphotericin B had a significantly higher cure rate (88%) than those treated with catheter retention plus amphotericin B (56%) (Table 2).

These data indicate that prompt catheter removal is crucial in the treatment of catheter-related candidemia. Until more conclusive data are available, prompt removal of central and peripheral catheters plus amphotericin B therapy should be instituted in patients with catheter-related candidemia.

▶ This study supports the approach used in Abstract 10–10, namely, prompt removal of the catheter in patients with catheter-related *Candida* infection. It should be noted that this retrospective review suggested that, to minimize complications, the catheter should be removed within a day of the positive blood culture, and that amphotericin B probably should be given; the additional utility of amphotericin B once the catheter has been removed is suggestive but not clear-cut. The optimum dose of amphotericin B is even more conjectural. These authors, working in a pediatric setting, are currently using a cumulative dosage of 15 mg/kg.—M.J. Barza, M.D.

TABLE 2.—Outcome of Catheter-Related *Candida* Sepsis in Relation to Catheter Removal and Amphotericin B Therapy in Patients in This Study and the Recent Literature

Category	Series	Population	Cures	Failures
Catheters removed* no amphotericin B	Thomas and Lang	Adult TPN	2/3	1/3
	Fleming et al.	Adult TPN	1/1	0/1
	Shapiro et al.	Pediatric cancer	1/1	0/1
	Present	Pediatric	10/15	5/15 (1 death)
	Total		14/20	6/20 (1 death)
Catheter removed* amphotericin B administered	Wang et al.	Pediatric	1/1	0/1
	Thomas and Lang	Adult TPN	1/1	0/1
	Sadiq et al.	Infants	3/4	1/4 (1 death)
	Sitzman et al.	Adult TPN	1/1	0/1
	Eppes et al.	Pediatric	12/12	0/12
	Present	Pediatric	5/7	2/7
	Total		23/26	3/26 (1 death)
Catheters retained; amphotericin B administered	Wade et al.	Adult cancer	2/3	1/3
	Eppes et al.	Pediatric	4/10	6/10 (1 death)
	Hendrick and Wilkinson	Adult cancer	0/1	1/1
	Schuman	Adults	1/1	0/1
	Hartman and Shochat	Pediatric cancer	3/4	1/4 (1 death)
	Present	Pediatric	4/6	2/6 (1 death)
	Total		14/25	11/25 (3 deaths)

Abbreviation: TPN, total parenteral nutrition.
*Catheters removed within 4 days of obtaining a blood culture subsequently positive for *Candida.*
(Courtesy of Dato VM, Dajani AS: *Pediatr Infect Dis J* 9:309–314, 1990.)

Endogenous *Candida* Endophthalmitis: Management Without Intravenous Amphotericin B

Brod RD, Flynn HW Jr, Clarkson JG, Pflugfelder SC, Culbertson WW, Miller D
(Univ of Miami)

Ophthalmology 97:666–674, 1990 4–5

Intravenously administered amphotericin B is often recommended as part of the treatment for endogenous *Candida* endophthalmitis (ECE), even when disseminated infection is not evident. Because of the systemic toxicity of amphotericin B, the need for systemic treatment in all ECE. Data were reviewed on 8 patients aged 30–79 years with culture-proven ECE who were treated successfully with vitrectomy, but without systemically administered amphotericin. Positive culture results were obtained from the vitreous in all patients. All had symptomatic visual loss in the involved eye. There were multiple predisposing conditions to ECE in 6 patients, including systemically administered antibiotics and/or corticosteroids within 3 months of onset of the ocular symptoms. The interval from onset of symptoms to presentation ranged from 3 days to 16 weeks (table).

Only 1 patient had *Candida* cultured from a source other than the eye (an infected foot ulcer). *Candida albicans* was cultured from the vitreous in 6 patients; *Candida tropicalis* was cultured from 2 patients. Vitrectomy was performed through a pars plana approach in 7 patients and through the limbus at the time of extracapsular cataract extraction and anterior membranectomy in 1. Amphotericin B was injected intravitreally at the time of vitrectomy in 7 patients, and 4 days post vitrectomy in 1. Flucytosine or ketoconazole was administered to 5 patients to supplement the local ocular therapy for ECE.

At follow-up averaging 11.8 months, 6 patients had improved and 2 had worsened visual acuity compared with the presenting and preoperative vision. Vision was better in those with a shorter interval between onset of symptoms and start of antifungal therapy. These findings suggest that intravenously administered amphotericin B is not necessary in patients with ECE limited to the eye.

► One must be careful not to draw from this study the inference that systemic treatment generally can be omitted in patients with endogenous *Candida* endophthalmitis. In fact, 5 of the 8 patients reported received systemic treatment (oral ketoconazole or flucytosine, admittedly not optimal treatment) and in 7 of the 8 patients there was no evidence of infection at any site but the eye. It is not mentioned whether blood cultures were done. Finally, the median interval between onset of symptoms and presentation was 2 weeks. One would imagine that patients with extraocular involvement of significance might have been sicker and have come for medical treatment sooner. Thus the patients reported here were at a relatively low risk for systemic infection outside of the eye.—M.J. Barza, M.D.

Duration of Symptoms, Initial Management, and Antifungal Therapy

Case No.	Interval from Onset Symptoms to Presentation (wks)	Initial Management (before antifungal therapy)	Systemic Antifungal Therapy	Intravitreal Antifungal Therapy
1	16	Topical and systemic steroids	Flucytosine	Amphotericin B, 5 μg (injected 4 days postvitrectomy)
2	1	Topical and systemic steroids	None	Amphotericin B, 10 μg
3	0.5	Topical steroids	None	Amphotericin B, 5 μg
4	8	None	Ketoconazole	Amphotericin B, 5 μg (at time of vitrectomy); repeat vitreous tap and injection, 12.5 μg; amphotericin B, 3 days later
5	2	Topical steroids	Ketoconazole	Amphotericin B, 5 μg
6	3	Topical and sub-Tenon's steroids	Flucytosine	Amphotericin B, 10 μg (at initial AC tap); amphotericin B 5 μg, and miconazole, 25 μg (at time of vitrectomy)
7	1.5	Treated for toxoplasmosis retinitis with antibiotics, topical and systemic steroids	None	Amphotericin B, 5 μg
8	2	None	Ketoconazole	Amphotericin B, 5 μg

Abbreviation: AC, anterior chamber.
(Courtesy of Brod RD, Flynn HW Jr, Clarkson JG, et al: *Ophthalmology* 97:666–674, 1990.)

Itraconazole Treatment of Coccidioidomycosis

Graybill JR, Stevens DA, Galgiani JN, Dismukes WE, Cloud GA, and the NAIAD Mycoses Study Group (Audie L Murphy Mem VA Hosp; Univ of Texas, San Antonio; Santa Clara Valley Med Ctr, San Jose; Stanford Univ; VA Med Ctr, Tucson; et al)

Am J Med 89:282–290, 1990 4–6

Amphotericin B and ketoconazole are widely used in the treatment of coccidioidomycosis. Ketoconazole is administered orally and is a less toxic alternative to amphotericin B, but it has significant limitations. Posttreatment relapse is high with this imidazole, and larger doses may cause intolerable nausea and vomiting. Data were reviewed on a trial of itraconazole, a potent triazole that appears to offer greater potency and less toxicity than ketoconazole.

The 49 patients who met study criteria were divided into 3 groups (Table 1): skin and soft tissue (14), chronic pulmonary (23), and osteoarticular disease (12). Most of the patients previously had relapse or treat-

TABLE 1.—Demographic Characteristics

	Principal Site of Disease			
	Osteoarticular*	Chronic Pulmonary†	Soft Tissue	Total
Number of patients	12	23	14	49
Median age	36	37	37	37
Range	19–68	18–68	15–73	15–73
Sex				
Male	10 (83)‡	14 (61)	11 (79)	35 (71)
Female	2 (17)	9 (39)	3 (21)	14 (29)
Race				
White	6 (50)	7 (31)	7 (50)	20 (41)
Black	3 (25)	2 (9)	2 (14)	7 (14)
Hispanic	2 (17)	12 (52)	0 (0)	14 (29)
Oriental	0 (0)	1 (4)	3 (22)	4 (8)
Native American	1 (8)	1 (4)	2 (14)	4 (8)
Immunosuppressive therapy	1 (8)	2 (9)	0 (0)	3 (6)
Underlying disease	5 (42)	11 (48)	4 (29)	20 (41)
Diabetes	1	6	1	8
Alcoholism	0	1	0	1
Systemic lupus	0	0	1	1
Neoplasm	3	0	0	3
Renal transplant	0	1	0	1
Rheumatoid arthritis	1	0	0	1
Nephritis	1	0	0	1
Atherosclerosis	1	0	0	1
Sarcoidosis	1	0	0	1
Cholelithiasis	1	0	0	1
Pulmonary fibrosis	0	1	0	1
Mitral stenosis	0	1	0	1
Emphysema	0	1	0	1

*Includes 4 patients with skin lesions.
†Includes 1 patient with skin lesions.
‡Values in parentheses are percentages.
(Courtesy of Graybill JR, Steven DA, Galgiani JN, et al: *Am J Med* 89:282–290, 1990.)

TABLE 2.—Patients Who Experienced Relapse After Previous Antifungal Treatment

Number of Relapses	Osteo-articular	Chronic Pulmonary	Skin, Soft Tissue	Total
Relapses (% of patients)	11 (92)	10 (43)	8 (57)	29 (59)
No details of treatment	1	0	0	1
Amphotericin B (courses)	4	6	3	13
Median (g)	4.7	2.0	1.5	
Range (g)	1.0–6.1	1.0–4.5	0.1–2.0	
Ketoconazole (courses)	8	8	8	24
Median dose (g)	200	780	162	
Range (g)	10–600	12–1,100	15–1,300	
No total dose given	1	5	3	9

(Courtesy of Graybill JR, Steven DA, Galgiani JN, et al: *Am J Med* 89:282–290, 1990.)

ment failure (Table 2). Those with chronic pulmonary or osteoarticular disease had higher overall disease severity scores than those with soft tissue disease.

Itraconazole, 100 or 200 mg, was given orally once a day to 12 patients; the remaining 37 patients were given 200 mg twice daily. This initial dosage was increased if patients were responding too slowly to lower doses. Treatment continued for up to 39 months. Of 44 patients who completed treatment with itraconazole, 25% had clinical remission, defined as a reduction of the pretreatment score by 50% or more (Table 3). All 3 groups responded slowly, with few experiencing remission before 10 months of treatment.

Nearly half of the patients had no toxic effects. The most common adverse reactions to itraconazole were nausea and vomiting (Table 4). Three patients left the protocol—1 because of intractable nausea and vomiting, 1 with leukopenia, and 1 with nephrotic syndrome. In most patients the treatment was tolerated at 400 mg/day, the highest permitted

TABLE 3.—Clinical Outcome of Patients at Completion of Treatment

	Osteo-articular	Chronic Pulmonary	Soft Tissue	Total (%)
With treatment	1	1	1	3
Without treatment	10	22	12	44 (100)
Remission	6	12	7	25 (57)
No relapse	4	12	5	21 (48)
Relapse	2	0	2	4 (9)
Failure	4	10	5	19 (43)
Clinical	3	8	5	16 (36)
Toxicity	1	2	0	3 (7)

(Courtesy of Graybill JR, Steven DA, Galgiani JN, et al: *Am J Med* 89:282–290, 1990.)

TABLE 4.—Possible Toxicities of Itraconazole

Total number of patients	49
Patients with no toxic effect	23
Number of toxic effects	
Nausea/vomiting	6
Edema	5
Rash	3
Diarrhea	3
Decreased libido	3
Pruritus	3
Chills/fever	3
Headache	2
Hallucinations/somnolence	2
Dizziness	2
Alopecia	2
Urinary frequency	2
Fatigue	2
Hypertension	2
Photophobia	1
Blurred vision	1
Leukopenia	1
Polyuria	1
Nephrotic syndrome	1
Palpitations	1
Proteinuria	1
SGOT > 3 × upper limits normal	1
Hypokalemia	1

Abbreviation: SGOT, serum glutamic oxaloacetic transaminase.
(Courtesy of Graybill JR, Stevens DA, Galgiani JN, et al: *Am J Med* 89:282–290, 1990.)

dose. These findings indicate that itraconazole has lower toxicity, and possibly greater efficacy, than the 2 drugs commonly used for treatment of nonmeningeal coccidioidomycosis.

▶ The rapid acceptance of fluconazole points out our major need for new antifungal agents. Itraconazole appears to be just such an agent on the horizon. In this study of nonmeningeal coccidioidomycosis, itraconazole was quite effective in inducing remission. It is important to note, however, that direct comparisons cannot be drawn between this study and the previous one by this group on the effectiveness of ketaconazole for treatment of similar patients. The definitions of response in this study were much more liberal than in the previous study, and this may account for the greater remission rates reported here than for ketaconazole. Similarly, we will need longer term follow-up to determine whether relapses after itraconazole therapy are as common as they are after ketaconazole. Only 6% of the patients treated with itraconazole needed to stop therapy because of drug toxicity. This contrasts with at least a 20% rate in patients receiving ketaconazole at 400 mg/day and a much higher rate at dosages of 800 mg or more daily.—M.S. Klempner, M.D.

A Comparative Double-Blind Study of Terbinafine (Lamisil) and Griseofulvin in Tinea Corporis and Tinea Cruris

Del Palacio Hernanz A, López Gómez S, González Lastra F, Moreno Palancar P, Iglesias Díez L (Carretera de Andalucía, Madrid)

Clin Exp Dermatol 15:210–216, 1990 4–7

Terbinafine (Lamisil) is a synthetic allylamine that is primarily fungicidal. The efficacy and safety of terbinafine in treating widespread tinea corporis and tinea cruris was compared with that of griseofulvin in a double-blind, randomized study. Ninety-two patients with culturally proved tinea corporis or tinea cruris, or both, received either terbinafine, 125 mg, or griseofulvin, 500 mg, orally twice daily for up to 6 weeks. Assessments were performed at weekly intervals during treatment and at follow-up 2 weeks post therapy.

The demographic characteristics and distribution of lesions were similar between groups, but the group given terbinafine had slightly higher mean clinical scores at baseline. At the end of therapy, the percentage of patients with negative microscopic findings and cultures was 78% in the terbinafine-treated group and 83% in the griseofulvin-treated group. At 2 weeks post therapy (follow-up), 93% and 95% of patients, respectively, had negative microscopic findings and cultures.

Clinically, the rate of decrease in erythema, desquamation, and pruritus was significantly faster in the patients given griseofulvin, and the treatment period with griseofulvin was shorter. Although there was a significant difference in favor of griseofulvin by the end of therapy, overall assessment at follow-up did not differ significantly between groups (table). Overall, effective therapy was noted in 77% of ter-

Combined Clinical and Mycological Evaluation

	End of therapy		Follow-up (overall assessment)	
Response	Terbinafine	Griseofulvin	Terbinafine	Griseofulvin
Complete cure	24	28	37	35
Mycological cure + minimal signs	7	9	0	1
Effective treatment	31 (65%)	37 (84%)	37 (77%)	36 (82%)
Mycological cure + improvement (Imp A or B)	6	0	3	0
Mycological failure + improvement (Imp C)	5	0	1	0
Failure	6	7	7	8
Ineffective treatment*	17 (35%)	7 (16%)	11 (23%)	8 (18%)
Total patients	48	44	48	44

*Ineffective treatment group includes premature termination of therapy because of adverse effects.

(Courtesy of Del Palacio Hernanz A, López Gómez S, González Lastra F, et al: *Clin Exp Dermatol* 15:210–216, 1990.)

binafine-treated patients and 82% of griseofulvin-treated patients. Relapses occurred after mycological cure in 3 patients given griseofulvin and 2 given terbinafine. Adverse effects of treatment occurred with the same frequency in both groups, and 5 patients given terbinafine and 6 given griseofulvin stopped treatment because of headaches or gastrointestinal side effects. One patient treated with terbinafine had unexpectedly increased liver enzymes activity after 6 weeks of treatment.

Terbinafine, 125 mg orally twice daily, is comparably safe and only slightly less effective than griseofulvin (1 g daily) in the treatment of widespread tinea corporis or tinea cruris, or both, although results of using both drugs were comparable on long-term follow-up. Further studies are recommended to establish the place of terbinafine in the management of fungal infections.

▶ One of the pleasures of preparing the YEAR BOOK is the opportunity to see articles from journals that I would not otherwise encounter. *Clinical and Experimental Dermatology* is not my usual reading material, and it was nice to come across a compound (terbinafine) that is a relatively new oral fungicidal agent against dermatophytes. I am not aware that it is yet available in the United States, but in this and several other European studies, it appears as safe and effective as griseofulvin in the treatment of tinea corporis or tinea cruris.—M.S. Klempner, M.D.

A Cluster of *Pneumocystis carinii* Pneumonia in Adults Without Predisposing Illnesses

Jacobs JL, Libby DM, Winters RA, Gelmont DM, Fried ED, Hartman BJ, Laurence J (New York Hosp–Cornell Med Ctr)

N Engl J Med 324:246–250, 1991 4–8

Pneumocystis carinii pneumonia is the most common infection complicating AIDS, but before 1981 it was a rare condition and involved small clusters of hospitalized patients with a predisposing or immunocompromising illness or children. During a 3-month period, a cluster of *P. carinii* was observed in 5 elderly patients without AIDS or other identifiable risk factors.

In all patients *P. carinii* was identified on bronchoscopy with bronchoalveolar lavage. Patient 1, a woman aged 78 years, with a history of chronic obstructive lung disease and congestive heart failure, was admitted to the hospital after sustaining minor trauma at home. Patient 2, a previously healthy man aged 66 years, had a 3-day history of fever, malaise, and frontal headache. Patient 3, a woman aged 73 years with a history of adult-onset diabetes mellitus, asthma, gastritis, and congestive heart failure, was admitted with a 3-week history of anorexia, nausea, and vomiting. Patient 4, a man aged 70 years, had a history of adult-onset diabetes mellitus and alcohol abuse. Surgery was performed for squamous cell carcinoma of the cervical esophagus. Patient 5, a woman aged 78 years with a history of aortic valve replacement and long-term anticoagulant therapy, was admitted after sustaining a head injury at home. Patients 1, 3, and 4 died in the hospital.

There was no evidence of undetected predisposing illness in the 5 patients, and the method of transmission is unclear. Hypothesis include an increased likelihood of exposure in the community or hospital, or simply increased susceptibility because of age.

Although rare, clusters of *P. carinii* have occurred in adults without predisposing illness. Bronchoalveolar lavage with staining for *P. carinii* should be performed on patients with undiagnosed pneumonia that is not responsive to empirical antibiotic therapy. This group of 5 older patients with *P. carinii* may be unique, or it may indicate a shift in the epidemiologic nature of *P. carinii.*

▶ One can only speculate whether this cluster of *P. carinii* pneumonia is related to increased community or nosocomial exposure. Based on previous clusters of *P. carinii* infection in immunocompromised patients, I have long been concerned about the nosocomial transmission of this organism. Some of these cases may represent such an event. Autopsy series have shown rates of *P. carinii* of .2%; therefore, the presence of organisms in this group of patients would appear to have pathophysiologic significance.—D.R. Snydman, M.D.

Recurrent Allergic Vulvovaginitis: Treatment With *Candida albicans* Allergen Immunotherapy

Rigg D, Miller MM, Metzger WJ (East Carolina Univ, Greenville, NC; Univ of Tennessee, Knoxville)

Am J Obstet Gynecol 162:332–336, 1990 4–9

Although recurrent vulvovaginal candidiasis is frequent in women who have recurrent infection, pain, and discharge, the cause is uncertain. The presence of *Candida albicans* in the vagina is not by itself an adequate explanation. There is some evidence for antigen-specific defects of T suppressor lymphocyte function in women with recurrent *Candida vaginitis.*

Candida extract was given for periods of 1–3 years to 18 women with recurrent vaginal candidiasis without associated systemic symptoms (Table 1). Immunotherapy was offered if there was a positive immediate skin test reaction or a late-phase cutaneous response to prick testing or intradermal skin testing. Some patients received prednisone before the start of immunotherapy.

The mean number of episodes occurring each year decreased from 17.2 to 4.3 after treatment (Table 2), and 3 women had complete remission. There was no improvement in 2 patients. Overall improvement was estimated at nearly 80%, a significant effect.

Immunotherapy may be especially promising for women with uncontrolled symptoms of candidal vulvovaginitis despite long-term antifungal

TABLE 1.—Characteristics of Patient Population

Patient	Age (yr)	Duration of symptoms (yr)	Atopy	Skin test response: Early	Skin test response: Late	Vaginal culture	Oral contraceptive use (yr)
1	32	2	Yes	Positive	NA	Positive	None
2	28	10	Yes	Positive	Negative	Positive	10
3	38	8	No	Positive	NA	Positive	None
4	27	8	No	Positive	Positive	Positive	9
5	24	9	No	Positive	Positive	Positive	9
6	28	7	Yes	Positive	Positive	Positive	6
7	38	7	Yes	Positive	NA	Positive	None*
8	30	2	No	Positive	NA	Positive	None
9	47	32	Yes	Positive	NA	Positive	None
10	37	10	No	Negative	Positive	Positive	12
11	29	1	Yes	Positive	NA	Positive	None
12	35	5	Yes	Positive	Positive	Positive	None
13	30	3	Yes	Positive	NA	Positive	None
14	48	15	Yes	Positive	Positive	Positive	None
15	32	3	No	Negative	Positive	Positive	None
16	30	7	Yes	Negative	Positive	Positive	None
17	36	17	No	Positive	NA	Positive	16
18	39	18	Yes	Positive	NA	Positive	None

Abbreviations: NA, not available; *Atopy*, more than 5 positive inhalant skin test results (prick) and a consistent history.
*Menstrual cycle related, midcycle.
(Courtesy of Rigg D, Miller MM, Metzger WJ: *Am J Obstet Gynecol* 162:332–336, 1990.)

treatment. The latter form of treatment carries a high risk of relapse and also, with ketoconazole, a significant risk of hepatitis.

▶ Women who experience frequent recurrences of vulvovaginal candidiasis despite antifungal therapy represent a difficult clinical problem. These authors approached it as a hypersensitivity disease and demonstrated efficacy of

TABLE 2.—Results of Therapy With *Candida* Allergen Immunotherapy

Patient	*Age (yr)*	*Cumulative dose (PNU)*	*Treatment (months)*	*Before*	*Incidence of candidiasis (episodes/yr)*	*% Improvement*
1	32	990,000	47	12	0.8	93.3
2	28	416,000	28	24*	0.3	98.8
3	38	276,000	16	24*	1	95.8
4	27	226,000	15	24*	24*	0
5	24	186,000	31	3	0.7	76.7
6	28	145,000	10	12	1	91.7
7	38	141,000	24	12	2	83.3
8	30	97,000	14	24†	4	83.3
9	47	96,000	17	12	2	83.3
10	37	96,000	10	4	0	100
11	30	51,000	11	24*	12	50.0
12	35	23,000	37	24*	1	95.8
13	30	200,000	51	12	2	83.3
14	48	99,000	11	24*	24*	0
15	32	NA	12	12	0	100
16	30	300,000	49	24*	0	100
17	36	128,000	30	24*	1	95.9
18	39	80,000	12	24*	2	91.6
Mean	33.8	—	—	17.2 ± 1.98‡	4.3 ± 1.8	79.0 ± 7.5

*Chronic persistent disease, with more than 2 episodes per month.
†Chronic symptoms with dyspareunia.
‡Difference is significant at $P < .0004$ by Wilcoxon signed rank sum test.
(Courtesy of Rigg D, Miller MM, Metzger WJ: *Am J Obstet Gynecol* 162:332–336, 1990.)

immunotherapy with a *Candida* extract. It is important to note that this was not a prospective randomized study, which will be required to confirm this result. Moreover, one suspects that combining immunotherapy with ketoconazole may be one arm of such a prospective study.—M.S. Klempner, M.D.

***Torulopsis glabrata* Vaginitis: Clinical Aspects and Susceptibility to Antifungal Agents**

Redondo-Lopez V, Lynch M, Schmitt C, Cook R, Sobel JD (Wayne State Univ)
Obstet Gynecol 76:651–654, 1990 4–10

Reports indicate that 7% to 16% of yeasts isolated from the vagina are *Torulopsis glabrata.* To determine the spectrum of lower genital disease and susceptibility to antifungal agents of *T. glabrata,* data on 33 patients from whom vaginal isolates of *T. glabrata* were obtained were reviewed retrospectively.

The patients represented a racially mixed, nonpromiscuous, middle-class population of women aged 22–72 years (mean age, 38.7 years) (table). Fourteen (42%) had symptomatic yeast vaginitis and 10 (30%) were asymptomatic. In the remaining 9 (27%) patients the importance of *T glabrata* was uncertain because of concomitant pathology. The clinical features of vaginitis caused by *T. glabrata* were clinically indistinguishable from those caused by *Candida species.* Most of the women had a frequent history of recent systemic antibacterial therapy and recent antimycotic therapy.

Antifungal susceptibility testing was performed on 39 *T. glabrata* strains isolated from 39 patients. Compared with *Candida albicans* iso-

Demographic Characteristics of Women With Positive Vaginal Cultures for *Torulopsis glabrata*

No. of patients	33
Age (yr)	38.7 (22–72)
Marital status	
Single	9
Married	13
Divorced	11
Ethnic origin	
White	17
Black	16
Contraception	
None	5
Tubal ligation	6
Vasectomy	4
Oral contraceptive	3
Condom	4
Hysterectomy	5
Unknown	6
Pregnancies/patient	2.3 (0–11)
Sexual partners/patient	1.2 (0–6)
Coitus/wk	1.0 (0–5.5)

(Courtesy of Redondo-Lopez V, Lynch M, Schmitt C, et al: *Obstet Gynecol* 76:651–654, 1990.)

lates, *T. glabrata* isolates tended to be less susceptible to all azole agents tested. Nevertheless, most of the isolates fell within the sensitive range. The most active azoles in vitro were miconazole and itraconazole and the least active were fluconazole and ketoconazole. The clinical response to antimycotic therapy was satisfactory in 67% of patients, but mycologic cure was achieved in only 25%. There was no correlation between the measured in vitro activity and the clinical response to antifungal therapy. Recurrent and often chronic *T. glabrata* vaginitis unresponsive to conventional therapy developed in 3 patients; responded to oral flucytosine therapy and another to topical treatment with boric acid.

Conventional topical or oral azoles treatment should be the first-line therapy for *T. glabrata* vaginitis. Patients with recurrent or chronic *T. glabrata* vaginitis may not respond to repeated courses of azoles, but topical or oral flucytosine or topical boric acid treatment may be helpful.

5 Parasitic Infections

Parasitologic Findings in Percutaneous Drainage of Human Hydatid Liver Cysts

Filice C, Di Perri G, Strosselli M, Pirola F, Brunetti E, Dughetti S, Concia E (Univ of Pavia-IRCCS Policlinico San Matteo, Pavia, Italy)
J Infect Dis 161:1290–1295, 1990 5–1

The diagnosis and treatment of cystic hydatid disease need to be improved. Percutaneous drainage under ultrasonographic guidance was undertaken in 12 patients with hydatid liver cysts and 1 patient with an abdominal cyst. The fluid was aspirated from the cyst and a series of examinations was performed on the fluid, including direct microscopic examination, staining for viability assessment, and culture. Through a catheter connected to the cavity, 95% ethanol solution corresponding to one third of the fluid aspirated was introduced into the cavity and slowly removed after 30 minutes. The procedure was repeated over the following days until parasites were no longer detected on 3 consecutive examinations. All patients received mebendazole, 3 g/day, for 10 days before to 1 month after the procedure.

Eight patients had cystic hydatid disease. Protoscolices were seen di-

Parasitologic Findings in 8 Patients With Cystic Hydatid Disease

Patients	Before infusion of alcohol	After infusion of alcohol		
		5 min	10 min	15 min
1-3, 5, 7, 8				
Presence of protoscolices	++	+	−	−
Flame cell activity	++	−	−	−
In vitro cultivation	++		−	−
Neutral red uptake †	85-100	1-3		
Methylene blue uptake †	0-15	97-99		
Rostellar hooks	+	+	++	++
4, 6				
Presence of protoscolices	−	+	−	−
Flame cell activity	−	−	−	−
In vitro cultivation	++	−	−	−
Neutral red uptake †		1-2		
Methylene blue uptake †		98-99		
Rostellar hooks	−	+	++	++

*++, highly positive; +, rare; −, negative.
†% of parasites stained: 10 minutes after alcohol infusion, intact protoscolices were no longer detected.
(Courtesy of Filice C, Di Perri G, Strosselli M, et al: *J Infect Dis* 161:1290–1295, 1990.)

rectly in 4 patients and after centrifugation in 2 (table). Although typical flame cell activity occurred in only 4 patients, viability was present in all specimens as evidenced by staining with neutral red (living organism) and by exclusion of methylene blue and eosin (dead organisms). In 2 patients with a steady low titer of specific antibodies and absence of protoscolices and rostellar hooks, culture of the cystic fluid proved the presence of the parasites.

After the intervention, symptoms disappeared promptly in all patients. Markedly increased specific serologic titers were seen within 7–10 days after the intervention in all patients, but the titers declined progressively within 6 months. None of the patients had increased blood alcohol levels during the intervention, and, except for 1 patient with mild maculopapular rash, no adverse reactions were noted. There was no regrowth of the cysts during a follow-up period of 6–31 months. Percutaneous drainage of hydatid cyst under ultrasonographic guidance, coupled with the subsequent introduction of a scolicidal alcohol solution, is therapeutically successful, safe, and feasible.

▶ With the continuing immigration into the United States from areas of the world with endemic hydatid disease, questions are raised concerning diagnosis and management. The possibility of drug therapy is of recent vintage, with the development of drugs such as mebendazole and particularly albendazole; however, the debate about the efficacy and safety of percutaneous vs operative drainage has remained. In this study, 8 of 13 patients with liver cysts were shown to have hydatid disease by direct examination or culture of fluid aspirated via a fine needle. Instillation of ethanol was well tolerated and appeared to sterilize the cyst, although all patients were also treated with mebendazole. Of interest, the patients had a rise in the specific antibody titer within 10 days of treatment, suggesting that the living parasite exerted an immunosuppressive effect, or that the procedure led to the release of antigen. Nonetheless, no significant allergic responses were detected except for a transient maculopapular rash in 1 patient. These investigators appear to have experience and the right stuff for this procedure. At present, I would probably send my patients to Pavia for needle aspiration unless I had available a skilled radiologist with a steady hand accustomed to needling lesions under direct vision. I have been waiting for a reasonable recommendation to provide to those inquiring about this disease.—G.T. Keusch, M.D.

Prevalence and Clinical Importance of *Entamoeba histolytica* in Two High-Risk Groups: Travelers Returning From the Tropics and Male Homosexuals

Weinke T, Friedrich-Jänicke B, Hopp P, Janitschke K (Free Univ of Berlin, Germany; Landesinstitut für Tropenmedizin; Robert Koch-Institut, Berlin)
J Infect Dis 161:1029–1031, 1990 5–2

Previous studies have reported a high prevalence of *Entamoeba histolytica* infection among homosexual men. Because studies in homosex-

Zymodeme Status and Evidence of Pathogenicity in 109 Travelers From the Tropics and 52 Homosexual Men With Proven *Entamoeba histolytica*

	Evidence of pathogenicity		
Patient status	Diarrhea, no. (%)	Diarrhea and detection of *Entamoeba histolytica* only, no. (%)	Positive serology, no. (%)
Travelers			
Pathogenic zymodeme	4/5 (80.0)*	4/5 (80.0)	4/5 (80.0)
Nonpathogenic zymodeme	17/56 (30.4)	3/56 (5.4)	0/56
Not tested	10/48 (20.8)	4/48 (8.3)	3/48 (6.3)
Homosexual men			
Pathogenic zymodeme	0/0	0/0	0/0
Nonpathogenic zymodeme	7/26 (26.9)	5/26 (19.2)	0/26
Not tested	6/26 (23.1)	3/26 (11.5)	0/26

*One patient without diarrhea at the time of examination had amebic liver abscess and had an episode of mucosanguineous diarrhea 3 months earlier.

(Courtesy of Weinke T, Friedrich-Jänicke B, Hopp P, et al: *J Infect Dis* 161:1029–1031, 1990.)

ual men have shown that there is no correlation between the presence or absence of *E. histolytica* and gastrointestinal symptoms, and no evidence of invasive amebiasis has been demonstrated, *E. histolytica* in this population is considered a commensal that need not be treated. The prevalence of amebiasis and *E. histolytica* was compared among homosexual men and travelers returning from the tropics.

The study population included 2,700 travelers (mean age, 34 years) who voluntarily submitted a stool specimen for routine microscopic examination after a stay in the tropics, and 320 homosexual men (mean age, 36 years) who came in for routine check-ups or were inpatients with infections associated with HIV. Patients with AIDS were excluded from the study. Most returning travelers were asymptomatic.

Fecal parasites were found in 827 travelers (31%) and 142 homosexual men (44%). *Entamoeba histolytica* was identified in 109 travelers (4%) and 52 homosexual men (16%). The difference was statistically significant. Five travelers had symptoms of invasive amebiasis and a pathogenic zymodeme of *E. histolytica*. Three other travelers with gastrointestinal symptoms had positive amebic serology, but zymodeme status was not determined. Thus the prevalence of invasive amebiasis among travelers returning from the tropics was .3%, and 8 (7.3%) of the 109 *E. histolytica* infections led to invasive amebiasis. None of the homosexual men had positive amebic serology, and none had pathogenic zymodeme patterns (table). The absence of a strain of *E. histolytica* with a pathogenic zymodeme in homosexual men confirms that *E. histolytica* in this population can be considered a harmless commensal that need not be treated.

▶ This study seems to confirm the reports, primarily from Sargeaunt and colleagues in London, that male homosexuals are infected with the "nonpathogenic" zymodemes of *E. histolytica* and are not at risk of symptomatic amebiasis. It is of epidemiologic interest that *E. histolytica* was found more commonly in the homosexual men, whereas *Giardia lamblia* was more common in the travelers. Only .3% of travelers contracted invasive amebiasis, caused in all cases studied by a "pathogenic" zymodeme. However, looked at another way, 7% of the travelers with *E. histolytica* infection had invasive illness. The authors point out the need to consider the potential risk of invasive amebiasis to homosexual men with recent travel to the tropics. Because travel to *E. histolytica* endemic regions is not uncommon among this group, acquired invasive amebiasis could lead to a focal outbreak via sexually transmitted infection. Although this has not happened to my knowledge, this study is a further rationale to introduce zymodeme analysis of *E. histolytica* into the clinical microbiology laboratory.—G.T. Keusch, M.D.

A *T. cruzi*–Secreted Protein Immunologically Related to the Complement Component C9: Evidence for Membrane Pore-Forming Activity at Low pH

Andrews NW, Abrams CK, Slatin SL, Griffiths G (New York Univ; Albert Einstein College of Medicine; European Molecular Biology Lab, Heidelberg, Germany)

Cell 61:1277–1287, 1990 5–3

Trypanosoma cruzi, the agent that causes Chagas' disease in humans, leaves the phagolysosome of a host cell soon after invasion and then multiplies freely in the cytosol. Phagosomes containing *T. cruzi* are acidic, and agents that raise phagosome pH significantly inhibit the parasites' escape into the cytosol. Thus a previously described low-pH active hemolysin secreted by *T. cruzi* might disrupt the phagosome membrane.

Trypanosoma cruzi supernatants are cytotoxic for nucleated cells at pH 5.5. These supernatants contain a protein that reacts with antibodies raised against reduced and alkylated human C9 (the ninth component of complement). The C9 cross-reactive protein (TC-TOX) copurifies with the cytolytic activity. Fractions enriched in TC-TOX are hemolytic, and they form ion channels in planar phospholipid bilayers at low pH. Immunocytochemical studies using antibodies against purified TC-TOX indicated that the protein is localized in the luminal space of phagosomes containing parasites.

The findings suggest that TC-TOX secreted into acidic phagosome compartments forms pores in the membrane that contribute to membrane disruption. Further studies may demonstrate actual insertion of TC-TOX into the bilayer, and they may clarify how membrane fragments are disposed of by the host cell. The parasite's method of protection from membrane damage in the acidic environment of the phagosome is also of interest.

▶ This beautiful paper is well worth reading. It describes the relationship between an acid pH active hemolysin in the protozoan *T. cruzi* and the ninth component of complement, and its possible role in rapid escape of the parasite from the phagolysosome. The more we understand the mechanisms of disease pathogenesis, the more likely we are to be able to use this information clinically. This is real nice science.—G.T. Keusch, M.D.

Cytokine Regulation of Antigen-Driven Immunoglobulin Production in Filarial Parasite Infections in Humans
King CL, Ottesen EA, Nutman TB (Natl Insts of Health, Bethesda, Md)
J Clin Invest 85:1810–1815, 1990 5–4

The production of high levels of IgE antibody is a characteristic response to infection from human filarial parasites. To define the immunoregulatory mechanisms underlying serum IgE levels found in patients with filariasis, polyclonal IgE production by peripheral blood mononuclear cells (PBMC) from 15 such patients was studied.

Ten of the patients had *Loa loa* and 5 had *Onchocerca volvulus*. Two patients were native to the endemic areas, and 13 had acquired their infections while working in endemic areas. Eight were studied before any treatment was given. The remaining patients had received at least 1 course of therapy, but their infection had not been completely eradicated.

Normal in vitro IgE production is <500 pg/mL. Ten of these patients had elevated spontaneous in vitro IgE production that ranged from 838 to 6,464 pg/mL. In 10 of 12 patients tested, the addition of filarial parasite antigen to PBMC cultures significantly stimulated polyclonal IgE production in an antigen dose-dependent manner. The simultaneous addition of anti-interleukin (IL)-4 demonstrated the essential role of IL-4 in the generation of this response, because antigen-stimulated IgE production was completely inhibited in all 10 patients studied (Fig 5–1). In these

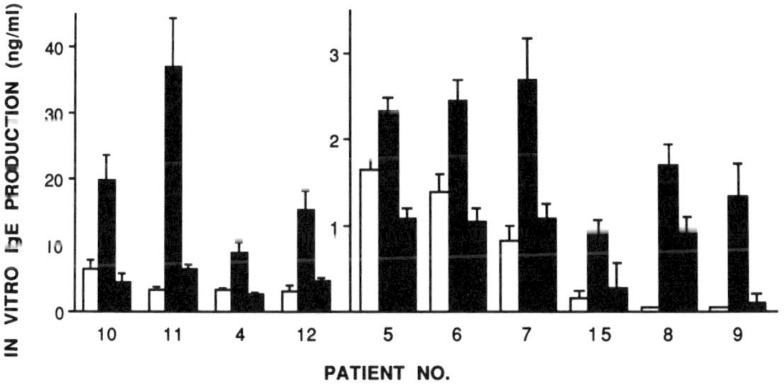

Fig 5–1.—Effect of anti-IL-4 on parasite antigen-induced IgE production. The ordinate indicates the amount of IgE produced in culture, and for patient nos. 10, 11, 4, and 12 the scale ranges from 0 to 40 ng/mL, whereas the scale for the other patients ranges from 0 to 3 ng/mL. Each bar represents the mean ± SEM IgE production of quadruplicate cultures in the presence of media alone *(open bars)* or after the addition of parasite antigen *(filled bars)*, or parasite antigen + anti-IL-4 *(shaded bars)*. Patients are presented in rank order of spontaneous in vitro IgE production. (Courtesy of King CL, Ottesen EA, Nutman TB: *J Clin Invest* 85:1810–1815, 1990.)

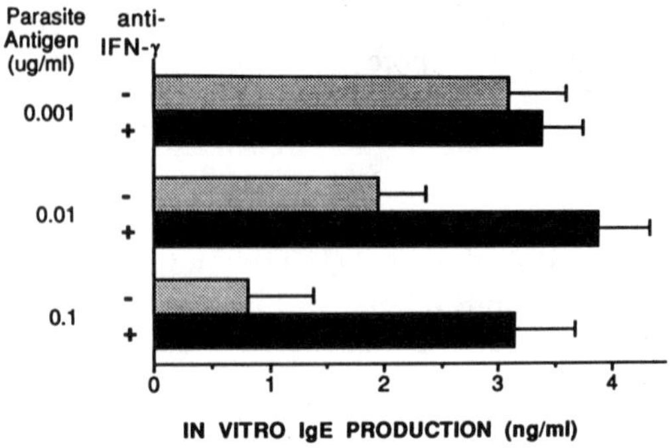

Fig 5–2.—Effect of anti-IFN-γ on the amount of IgE induced by different concentrations of parasite antigen. Each bar represents the mean ± SEM IgE production of 5 patients with loiasis. *Shaded bars* represent cultures with parasite antigen alone, and *dark bars* represent paired cultures with both parasite antigen and anti-IFN-γ. (Courtesy of King CL, Ottesen EA, Nutman TB: *J Clin Invest* 85:1810–1815, 1990.)

same patients, the addition of anti-interferon-γ to the cultures significantly augmented filarial antigen-stimulated IgE production by 33% to 1,238%. Parasite antigen-induced IgE production was completely inhibited by addition of 10–1,000 units of recombinant human interferon-γ per mL to PBMC (Fig 5–2).

Interleukin-4 and interferon-γ are important mediators for the regulation of parasite antigen-stimulated IgE production in humans. Parasite antigen-induced in vitro IgE production by PBMC from patients with filariasis is IL-4 dependent. Further, recombinant human interferon-γ, at concentrations of 10–100,000 units per mL, thoroughly inhibits parasite antigen-induced IgE production in vitro.

▶ It has long been known that helminth infection is associated with elevated IgE levels. This study contributes to the understanding of the mechanism by demonstrating that interleukin-4 induced by filaria, including *Onchocera volvulus* and *Loa loa,* is involved, and that there is a continuing influence of regulatory pathways through interferon-γ during the helminthic infection. It is still not clear what IgE does to the host or the pathogen.—G.T. Keusch, M.D.

Modulation of In Vitro Monocyte Cytokine Responses to *Leishmania donovani:* Interferon-γ Prevents Parasite-Induced Inhibition of Interleukin 1 Production and Primes Monocytes to Respond to Leishmania by Producing Both Tumor Necrosis Factor-α and Interleukin 1

Reiner NE, Ng W, Wilson CB, McMaster WR, Burchett SK (Univ of British Columbia; Vancouver Gen Hosp; Univ of Washington; Children's Hosp and Med Ctr, Seattle)

J Clin Invest 85:1914–1924, 1990 5–5

Cytokines produced by mononuclear cells are important regulatory and effector molecules. Evidence suggests that there is a role at least for

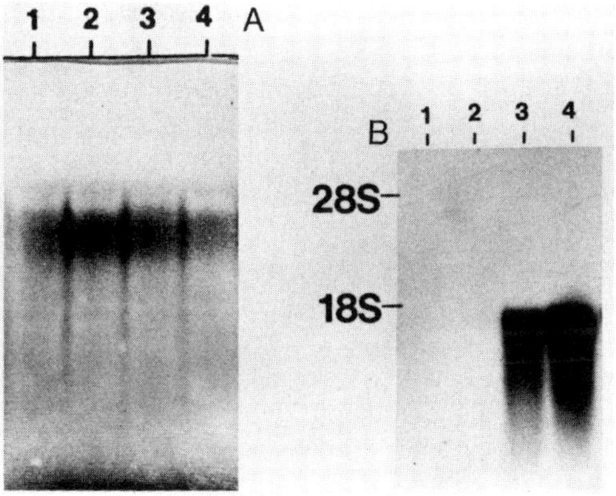

Fig 5–3.—Northern blot analysis of interleukin 1 β mRNA in human monocytes. Monolayers of freshly isolated monocytes treated as indicated below for ~16 hours were washed and lysed in guanidium isothiocyanate. Total cytoplasmic RNA, 5 μg, was fractionated on a 1.2% agarose formaldehyde gel and transferred to Hybond-N and hybridized with ^{32}P-labeled cDNA insert of pHu interleukin 1β (**B**). Lane 1, unstimulated monocytes; lane 2, *Leishmania*-infected monocytes; lane 3, monocytes stimulated with *S. aureus;* lane 4, monocytes treated with lipopolysaccharide (1 μg/mL). **A,** gel stained with acridine orange. (Courtesy of Reiner NE, Ng W, Wilson CB, et al: *J Clin Invest* 85:1914–1924, 1990.)

tumor necrosis factor-α (TNF-α) and interferon-γ (IFN-γ) in host defense against *Leishmania* species. The production of TNF-α and interleukin 1 was examined by resting and IFN-γ-primed peripheral blood monocytes infected in vitro with *Leishmania donovani.*

Amastigotes of the Sudan strain 2S of *L. donovani* were isolated from the spleens of male Syrian hamsters. During challenge with *Leishmania,* monocytes produced neither interleukin 1 nor TNF-α. Although preinfected cells synthesized normal amounts of TNF-α, they had reduced interleukin 1 production in response to stimulation with *Staphylococcus aureus* or lipopolysaccharide. Induction by *S. aureus* or lipopolysaccharide of interleukin-1β mRNA accumulation in infected cells was normal despite lessened intracellular or supernatant interleukin 1 protein and bioactivity. Inhibition of interleukin 1 production by *Leishmania* therefore probably reflected reduced translation of interleukin 1 β mRNA. Pretreatment of cells with IFN-γ abrogated infection-induced inhibition of interleukin 1 production and primed cells for interleukin 1 and TNF-α production on later exposure to *Leishmania* (Fig 5–3).

Leishmania donovani has evolved the ability to infect mononuclear phagocytes without stimulating the production of 2 potentially host-protective monokines. Interferon-γ's ability to prime monocytes to produce TNF-α and interleukin 1 in response to *Leishmania* infection and to prevent inhibition of interleukin 1 production may have implications for immunotherapy with this lymphokine.

▶ There is increasing evidence in the case of leishmaniasis that cytokines are important to the host response, and that administration of interferon-α may potentiate beneficial responses. There is still a paucity of clean data in humans to address the role of the interferon itself, however, and the therapeutic use of this cytokine remains experimental. The finding reported in this paper that *L. donovani* prevents the transcriptional activation of interleukin-1 is of general interest. Specific cytokine responses to different infectious agents may explain, in part, the variable patterns of host response to infectious agents and the presentation of disease. In addition, in this investigation, the infecting organism induced a more general unresponsiveness to other interleukin-1 regulatory stimuli, and it is possible that further study may well reveal a common regulatory pathway amenable to therapeutic manipulation. The possibility of direct clinical relevance of this sort of research is always a part of the potential payoff from basic science, especially when the clinically prepared mind is at work. If this sounds like a plug for the continued involvement of physicians in basic research, you win the golden ring. If only Congress had the YEAR BOOK OF INFECTIOUS DISEASES available and could both read the lines and between them!—G.T. Keusch, M.D.

Longitudinal Study of *Giardia lamblia* Infection in a Day Care Center Population

Rauch AM, Van R, Bartlett AV, Pickering LK (Univ of Texas, Houston; Johns Hopkins Univ)

Pediatr Infect Dis 9:186–189, 1990 5–6

Previous studies have suggested that excretion of *Giardia lamblia* is common among asymptomatic carriers younger than age 3 years in the daycare center (DCC) environment. Treatment of asymptomatic carriers remains controversial. The incidence of symptomatic and asymptomatic *G. lamblia* infection in a DCC population was determined in a 15-month longitudinal study. A total of 2,727 stool specimens collected weekly from 82 children aged 1–24 months was evaluated for rotavirus and *G. lamblia*. Stool specimens also were cultured for bacterial enteropathogens in children with diarrhea.

Forty-eight episodes of *Giardia* infection were detected in 27 of 82 DCC children (33%), compared with 57 episodes of rotavirus infection in 37 of these same children (45%). *Giardia* infection occurred in 14 of the 15 months of the study, and the mean duration of infection was 2 weeks. Only 6 of the 48 episodes of *Giardia* (12%) were associated with symptoms, and there was no correlation between the diarrheal episodes and detection of *Giardia* in collected stool specimens.

Two outbreaks of giardiasis occurred in 1 of the 6 DCC rooms. Both outbreaks were associated with overcrowding, and all but 1 of the 12 children involved had no diarrhea. Neither outbreak was associated with the introduction of a new *Giardia*-positive child into the affected room. It appears that infection in asymptomatic carriers is well tolerated, and that routine treatment or exclusion of these children from the DCC is not warranted. Children with symptomatic giardiasis can return to the DCC once the diarrhea has resolved.

▶ *Giardia lamblia* is one of the more energetic parasites to watch under the microscope, with its big "eyes" looking back at you. It was the first enteric pathogen to be visualized (way back in the 17th century and beautifully described by van Leeuwenhoek), but its pathogenic potential remains a controversy to this day. In this study, a third of the children in a DCC became infected for a mean duration of 2 weeks, but only a few (12%) had diarrhea, and there was no evidence of a relationship between infection and diarrheic episodes. Although the study provides proof of the contagiousness of *Giardia* in a closed setting such as DCCs, does it also show that the parasite is not a pathogen? Probably not, because there are ample demonstrations of the virulence of *G. lamblia* in humans. More likely, strain differences exist with varying pathogenicity. For example, our laboratory has found that different *Giardia* isolates or parasite clones isolated from a single *Giardia* strain are markedly different in their ability to attach to tissue culture cells and in expression of putative virulence factors such as adhesions. The relevant comparison may be to *Entamoeba histolytica,* with its pathogenic and nonpathogenic zymodemes (see Abstract 5–2), and not to *Entamoeba coli,* which appears to be truly nonpathogenic. In addition, it may be just the first few postweaning infections with *Giardia* that are associated with symptoms, as others have shown in retrospective analysis of prospective data in Guatemala (1). It would be impossible to ascertain the previous experience of children with the parasite in the present study, however. In any event, the authors' conclusion to withhold routine treatment and not to exclude children with asymptomatic infections from attending day care seems appropriate.— G.T. Keusch, M.D.

Reference

1. Farthing MJ, et al: *Am J Clin Nutr* 43:395, 1986.

6 Mycobacterial Infections

A 62-Dose, 6-Month Therapy for Pulmonary and Extrapulmonary Tuberculosis: A Twice-Weekly, Directly Observed, and Cost-Effective Regimen

Cohn DL, Catlin BJ, Peterson KL, Judson FN, Sbarbaro JA (Denver Dept of Health and Hosps; Univ of Colorado)

Ann Intern Med 112:407–415, 1990 6–1

There have been rapid changes in the drugs used for chemotherapy and in the duration of chemotherapy in the treatment of tuberculosis. The efficacy and toxicity of a 62-dose, 4-drug, 6-month directly observed regimen for treating pulmonary and extrapulmonary tuberculosis were evaluated. In the open, nonblinded clinical trial 160 patients from a metropolitan tuberculosis clinic were treated.

The treatment regimen consisted of isoniazid, rifampin, pyrazinamide, and streptomycin given daily for 2 weeks and then twice weekly in higher doses for another 6 weeks. Isoniazid and rifampin were then given twice

TABLE 1.—Sixty-Two Dose, 4 Drug, 6-Month Therapy for Tuberculosis (Denver Metro Clinic Regimen)

First 2 weeks*
- **isoniazid, 300 mg†**
- **rifampin, 600 mg**
- **pyrazinamide, 1.5 g if ≤ 50 kg body weight; 2.0 g if 51 to 74 kg; 2.5 g if ≥ 75 kg**
- **streptomycin, 750 mg if ≤ 50 kg body weight; 1.0 g if > 50 kg**

Week 3 through week 8 (twice weekly)‡
- **isoniazid, 15 mg/kg body weight**
- **rifampin, 600 mg**
- **pyrazinamide, 3.0 g if ≤ 50 kg body weight; 3.5 g if 51 to 74 kg; 4.0 g if ≥ 75 kg**
- **streptomycin, 1.0 g if ≤ 50 kg body weight; 1.25 g if 51 to 74 kg; 1.5 g if > 75 kg**

Week 9 through week 26 (twice weekly)
- **isoniazid, 15 mg/kg body weight**
- **rifampin, 600 mg**

*All medications given as 1 daily dose for 14 consecutive days.

†Isoniazid, rifampin, and pyrazinamide were given by mouth as 300, 600, and 500 mg capsules, respectively, and streptomycin was given intramuscularly.

‡If *Mycobacterium, tuberculosis* isolates were resistant to isoniazid, regimen was changed to rifampin, pyrazinamide, and streptomycin twice weekly (regimen B); if resistant to streptomycin, regimen remained as above without streptomycin (regimen C).

(Courtesy of Cohn DL, Catlin BJ, Peterson KL, et al: *Ann Intern Med* 112:407–415, 1990.)

TABLE 2.—Demographic and Clinical Characteristics of 125 Evaluable Patients With Pulmonary and Extrapulmonary Tuberculosis

Characteristic	Patients, *n* (%)
Gender	
Male	87(70)
Female	38(30)
Race or ethnicity	
Hispanic	41(33)
White	30(24)
Southeast or other Asian	29(23)
Black	21(17)
Native American	4(3)
Site of disease	
Pulmonary only	101(81)
Pulmonary and extrapulmonary*	7(6)
Extrapulmonary only†	17(13)

*Pleural, 3 patients; otitis media, 2 patients; peritoneal, 1 patient, genitourinary, 1 patient.

†Lymphatic, 7 patients; pleural, 3 patients; musculoskeletal, 2 patients; endometrial, 2 patients; peritoneal, 1 patient; pericardial, 1 patient; genitourinary, 1 patient.

(Courtesy of Cohn DL, Catlin BJ, Peterson KL, et al: *Ann Intern Med* 112:407–415, 1990.)

weekly for 18 weeks, thereby completing 62 doses (Table 1). All therapy was directly observed by a nurse or an outreach worker.

Thirty-five patients were excluded from the analysis. Among the 125 evaluable patients, 81% had pulmonary tuberculosis, 6% had both pulmonary and extrapulmonary disease, and 13% had extrapulmonary disease only (Table 2). More than half of the patients (57%) had a history of alcoholism.

The median time at which sputum cultures became negative in patients with pulmonary tuberculosis was 4.6 weeks (range, 1–19 weeks). Of these patients 40% were culture negative after only 4 weeks of therapy

TABLE 3.—Time for Conversion to Negative Sputum Cultures in 100 Patients With Pulmonary Tuberculosis

Week of Therapy	Cumulative Percentage of Patients Who Were Culture Negative (95% CI)
4	40 (30.4 to 49.6)
8	75 (66.5 to 83.5)
12	94 (89.3 to 98.7)
16	97 (93.7 to 100)
20	100

Note: Excludes 4 culture-negative pulmonary patients and 4 patients who had diagnostic resections of tuberculomas. For 100 patients median time to achieve negative culture was 4.6 weeks (range, 1 to 19 weeks).

(Courtesy of Cohn DL, Catlin BJ, Peterson KL, et al: *Ann Intern Med* 112:407–415, 1990.)

and 94% were culture negative after 12 weeks (Table 3). There were no treatment failures, and only 2 patients had relapses, 1 at 6 and 1 at 56 months after completing therapy. Side effects included cutaneous abnormalities in 6% of the patients, nausea in 4%, dizziness in 1%, twofold or greater elevations in levels of aspartate aminotransferase in 17%, and 1.5-fold or greater elevations in levels of alkaline phosphatase in 27%. Hyperuricemia also was common (64%), but none of the patients reported arthralgia or gouty arthritis, and levels of uric acid always returned to normal after withdrawal of pyrazinamide.

This 62-dose, 4-drug, 6-month, largely twice-weekly regimen was efficacious and relatively safe for treating pulmonary and extrapulmonary tuberculosis. Compared with other antituberculous chemotherapy protocols, this regimen costs the least and requires the fewest patient visits, thereby making it the most cost effective. Furthermore, this regimen is well suited for patients in whom directly observed therapy is indicated.

USPHS Tuberculosis Short-Course Chemotherapy Trial 21: Effectiveness, Toxicity, and Acceptability: The Report of Final Results

Combs DL, O'Brien RJ, Geiter LJ (Ctrs for Disease Control, Atlanta)
Ann Intern Med 112:397–406, 1990 6–2

Characteristics of Eligible Patients by Regimen

Characteristic	Patients* Assigned to the 6-Month Regimen	Patients* Assigned to the 9-Month Regimen	*P* Value
	%	%	
Racial or ethnic minority	81	79	0.52
Male	78	77	0.65
Born in the United States	76	76	0.74
Cavitary disease	66	72	0.05
Cavity > 4 cm	7	8	0.61
Pleural disease	2	4	0.02
Concurrent diagnosis at entry to study	37	41	0.25
Substance abuse	61	63	0.50
No transportation to clinic	29	29	0.93
Enrollment culture with more than 50 colonies	15	14	0.82
Assigned to ethambutol	26	25	0.67

*Mean age (± standard error) at enrollment of patients assigned to 6-month regimen was 40.9 years and mean age of patients assigned to 9-month regimen was 41.4 years.

(Courtesy of Combs DL, O'Brien RJ, Geiter LJ: *Ann Intern Med* 112:397–406, 1990.)

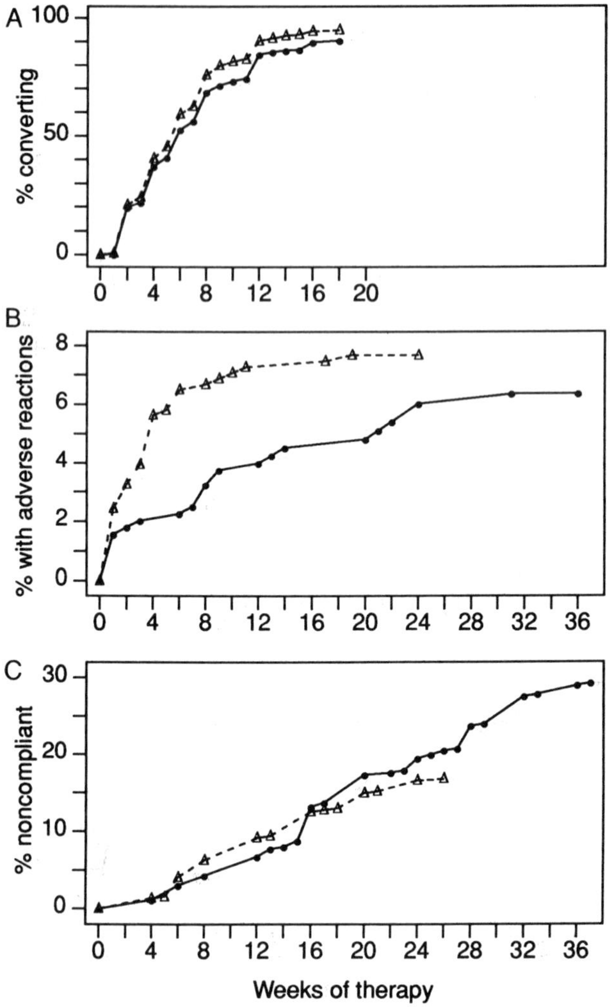

Fig 6–1.—A shows rate of bacteriologic sputum conversion by regimen. Breslow = 4.06; $P = .04$. B shows rate of adverse reactions to regimen. Breslow = 2.68; $P = .10$. C shows rate of noncompliance by regimen. Breslow = 1.06; $P = .30$. Broken lines with triangles represent patients on 6-month regimen and solid lines with circles represent patients on 9-month regimen. (Courtesy of Combs DL, O'Brien RJ, Geiter LJ: *Ann Intern Med* 112:397–406, 1990.)

Previous trials have shown that 6 months of treatment with isoniazid and rifampin are inadequate. The addition of ethambutol has not proved helpful, but the addition of streptomycin and pyrazinamide for the first 2 to 3 months has lowered relapse rates. A nonblinded but randomized trial was conducted at 22 tuberculosis clinics to compare a 6-month treatment regimen in 617 patients with a 9-month regimen in 445 others. Characteristics of both groups are shown in the table. Patients self-administered isoniazid and rifampin daily, and those treated for 6 months added pyrazinamide for the first 8 weeks.

Arthralgia was more frequent in the 6-month regimen, but there were

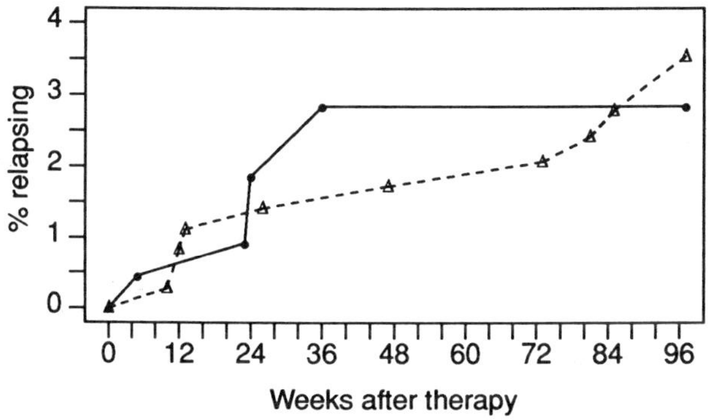

Fig 6–2.—Rates of confirmed relapses, by regimen. Breslow = .03; P = .86. *Dashed lines* with *triangles* represent patients on 6-month regimen and *solid lines* with *circles* represent patients on 9-month regimen. (Courtesy of Combs DL, O'Brien RJ, Geiter LJ: *Ann Intern Med* 112:397–406, 1990.)

no other significant treatment-related differences in clinical side effects. A high level of uric acid was more frequent in the 6-month treatment group. Rates of noncompliance were similar in the 2 regimens (Fig 6–1). Relapse rates also were similar (Fig 6–2). Relapse was less frequent in the 9-month treatment group, but not significantly so. Significantly more patients completed 6-month treatment successfully. Patients who took Rifater, a combination tablet including isoniazid, rifampin, and pyrazinamide, had higher conversion rates than patients who took the same drugs separately, but they also had more frequent adverse reactions. This 6-month antituberculous regimen appears to be as effective as a 9-month course.

▶ Although these 2 studies used somewhat different regimens, which are detailed in the abstract, they both document that 6 months of antituberculous chemotherapy is as good as longer courses of treatment. This is true even in patients who have extrapulmonary disease. It may be that we have finally reached the limit of short-term therapy, because previous studies of 3 months and 5 months of chemotherapy have resulted in unacceptably high relapse rates of 11% to 40% (1).—M.S. Klempner, M.D.

Reference

1. Tuberculosis Research Centre (Madras), National Tuberculosis Institute (Bangalore): *Am Rev Respir Dis* 27:33, 1986.

Tuberculous Meningitis: Short Course of Chemotherapy

Alarcón F, Escalante L, Pérez Y, Banda H, Chacón G, Dueñas G (Eugenio Espejo Hosp, Quito, Ecuador; Natl Inst of Hygiene and Tropical Medicine, Quito)

Arch Neurol 47:1313–1317, 1990 6–3

Tuberculous meningitis is the most common form of infection of the CNS in developing countries such as Ecuador. The clinical and therapeutic efficacy of a short course of chemotherapy was studied in 28 patients

Clinical and Neurologic Manifestations on Admission in 28 Patients With Tuberculous Meningitis

	Diagnostic Categories*		Total No. of	
	Definite	Probable	Cases	Percentage
Neurological signs and symptoms	22	6	28	100
Headache	20	6	26	92.8
Apathy / irritability	7	1	8	28.5
Confusion / stupor	2	4	6	21.4
Stupor	2	0	2	7.1
Coma	10	2	12	42.8
Meningeal irritation	20	6	26	92.8
Cranial nerve palsy	4	2	6	21.4
Gastrointestinal symptoms	15	5	20	71.4
Abdominal pain	12	5	17	60.7
Vomiting	14	1	15	53.5
Weakness / anorexia	14	6	20	71.4
Constipation	14	6	20	71.4
Respiratory symptoms	6	4	10	35.7
Respiratory signs	11	6	17	60.7
Fever	19	6	25	89.2
Weight loss	5	5	10	35.7
Fatigue	5	6	11	39.2

*Diagnostic categories for tuberculous meningitis.
(Courtesy of Alarcón F, Escalante L, Pérez Y, et al: *Arch Neurol* 47:1313–1317, 1990.)

with tuberculous meningitis. All received isoniazid, 10 mg/kg; rifampin, 15 mg/kg; and pyrazinamide, 30 mg/kg, orally each day for 2 months, followed by isoniazid and rifampin for the next 4 months. The follow-up period ranged from 24 to 36 months.

The CSF diagnosis was based on identification of *Mycobacterium tuberculosis* by direct smear in 53.5% of patients and by culture in Lowenstein-Jensen medium in 57%, detection of antibacille Calmette-Guerin antibodies by enzyme-linked immunosorbent assay in 83.3%, and dosification of adenosine deaminase activity in 74%. Moreover, the diagnosis was supported by bacteriologic analyses of other tissue or body fluids. Based on these tests, 78.5% of patients had a definite diagnosis of tuberculous meningitis, and 21.4% had a diagnosis of probable tuberculous meningitis.

Headache and meningeal signs were the most important neurologic manifestations and were also the last to disappear (table). Other important factors were gastrointestinal symptoms and fever. Nine patients (32.1%) died. Mortality was associated with British Research Council stage 3 classification, delayed onset of treatment, prolonged duration (more than 3 weeks) of disease before admission, age older than 40 years, and abnormal CT scan.

Only 3 of the 19 patients who survived for 18 months after completion of therapy had neurologic sequelae. Morbidity and mortality with the short course of therapy were comparable to rates in longer course therapies. Treatment had to be stopped temporarily in 4 patients because of increased levels of hepatic enzymes.

These data suggest that a 6-month course of antituberculous therapy is a good and acceptable therapeutic option for tuberculous meningitis. The findings also suggest that early diagnosis and prompt treatment with antituberculous drugs are more important than the regimen of drugs applied or the duration of therapy.

▶ I was struck by the severity of illness in the patients with tuberculous meningitis in this series. As shown in the table, almost 50% of the patients were either stuporous or comatose. This is in contrast to my perception of a more chronic presentation of tuberculous meningitis in the United States. Nevertheless, this 3-drug, 6-month course of therapy seemed to be as effective as previous reports of longer term therapy. Moreover, the relative infrequency (16%) of long-term neurologic sequelae is encouraging. It's also worth noting that steroids were given to all patients with impairment of consciousness at presentation, focal neurologic abnormalities, or evidence of increased intracranial pressure.—M.S. Klempner, M.D.

Pulmonary and Disseminated Infection Due to *Mycobacterium kansasii:* A Decade of Experience

Lillo M, Orengo S, Cernoch P, Harris RL (Methodist Hosp, Houston; Baylor College of Medicine, Houston)
Rev Infect Dis 12:760–767, 1990 6–4

Because the nontuberculous mycobacteria can be true pathogens or contaminants, their clinical significance is difficult to determine. Of the nontuberculous mycobacteria, *Mycobacterium kansasii* is clinically and antigenically most closely related to *M. tuberculosis*. *Mycobacterium kansasii* is an unlikely contaminant because it is difficult to isolate from the environment, and its pulmonary isolation usually represents disease in previously damaged lungs.

TABLE 1.—Clinical Significance of *Mycobacterium kansasii* Pulmonary Isolates

Classification	No. of patients	Percentage of total
Disease	30	63.8
Probable disease	6	12.8
Possible disease	8	17.0
Contamination/colonization	3	6.4
Total	47	100.0

(Courtesy of Lillo M, Orengo S, Cernoch P, et al: *Rev Infect Dis* 12:760–767, 1990.)

TABLE 2.—Clinical Profiles of Patients With Disseminated *Mycobacterium kansasii* Infection

Patient no.	Age (y)/ sex/race	Underlying diseases/ immunosuppressive therapy	Pulmonary exposure(s)	Site(s) of isolation
1	30/F/W	Renal transplant, postsplenectomy, cyclophosphamide, prednisone	Smoking	Joint
2	47/M/H	Metastatic clear cell cancer, silicosis, diabetes, alcohol abuse, prednisone	Smoking, welding, sandblasting	Lung, lymph node
3	48/M/W	Well-differentiated lymphoma, neutropenia	Smoking	Bone marrow
4	54/M/W	Hairy cell leukemia, cyclophosphamide, vincristine, prednisone	None	Lung, pleura, lymph node
5	40/M/W	AML in remission, alcohol abuse, cytarabine, thioguanine	Smoking	Bone marrow
6	64/M/W	CML, diabetes, prednisone	Smoking	Lung, skin, bone
7	72/F/W	Breast cancer, alcohol abuse	Smoking	Spleen
8	65/M/W	Vasculitis, renal failure, prednisone	Welding	Bone marrow, spleen, skin

Abbreviations: W, white; *H,* hispanic; *AML,* acute myelogenous leukemia; *CML,* chronic myelogenous leukemia.
(Courtesy of Lillo M, Orengo S, Cernoch P, et al: *Rev Infect Dis* 12:760–767, 1990.)

During a 10-year period *M. kansasii* was isolated from 55 patients (mean age, 60 years); 47 patients had pulmonary infection (Table 1) and 8 had disseminated infection (Table 2). Most patients with pulmonary *M. kansasii* infection had underlying pulmonary disease, which was often as-

TABLE 3.—In Vitro Drug Susceptibility of *Mycobacterium kansasii* Isolates From Patients With Pulmonary or Disseminated Disease

Rank	Antibiotic	Concentration (μg/mL)	Percentage susceptible
1	Rifampin	1.0	72
		5.0	90
2	Streptomycin	2.0	34
		10.0	77
3	Ethionamide	2.5	35
		5.0	65
4	Ethambutol	5.0	36
		10.0	58
5	Isoniazid	0.2	8
		1.0	47
6	*p*-Aminosalicylic acid	2.0	11
		10.0	36
7	Cycloserine	10.0	23
		20.0	36

(Courtesy of Lillo M, Orengo S, Cernoch P, et al: *Rev Infect Dis* 12:760–767, 1990.)

sociated with a history of smoking. Seventy percent of the patients had nonpulmonary comorbid illnesses.

Clinical and radiographic pulmonary findings (e.g., cough and production of sputum) resembled those of pulmonary tuberculosis. Some patients also had hemoptysis, chest pain, fever, and weight loss. All 8 patients with disseminated infection were severely immunocompromised and often had pulmonary predispositions as well. Findings in these patients included infiltrates, hilar adenopathy, and mass lesions, but cavitation and pleural scarring were uncommon.

Culture of expectorated sputum from patients with pulmonary disease had a 75% yield of the organism, and acid-fast bacillus smear, 25%. Bronchoscopy, performed in 26 patients, had a 76.9% yield by culture. In patients with disseminated disease *M. kansasii* was isolated from biopsy specimens. Some of these patients also had positive sputum cultures.

Although antituberculous drugs are less active in vitro against *M. kansasii* than against *M. tuberculosis,* most patients responded to a regimen containing rifampin (Table 3). No deaths were directly related to *M. kansasii* pulmonary disease; instead, patients died of their underlying diseases.

▶ A thorough review of an infection that is uncommon in most parts of the United States. Nationwide, *M. kansasii* accounts for about 3% of isolates of pathogenic mycobacteria. The authors point out that the geographic distribution is like an inverted T, extending from Florida to California and from Texas up to Illinois.—M.J. Barza, M.D.

The Pathogenicity of *Mycobacterium tuberculosis* During Chemotherapy

Clancy LJ, Kelly P, O'Reilly L, Byrne C, Costello E (Peamount Hosp, Dublin; Veterinary Research Lab, Dublin)

Eur Respir J 3:399–402, 1990 6–5

The most common method of transmitting tuberculosis is the inhalation of aerosolized sputum from a patient with pulmonary tuberculosis. Two weeks after the start of chemotherapy patients are considered to be noninfectious to others, even though sputum may remain positive on smear and culture. It has been suggested that antituberculous chemotherapy brings about a change in pathogenicity. This hypothesis was tested in a guinea pig model.

Twenty-nine sputum samples from 21 patients receiving triple therapy were prepared for subcutaneous injection into the animals' thighs. After 8 weeks the guinea pigs were killed and autopsies were performed. The presence and extent of tuberculosis was classified and the lesions were analyzed in relation to 3 parameters: duration of chemotherapy, direct smear positivity, and culture positivity.

There was a relationship between the duration of treatment and the absence of tuberculous lesions in inoculated guinea pigs, but the ability of the sputum to produce lesions was also associated with the degree of positivity of the sputum. Multiple regression analysis showed that the correlation between severity of the guinea pig lesions was strongest with culture positivity.

Although it is difficult to extrapolate from guinea pig models to man, it does appear that patients who continue to cough and remain sputum positive, particularly culture positive, produce pathogenic bacilli. Modern chemotherapy reduces cough and rapidly and dramatically reduces the number of bacilli in the sputum of patients with tuberculosis, but there is a risk that immunocompromised individuals may be infected. Thus the belief that a change in pathogenicity occurs during treatment is not supported.

▶ The reason that medicine is a science as well as an art is nicely illustrated here. It is a common belief that effective chemotherapy regimens for *Mycobacterium tuberculosis* quickly renders the organism avirulent, and that even if the organism is seen in sputum in the treated patient, it is of no great concern. This study suggests that this is not the case; rather, it is the number of organisms in sputum and their viability that are most relevant to transmission potential (at least to guinea pigs). Because viability is more difficult to monitor, needing culture methods that are relatively slow to yield information, the clinician (and the hospital epidemiologist) may have to depend on the classic method of AFB staining of sputum and microscopy to determine the risk each patient poses. Perhaps the polymerase chain reaction or another method will come along to detect bacillary load in a more quantitative manner, but until then we must rely on "old time" standard signs to evaluate the risk of a patient transmitting infection (coughing, open cavities, and AFB smears) rather than an arbitrary duration of chemotherapy.—G.T. Keusch, M.D.

Smear-Negative, Culture-Positive Pulmonary Tuberculosis: Six-Month Chemotherapy With Isoniazid and Rifampin

Dutt AK, Moers D, Stead WW (Arkansas Dept of Health, Little Rock)

Am Rev Respir Dis 141:1232–1235, 1990 6–6

Sputum-smear-positive pulmonary tuberculosis is controlled with a 9-month chemotherapy regimen of isoniazid (INH) and rifampin (RIF) in 95% of cases, even in patients with many *Mycobacterium tuberculosis* bacilli in their smears. Because it seemed likely that a shorter treatment regimen would suffice in patients with less severe disease, the treatment period for patients meeting certain eligibility criteria was reduced to 6 months. Patients with at least 1 positive sputum culture for *M. tuberculosis* but no organisms in at least 3 sputum smears are started on 300 mg of INH and 600 mg of RIF daily for 1 month, followed by 900 mg of INH and 600 mg of RIF twice weekly for another 5 months. The shortened regimen has been in use for 9 years.

To date, 286 patients, aged 18–99 years, with an average age of 68.2 years, have been treated with the shortened treatment regimen. Three fourths of these patients were older than age 60 years. Sixty-eight patients (24%) had associated medical conditions as risk factors (e.g. present or past malignancies, alcoholism, and diabetes mellitus). Patients were examined every month for the first year and every 3 months for the second year. The total follow-up period was 18 months.

Twenty-one patients died during the 6-month treatment period from nontuberculous causes. Eight patients moved to another state, and 4 patients were lost to follow-up. Drug side effects required a change in treatment for 33 patients (11.5%). However, only 8 (2.8%) patients had life-threatening side effects. The other 25 patients had minor side effects caused by drug intolerance. Four patients had to have a change in drug treatment because of drug resistance to INH. There was only 1 treatment failure. A total of 211 patients completed the full 6-month protocol.

During a follow-up period of 3–107 months, 5 patients (2.4%) relapsed bacteriologically 3–73 months after completion of drug therapy

Follow-Up of 211 Patients After Completion of Therapy

Follow-up (*months*)	Patients (*n*)	Relapse (*n*)	Relapse (*months*)	Non-TB Deaths	Moved	Remaining Disease-free
1–12	38	1	3	17	5	15
13–24	50	—		14	1	35
25–36	25	1	29	—	—	24
37–48	31	1	37	3	—	27
49–60	31	1	60	—	—	30
61–72	14	—		—	—	14
73–107	22	1	73	—	—	21
Total	211	5 (2.4%)		34	6	166

(Courtesy of Dutt AK, Moers D, Stead WW: *Am Rev Respir Dis* 141:1232–1235, 1990.)

(table). All relapses were associated with drug-susceptible organisms, and patients were retreated with the same drugs for a full 9-month course. Thirty-four patients died during follow-up of nontuberculous causes. The remaining 166 patients were followed for the full 18 months. The overall success rate of the 6-month treatment regimen was 97%. Thus, a 6-month regimen of INH/RIF appears to be adequate for most cases of smear-negative, culture-positive pulmonary tuberculosis.

▶ It makes sense that a highly effective bactericidal regimen would be effective in a shorter duration for individuals with evidence of low level (paucibacillary) *M. tuberculosis* infection, and the authors have shown this. It is a bit disconcerting that in almost 12% the regimen had to be changed because of side effects, albeit only 2.8% had severe complications. Of the 42 patients (15%) not completing therapy for some reason, only 4 had documented resistance to isoniazid requiring the addition of other drugs. In only 1 of 211 patients with sensitive organisms did therapy fail, using a most conservative criterion of failure (positive smear in the fifth month), and this probably resulted from noncompliance. In addition, there were only 5 (2.4%) bacteriologic relapses, requiring a second 9-month course of the same drugs. However, in the decade since this study was initiated, HIV has come upon the scene. This means that now all patients with proven (or highly suspicious) tuberculosis should be asked to submit to HIV testing. If findings are positive, the question will no longer be whether or not a short course may be given but, rather, what will be the most effective way of providing needed maintenance chemotherapy following the standard course of treatment.—G.T. Keusch, M.D.

7 Infections in the Compromised Host

Trimethoprim-Sulfamethoxazole Prophylaxis in the Management of Chronic Granulomatous Disease

Margolis DM, Melnick DA, Alling DW, Gallin JI (Natl Inst of Allergy and Infectious Diseases, Bethesda, Md)

J Infect Dis 162:723–726, 1990 7–1

Chronic granulomatous disease (CGD) is a rare disorder of leukocyte function. Since the 1970s, long-term prophylactic trimethoprim-sulfamethoxazole (TMP-SMX) therapy has been widely used in patients with CGD to reduce the incidence of life-threatening episodes. However, some studies in cancer patients have reported that the daily use of TMP-SMX is associated with an increased incidence of severe systemic fungal infections.

A comparison was made of the rate of fungal and nonfungal infections in 36 treated and untreated patients with CGD who had at least 1 year of follow-up. Twenty patients had autosomal disease and 16 had X-linked disease. A direct comparison of infection rates was possible in 4 patients with X-linked disease and 7 with autosomal disease. The remaining 25 patients were followed unpaired (table). Most patients had begun prophylactic TMP-SMX treatment in the early 1980s.

Prophylaxis with TMP-SMX decreased the rate of nonfungal infection from 7.1 to 2.4/100 patient-months for patients with autosomal CGD and from 15.8 to 6.9/100 patients-months for those with X-linked disease. There was no significant difference in the incidence of fungal infection with or without TMP-SMX prophylaxis for patients with either X-linked or autosomal CGD. The incidence of fungal infection with TMP-SMX decreased from 1.5 to .3/100 patient-months for paired patients with autosomal disease and from 2.8 to .4/100 patient-months for the unpaired autosomal group. For those with X-linked disease, incidences of fungal infection with and without prophylaxis were 1.7 and .2 fungal infections per 100 patient-months, respectively. These findings confirm that the use of TMP-SMX prophylaxis decreases the incidence of nonfungal infections in patients with CGD without increasing the rate of fungal infections.

▶ It has been standard practice for more than 15 years to give patients with CGD prophylactic TMP-SMX to try to prevent the severe recurrent bacterial in-

Infectious Episodes of Chronic Granulomatous Disease With and Without Trimethoprim-Sulfamethoxazole (TMP-SMX) Prophylaxis

						No. of infections					
			Months at risk			Nonfungal			Fungal		
Data, type of inheritance	No. of patients	TMP-SMX	Total	Mean*	Range	Total	Mean*	Range	Total	Mean*	Range
Paired†											
X-linked	4	On	270	34.6	2–148	34	3.0	1–31	3	0.4	0–3
	4	Off	38	7.7	2–16	5	1.2	1–2	3	0.4	0–3
Autosomal	7	On	382	52.7	28–72	8	0.9	0–3	1	0.1	0–1
	7	Off	261	20.3	1–141	17	1.8	1–9	3	0.3	0–1
Unpaired†											
X-linked	12	On	831	47.3	3–216	33	1.9	0–7	3	0.2	0–1
Autosomal	11	On	668	56.0	29–180	28	1.6	0–12	3	0.2	0–2
	2	Off	71	24.4	15–34	5	1.5	1–3	2	0.4	0–2
Total	36										

*Geometric mean.
†Paired data are for patients followed both with and without antibiotic prophylaxis; unpaired data are for patients followed only with or without antibiotic prophylaxis.
(Courtesy of Margolis DM, Melnick DA, Alling DW, et al: *J Infect Dis* 162:723–726, 1990.)

fections that plague these patients. Several retrospective studies have confirmed the utility of this approach. The large experience at the NIH with these patients adds further confirmation and reassures us that the incidence of fungal infections does not increase in these patients as a result of TMP-SMX prophylaxis.—M.S. Klempner, M.D.

Gram-Positive Bacteraemia in Granulocytopenic Cancer Patients

EORTC International Antimicrobial Therapy Cooperative Group (Univ of Genova, Italy)

Eur J Cancer 26:569–574, 1990 7–2

In the 4 EORTC International Antimicrobial Therapy Cooperative Group trials, the frequency of gram-positive isolates increased significantly from 29% of single-organism bacteremia in trial I (1973–1976) to 41% in trial IV (1983–1985) (Table 1). In trial IV, 90 febrile, neutropenic patients with cancer were randomized prospectively to receive either azlocillin plus a long course (9 or more days) of amikacin, or ceftazidime plus a short course (3 days) of amikacin, or ceftazidime plus a long course of amikacin (Table 2). Without modification of the allocated antibiotics, the overall response rates of gram-positive bacteremias were similar in all 3 groups. However, azlocillin plus amikacin was significantly more effective than ceftazidime plus 3 days of amikacin therapy in patients with prolonged and severe neutropenia. The overall response rate for these infections was significantly lower than that seen in trial I, but this was not associated with higher mortality. Treatment response was significantly influenced by susceptibility of the infecting strain to the β-lactam. Multivariate analysis demonstrated that increasing age, presence of a central venous catheter, and resistance to β-lactam adversely affected

TABLE 1.—Gram-Positive Bacteria Causing Septicemias in Trials II, III, and IV

Microorganism	Trial II	Trial III	Trial IV
Staph. aureus	10 (27%)	14 (25%)	25 (28%)
Staph. epidermidis	9 (24%)	24 (41%)	18 (20%)
Other gram-positive bacteria	18 (49%)	20 (34%)	47 (52%)
Total	37 (100%)	58 (100%)	90 (100%)

Note: Overall $P = .07$.

(Courtesy of EORTC International Antimicrobial Thereapy Cooperative Group: *Eur J Cancer* 26:569–574, 1990.)

TABLE 2.—Trial IV: Characteristics of Patients*

	Azlocillin plus amikacin	Ceftazidime plus amikacin (3 days)	Ceftazidime plus amikacin (long)
No. of patients	37	23	30
Age (yr)			
Median (range)	28 (2–79)	42 (3–76)	38 (1–69)
Mean	35	40	34
M/F	23/14	12/11	12/18
Underlying diseases:			
Leukaemia	21 (57%)	11 (47%)	19 (63%)
Lymphoma	3 (8%)	2 (9%)	5 (17%)
Solid tumour	2 (5%)	2 (9%)	4 (13%)
Others	11 (30%)	8 (35%)	2 (7%)
Patients at randomization with:			
Granulocytes < 100/μl	22 (59%)	13 (57%)	16 (53%)
Shock	0	1	2
Central catheter	16 (43%)	11 (48%)	9 (30%)

*No significant differences between groups.
(Courtesy of EORTC International Antimicrobial Therapy Cooperative Group: *Eur J Cancer* 26:569–574, 1990.)

outcome. Future research should aim at improving the outcome of gram-positive bacteremia in neutropenic patients.

β-Lactam Regimens for the Febrile Neutropenic Patient

Bodey GP, Fainstein V, Elting LS, Anaissie E, Rolston K, Khardori N, Kantarjian H, Plager C, Murphy WK, Holmes F, Cabanillas F (Univ of Texas, Houston)
Cancer 65:9–16, 1990 7–3

The ideal antibiotic regimen in the initial management of fever in neutropenic patients remains to be established. In a prospective, randomized study 535 evaluable febrile episodes in 456 cancer patients with neutropenia were treated with ticarcillin-clavulanate plus vancomycin (TV), ceftazidime plus vancomycin (CV), or all 3 antibiotics (TCV). Treatment was continued for a minimum of 7 days, or for 4 days after resolution of all signs and symptoms of infection.

The TCV regimen was significantly more effective than TV, considering all evaluable episodes (Table 1), documented infections, septicemias (particularly those caused by gram-negative organisms) (Tables 2 and 3), gram-negative infections (Table 4), infections in patients with persistent

TABLE 1.—Overall Results of Therapy

Type of episode	TV		CV		TCV		
	Episodes	Percent cure	Episodes	Percent cure	Episodes	Percent cure	*P* value*
Evaluable episodes	205	70	107	77	223	81	0.01
Fever of unknown origin	99	78	54	80	121	83	NS
Documented infection	106	63	53	74	102	78	0.02
Organism identified	74	68	30	83	59	92	0.003
Organism not identified	32	50	23	65	43	60	NS

**P* values represent comparisons between TV and TCV; all other comparisons were not significant.
(Courtesy of Bodey GP, Fainstein V, Elting LS, et al: *Cancer* 65:9–16, 1990.)

severe neutropenia (<100 neutrophils/mm^3) (Table 5), and in patients whose neutrophil count decreased during therapy. The efficacy of the CVregimen was intermediate between TV and TCV, but the differences between CV and TCV were not significant. Side effects to the antibiotic regimen, most commonly skin rashes, were infrequent and occurred with similar frequency in all 3 regimens (Table 6). The combination of TCV is

TABLE 2.—Results of Therapy by Site of Infection

	TV		CV		TCV	
Site	Episodes	Percent cure	Episodes	Percent cure	Episodes	Percent cure
Septicemia	38	58	17	76	29	86
Pneumonia	16	38	14	50	27	59
Urinary tract	16	100	6	100	11	100
Skin/soft tissue	17	82	6	67	22	91
Head and neck	16	50	8	88	11	64
Other	3	33	2	100	2	50
Total	106	63	53	74	102	78

(Courtesy of Bodey GP, Fainstein V, Elting LS, et al: *Cancer* 65:9–16, 1990.)

an effective regimen for febrile neutropenic patients and should be preferred to CV or TV.

▶ I chose the article reviewed in Abstract 7–2 mostly because it concerns sepsis with gram-positive organisms in all 4 of the previous EORTC studies of granulocytopenic cancer patients. These studies, which span almost 20 years, provide an important perspective on antibiotic use in immunocompromised patients. It is clear that gram-positive organisms account for an increasing number of episodes of sepsis. It is also clear that mortality caused by gram-positive bacteremia in these patients is relatively low (4%) compared to the mortality associated with gram-negative bacteremia (12%). Several more recent studies using empiric specific anti-gram-positive therapy (e.g., vancomycin or teicoplanin) have been reported (1), and most have found favorable results. These include an improved overall response rate, more rapid resolution of fever, reduction in the use of amphotericin B, and reduction in subsequent infections.

Although the authors of this report cite the low mortality of gram-positive bacteremia as a reason to document it before beginning specific anti-gram-positive therapy, I do not subscribe to this approach. I believe the pendulum has swung more in favor of incorporating specific anti-gram-positive therapy at the

TABLE 3.—Response in Gram-Negative Septicemias

	TV		CV		TCV	
Organism	Episodes	Cures	Episodes	Cures	Episodes	Cures
Escherichia coli	7	3	2	2	2	2
Klebsiella sp	5	2	3	1	2	2
Pseudomonas aeruginosa	1	1	2	2	2	1
Pseudomonas sp	2	1	0	—	1	1
Enterobacter sp	2	0	1	0	0	—
Serratia sp	2	2	0	—	0	—
Aeromonas sp	1	0	1	1	0	—
Citrobacter sp	1	0	0	—	1	0
CDC group V E2	1	1	0	—	0	—
Total	22	10 (45%)	9	6 (67%)	8	6 (75%)

Abbreviation: CDC, Centers for Disease Control.
(Courtesy of Bodey GP, Fainstein V, Elting LS, et al: *Cancer* 65:9–16, 1990.)

TABLE 4.—Response to Therapy According to Infecting Organism

	TV		CV		TCV	
Organism	Episodes	Cures	Episodes	Cures	Episodes	Cures
Gram-positive	21	20 (95%)	10	10 (100%)	32	31 (97%)
Staphylococcus aureus	9	9	3	3	10	9
Staphylococcus epidermidis	5	4	3	3	8	8
Other	7	7	4	4	14	14
Gram-negative	43	26 (60)	14	9 (64)	20	18 (90)
Escherichia coli	19	13	4	4	6	6
Klebsiella sp	8	4	3	1	3	3
Pseudomonas aeruginosa	5	4	5	3	6	5
Enterobacter sp	4	1	1	0	0	—
Other	7	4	1	1	5	4
Anaerobes	1	0	0	—	1	1
Polymicrobial	8	4	6	5	6	4

(Courtesy of Bodey GP, Fainstein V, Elting LS, et al: *Cancer* 65:9–16, 1990.)

TABLE 5.—Response Related to Neutrophil Count in Documented Infections

Initial neutrophil count/μl	Trend	TV Episodes	TV Percent cures	CV Episodes	CV Percent cures	TCV Episodes	TCV Percent cures	*P* value*
<100	Total	68	56	29	76	59	80	0.008
	Unchanged	33	33	11	55	23	74	0.003
	Increased	35	77	18	89	36	84	NS
101–1000	Total	25	72	17	71	30	77	NS
>1000	Total	13	85	7	71	13	77	NS
Total	Decreased	51	45	25	56*	47	77†	0.003
	Increased	55	80	28	89	55	80	

* *P* values represent comparisons between TV and TCV.
†Comparison of CV versus TCV, *P* = .10.
(Courtesy of Bodey GP, Fainstein V, Elting LS: *Cancer* 65:9–16, 1990.)

TABLE 6.—Toxicities Associated With Antibiotic Therapy

	TV	CV	TCV
Rash	2.9	4.2	3.4
Red neck syndrome	0.4	0	2.5
Clostridium difficile colitis	0.4	0.8	0.4
Diarrhea	0	0	1.2
Renal abnormalities	0.4	0	0
Bronchospasm	0	0.8	0

Note: Expressed as percent of total episodes.
(Courtesy of Bodey GP, Fainstein V, Elting LS, et al: *Cancer* 65:9–16, 1990.)

time of initial fever in these patients. The paper by Bodey et al. (Abstract 7–3) supports this approach and goes one step further by demonstrating that the double β-lactam regimen (timentin and ceftazidime) plus vancomycin was the preferred antibiotic treatment.— M.S. Klempner, M.D.

Reference

1. Shenep JL, et al: *N Engl J Med* 319:1053, 1988.

Increased Risk of Pneumococcal Infections in Cardiac Transplant Recipients

Amber IJ, Gilbert EM, Schiffman G, Jacobson JA (Univ of Utah; VA Med Ctr, Salt Lake City; LDS Hosp, Salt Lake City; State Univ of New York Health Sciences Ctr, Brooklyn)

Transplantation 49:122–125, 1990 7–4

A preliminary observation of the increased incidence of pneumococcal infection in heart transplant recipients prompted a prospective surveillance and retrospective chart review to determine whether cardiac transplant patients are at increased risk of pneumococcal infection. Of the 129 patients who received cardiac transplants between March 1985 and December 1987, pneumococcal infection developed in 5, for an estimated incidence of 36 cases per 1,000 patient-years. All 5 patients were male (mean age, 44 years), and none had previous pneumococcal vaccination.

Pneumococcal infections occurred within a mean of 58 days after transplantation. Pneumococcal pneumonia developed in 3 patients, bacteremia with empyema in 1, and bacteremia alone in 1. All 5 patients had an adequate number of neutrophils, but both patients with bacteremia had extremely low lymphocyte counts at the time of infection. The occurrence of pneumococcal infection did not correlate with age, sex, immunosuppression, or rejection episodes. All 5 patients recovered from their infection.

Serum antibody levels to 12 pneumococcal antigens were measured in 6 unvaccinated uninfected patients before and after cardiac transplantation (table). Protective levels of antibody, defined as at least 300 ng of

Geometric Mean Antibody Concentrations to 12 Pneumococcal Antigens in 6 Unvaccinated Cardiac Transplant Patients[a]

Serotype	Pretransplant	Posttransplant
1	868	82[b]
3	231	64[b]
4	269	29[b]
6A	413	219[b]
7F	459	146[b]
8	1029	421[b]
9N	156	46[b]
12F	1459	997
14	461	225
18C	946	272[b]
19F	370	109
23F	1048	252[b]

[a]Expressed as nanogram of antibody nitrogen per milliliter serum (Schiffman G, et al: *J Immunol Methods* 33:133, 1980.)

[b]$P < .05$.

(Courtesy of Amber IJ, Gilbert EM, Schiffman G, et al: Transplantation 49:122–125, 1990.)

anticapsular antibody nitrogen per mL of serum, were 8.7 pneumococcal serotypes before transplantation and 6.5 afterward. Pneumococcal pneumonia subsequently developed in 1 of these 6 patients.

Cardiac transplant patients are at increased risk of serious pneumococcal infections. Vaccinating transplant candidates before transplantation may provide protection against pneumococcal infection after transplantation.

▶ As cardiac transplantation is more widely used for the treatment of end-stage congestive heart failure, many infectious disease specialists are becoming involved in developing protocols for the prevention and treatment of infectious complications. In addition to cytomegalovirus, a predisposition toward infections with *Legionella, Aspergillus, Candida, Nocardia, Cryptococcus,* and *Toxoplasma gondii* have been well recognized. Unfortunately, none of these can be prevented. This is a small study but it demonstrates a 7- to 30-fold increase in the risk of pneumococcal infections in cardiac transplant patients compared to the general population. Because protective antibody titers declined after transplantation, the authors suggest that pretransplant vaccination with the polyvalent pneumococcal vaccine might be worth while. Pneumococcal vaccination has such a low incidence of complications that this seems a reasonable recommendation for all cardiac transplant recipients.—M.S. Klempner, M.D.

Opportunistic Viral Hepatitis in Liver Transplant Recipients

Markin RS, Langnas AN, Donovan JP, Zetterman RK, Stratta RJ (Univ of Nebraska)

Transplant Proc 23:1520–1521, 1991 7–5

Opportunistic viral hepatitis that involves the hepatic allograft after orthotopic liver transplant is a major source of morbidity. The incidence of opportunistic viral hepatitis was determined in liver transplant recipients. The factors important in diagnosing opportunistic viral hepatitis in these patients, effective prophylactic treatment, and the immunosuppressive regimens conducive to the development of opportunistic viral hepatitis were also investigated.

In all, 402 liver transplants were performed in 348 patients between 1985 and 1990. Thirty-two patients died within 1 month of transplantation. None had opportunistic viral hepatitis. Seventy-two opportunistic viral infections that arose in the allograft were documented by biopsy or culture in 62 patients, for an incidence of 19.6%. There were 51 cytomegalovirus, 6 Epstein-Barr virus, 2 herpes simplex virus, 1 herpes zoster, and 2 adenovirus infections. Sixty-seven infections occurred in the first 3 months after orthotopic liver transplantation. The mean duration of infection was 47 days (range, 4–300 days).

Cytomegalovirus hepatitis is the most frequent viral pathogen to infect the liver allograft. Its incidence is believed to be related to the endemic nature of the virus. Less common causes of opportunistic viral infection include Epstein-Barr virus, herpes simplex virus, and adenovirus. The incidence of opportunistic viral hepatitis after transplantation varies with the type of infection and the patient's clinical condition.

▶ This large study of opportunistic viral hepatitis following liver transplantation makes several important points. The overall incidence of opportunistic viral hepatitis was 19.6%. Infections with cytomegalovirus (51), herpes simplex virus, herpes zoster, and adenovirus were all diagnosed by culture, and the 6 cases of Epstein-Barr virus hepatitis were diagnosed serologically. There were 72 opportunistic viral infections. A single course of gancyclovir was effective treatment in 43 of the 51 patients with cytomegalovirus infection; 4 of the 8 patients who were retreated also responded. This is a higher than anticipated response rate and encourages us to be aggressive in attempts to make an early virologic diagnosis in liver transplant patients suspected of having superimposed opportunistic viral hepatitis.—M.S. Klempner, M.D.

Immunomodulatory and Antimicrobial Efficacy of Intravenous Immunoglobulin in Bone Marrow Transplantation

Sullivan KM, Kopecky KJ, Jocom J, Fisher L, Buckner CD, Meyers JD, Counts GW, Bowden RA, Petersen FB, Witherspoon RP, Budinger MD, Schwartz RS, Appelbaum FR, Clift RA, Hansen JA, Sanders JE, Thomas ED, Storb R (Fred Hutchinson Cancer Research Ctr, Seattle; Univ of Washington; Miles Inc, Berkeley, Calif)

N Engl J Med 323:705–712, 1990 7–6

Two major complications of allogeneic bone marrow transplantation are graft-vs.-host disease (GVHD) and infection. Treatment with intravenous immunoglobulin is beneficial in several immunodeficiency and autoimmune disorders. Its antimicrobial and immunomodulatory roles after

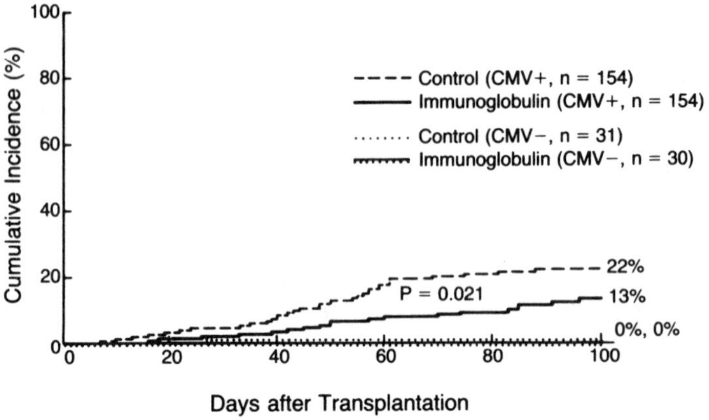

Fig 7–1.—Cumulative incidence of interstitial pneumonia in immunoglobulin and control groups according to serologic status for cytomegalovirus (CMV) before transplantation. Difference between seronegative and seropositive patients was significant, as was difference between seropositive controls and seropositive immunoglobulin recipients. (Courtesy of Sullivan KM, Kopecky KJ, Jocom J, et al: *N Engl J Med* 323:705–712, 1990.)

marrow transplantation were studied in 382 patients who were enrolled in a randomized, controlled trial. Transplant recipients who received immunoglobulin were compared with control subjects who did not.

Control patients who were seronegative for cytomegalovirus and received seronegative blood products remained uninfected. Interstitial pneumonia did not develop in any of the 61 evaluable seronegative patients who received screened blood. However, among the 308 seropositive patients evaluated, interstitial pneumonia developed in 22% of controls and 13% of immunoglobulin recipients (Fig 7–1). Control patients had an increased risk of gram-negative septicemia and local infection and received 51 more units of platelets than did the immunoglobulin recipients. Data on infections are summarized in the table.

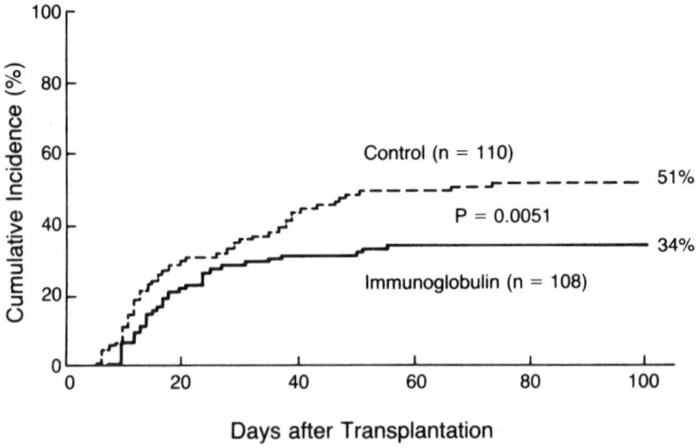

Fig 7–2.—Cumulative incidence of acute GVHD grades II through IV in patients aged 20 years or older. (Courtesy of Sullivan KM, Kopecky KJ, Jocom J, et al: *N Engl J Med* 323:705–712, 1990.)

Posttransplantation Infections in Study Groups

Infection	Control Group		Immunoglobulin Group		Relative Risk* (P Value†)
	No. of Infections	Rate per 100 Patient-Days	No. of Infections	Rate per 100 Patient-Days	
Patient-days at risk	13,878		13,415		
Septicemia					
Gram positive	19	0.14	14	0.10	1.69 (NS)
Gram negative	33	0.24	11	0.08	2.65 (0.0039)
Fungal	16	0.12	13	0.10	1.32 (NS)
Other	0	—	1	—	—
Any organism	68	0.49	39	0.29	2.15 (0.0022)
Bacteremia					
Gram positive	122	0.88	121	0.90	0.98 (NS)
Gram negative	38	0.27	41	0.31	0.88 (NS)
Fungal	13	0.09	16	0.12	0.83 (NS)
Any organism	173	1.25	178	1.33	0.97 (NS)
Local infection					
Gram positive	27	0.19	18	0.13	1.32 (NS)
Gram negative	12	0.09	9	0.07	0.96 (NS)
Fungal	22	0.16	10	0.07	1.82 (NS)
Viral	43	0.31	33	0.25	1.36 (NS)
Other	3	—	2	—	—
Clinical only	37	0.27	22	0.16	1.46 (NS)
Any organism	144	1.04	94	0.70	1.36 (0.029)

Abbreviation: NS, not significant.
Note: Infection occurring from day 0 through day 100 or until discharge home.
*Expressed as ratio of value for controls to value for immunoglobulin recipients, determined by proportional hazards regression analysis testing for greater relative risk (greater than 1) of infection among controls after adjustment for age, status for cytomegalovirus, use or nonuse of laminar-airflow isolation, and type of transplant.
†By 2-sided significance tests.
(Courtesy of Sullivan KM, Kopecky KJ, Jocom J, et al: *N Engl J Med* 323:705–712, 1990.)

Immunoglobulin did not change survival or the risk of relapse. Patients aged 20 years and older, however, had a reduction in the incidence of acute GVHD and of death from transplant-related causes after transplantation of HLA-identical marrow. When compared to immunoglobulin recipients, the incidence of GVHD was significantly increased in control subjects aged 20 years or older (Fig 7–2).

Passive immunotherapy with intravenous immunoglobulin can reduce the risk of acute GVHD after bone marrow transplantation. Associated interstitial pneumonia and infections after transplantation also appear to be decreased by such treatment.

▶ This is the second study that demonstrates a reduction in GVHD in bone marrow transplant patients who are given prophylactic immunoglobulin therapy—strong evidence that immune globulin has an immunomodulatory effect (1). In addition, a decrease in interstitial pneumonia was also demonstrated, although cytomegalovirus pneumonia itself could not be shown to be significantly decreased in globulin-treated patients. This may have been the result of the low rate of cytomegalovirus pneumonia. Rates of bacterial sepsis also were decreased in globulin recipients; however, the definition of "sepsis" included bacteremia with either hypotension or local infection with the same organism in the bloodstream.

The use of prophylactic immunoglobulin has been associated with a number of beneficial effects in marrow transplantation. However, because of the enormous dose required and lack of effect on overall survival, the cost effectiveness of this approach requires evaluation.—David R. Snydman, M.D.

Reference

1. 1988 Year Book of Infectious Diseases, pp 91–92.

Increased Incidence of Lymphoproliferative Disorder After Immunosuppression With the Monoclonal Antibody OKT3 in Cardiac-Transplant Recipients

Swinnen LJ, Costanzo-Nordin MR, Fisher SG, O'Sullivan EJ, Johnson MR, Heroux AL, Dizikes GJ, Pifarre R, Fisher RI (Loyola Univ, Maywood, Ill; Hines VA Hosp, Hines, Ill)

N Engl J Med 323:1723–1728, 1990 7–7

A sharp increase in the incidence of posttransplantation lymphoproliferative disorder was noted in heart transplantation patients in association with use of the monoclonal antibody OKT3. Data on 154 patients who underwent heart transplantation in a 6-year period were reviewed to identify factors that predict the development of this disorder. Of the patients, 79 received OKT3 prophylactically or for treatment of rejection, and 86 received prophylaxis with antithymocyte globulin. All patients received methylprednisolone, azathioprine, prednisone, and cyclosporine.

Characteristics of Patients With Posttransplantation Lymphoproliferative Disorder (PTLD)

Patient No.	Cumulative OKT3 Dose	Time to PTLD	Pathological Findings	Immunophenotype	Immunogenotype	Clinical Status (Time from Diagnosis)
	mg	*mo*				
1	None	50	DUL	M	M	Dead (5 mo)
2	70	13	DLCL	—	—	Alive in CR (42 mo)
3	70	8	DLCL	M	M	Alive in CR (20 mo)
4	70	18	IBL	M	M	Dead (10 wk)
5	75	3.5	IBL	P	P	Dead (21 days)
6	120	2	IBL	P	—	Dead (4 days)
7	120	1	IBL	P	—	Dead (18 days)
8	120	1	IBL	P	M	Dead (21 days)
9	135	1	IBL	P	—	Dead (postmortem diagnosis)
10	105	1.5	DM	P	M	Alive in CR (4 mo)

Abbreviations: DUL, diffuse undifferentiated lymphoma; *M,* monoclonal; *DLCL,* diffuse large-cell lymphoma; *CR,* complete remission; *IBL,* immunoblastic lymphoma; *P,* polyclonal; *DM,* diffuse mixed (polymorphic B-cell) lymphoma according to the classification scheme of Frizzera G, et al: *Cancer Res* 41:4262–4279, 1981.

(Courtesy of Swinnen LJ, Costanzo-Nordin MR, Fisher SG, et al: *N Engl J Med* 323:1723–1728, 1990.)

Statistical analysis of the results included univariate analyses and multivariate analysis by logistic regression.

Posttransplantation lymphoproliferative disorder occurred in 1 (1.3%) of 75 patients who did not receive OKT3, compared with 11.4% of patients who did receive it. The disorder was 9 times more likely to develop in the OKT3-treated group (table). Use of OKT3 was shown by multivariate analysis to be the only factor having a significant association with development of the disorder. Increasing doses of this agent significantly increased risk; of 65 patients whose overall dose was 75 mg or less, the disorder developed in only 4 patients compared with 5 of 14 patients who received more than 75 mg. There were 7 deaths attributed to the disorder.

In heart transplant patients, especially those who have had cumulative doses of more than 75 mg, OKT3 increases the incidence of posttransplantation lymphoproliferative disorder. The use of prophylactic OKT3 should be reassessed, particularly as the value of prophylactic immunotherapy is yet to be firmly established. All patients who have received OKT3 should be monitored closely for signs of posttransplantation lymphoproliferative disorder.

▶ One of the remarkable findings in this study is the rapidity of onset of the posttransplant lymphoproliferative syndrome in this group of heart transplant patients who received OKT3. Onset in 50% was sooner than 3 months after transplant, and the course in these patients was quite fulminant. The time to onset of posttransplant lymphoproliferative syndrome was inversely related to the dose of OKT3. The management of these patients is still controversial. High-dose acyclovir and withdrawal of immunosuppression have been advocated by some investigators. However, when disease is widespread and monoclonal in nature, the mortality rate is high.—D.R. Snydman, M.D.

C4B Deficiency: A Risk Factor for Bacteremia With Encapsulated Organisms

Bishof NA, Welch TR, Beischel LS (Children's Hosp Med Ctr, Cincinnati)
J Infect Dis 162:248–250, 1990 7–8

C4 is a polymorphic protein that is necessary for antibody-mediated complement activation and host defense against invading microorganisms. Most individuals have 2 C4 isotopes, C4A and C4B, the products of 2 distinct genetic loci on chromosome 6. These 2 isotopes have very different in vitro activities. Because isolated C4B deficiency has been noted in approximately 2% of whites, the hypothesis that such a deficiency would impair the immune response to infection with carbohydrate-encapsulated bacteria was tested in 50 children who were positive for *Streptococcus pneumoniae, Hemophilus influenzae,* or *Neisseria meningitidis.* Also included in the study were 100 black and 100 white children whose blood cultures were negative for these 3 pathogens. Plasma samples from all of the children were analyzed for C4B deficiency.

Incidence of C4B Deficiency in Bacteremic and Nonbacteremic Children

Patients	Nonbacteremic	Bacteremic	*P*	Odds ratio
White	2% (2/100)	14% (4/29)	.02	7.8
Black	7% (7/100)	5% (1/21)	>.5	0.7

(Courtesy of Bishof NA, Welch TR, Beischel LS: *J Infect Dis* 162:248–250, 1990.)

In whites who were not bacteremic, the incidence of homozygous C4B deficiency was 2%, similar to rates reported in previous studies in healthy populations. The incidence of 7% among blacks who had negative blood cultures was also similar to the rate reported in a previous population-based study. Of the bacteremic patients, 10% were homozygous C4B-deficient, but the incidence was significantly higher in whites (14%) than in blacks (5%) (table). The bacteremic children with C4B deficiency did not have significantly higher rates of hospitalization, longer hospital stays, or diagnoses different from those in C4B-competent patients.

Various complement deficiencies are associated with an increased risk of infection. These findings suggest another specific disease association. Total C4B deficiency, at least in whites, is a risk factor for invasive infection with these 3 encapsulated organisms.

▶ We normally think of deficiencies in C3, 5, 6, 7, and 8 as being associated with an increased incidence of bacterial infections. This is especially true of the late component deficiencies, with an increased incidence of *Neisseria* infections. In this study the authors document a markedly increased incidence of encapsulated bacterial infections in patients deficient in 1 of the isotypes of C4 (e.g., C4B). This newly recognized association should be added to the list of complement-deficiency states that should be measured when a patient presents with recurrent pneumococcal, neisserial, or *Hemophilus influenzae* bacteremia.—M.S. Klempner, M.D.

Immunoglobulin G Subclass Deficiency and Pneumococcal Infection After Allogeneic Bone Marrow Transplantation

Sheridan JF, Tutschka PJ, Sedmak DD, Copelan EA (Ohio State Univ, Columbus)

Blood 75:1583–1586, 1990 7–9

Pneumococcal infection in long-term survivors of allogeneic bone marrow transplantation (ABMT) is common. These patients typically have impaired opsonic activity for *Streptococcus pneumoniae* and low serum antibody levels for capsular polysaccharide. Previous studies have demonstrated a correlation between serum IgG subclass levels and infection severity. The purpose of this retrospective study was to measure the serum IgG sublcass levels in long-term survivors of ABMT with and without pneumococcal infections.

Serum IgG subclass levels were measured in 25 patients with leukemia

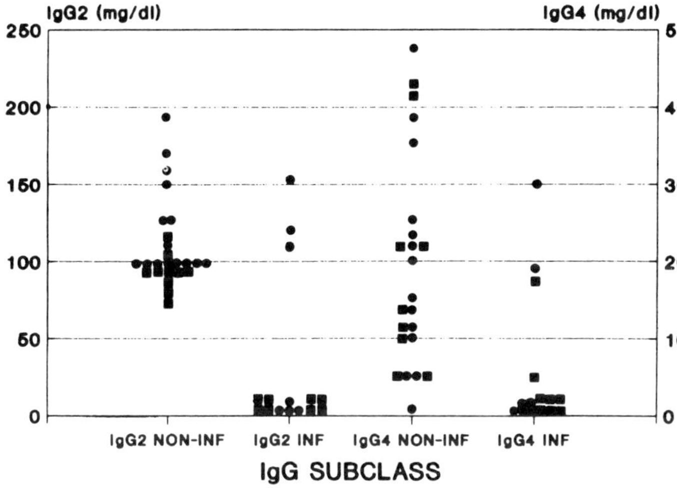

Fig 7–3.—Individual serum IgG2 and IgG4 subclass levels from BMT patients with bacterial infections and noninfected control BMT patients. For patients with infections, samples were assayed during infection *(circle)* or postinfection *(square)*. Noninfected patient samples were assayed during the same periods posttransplantation. The median time post BMT for the "during infection" sample was 7.6 months, whereas the "post-infection" sample was collected 12.9 months after transplantation. (Courtesy of Sheridan JF, Tutschka PJ, Sedmak DD, et al: *Blood* 75:1583–1586, 1990.)

before and after undergoing ABMT. All patients received bone marrow from an HLA-identical sibling after conditioning chemotherapy with busulfan and cyclophosphamide. Intravenous infusions of a commercial Ig preparation were administered every 2 weeks until day 120 after ABMT. Serum IgG1, IgG2, IgG3, and IgG4 levels were measured by end point radial immunodiffusion assay.

Nine patients had pneumococcal infections at least 6 months after undergoing ABMT. Serum IgG1 and IgG3 levels changed only slightly during the observation period. The differences in IgG1 and IgG3 levels between patients with and without pneumococcal infection were not statistically significant at any point during the observation period. Immunoglobulin G2 levels declined with time in both patients with and without pneumococcal infections. Serum IgG4 levels in the 16 noninfected patients varied very little over time, whereas they had significantly declined in the 9 patients with infection. After infection, none of the 8 evaluated patients had detectable levels of IgG2, and only 2 patients had detectable levels of IgG4 (Fig 7–3). In contrast, all 16 patients without infection had IgG2 levels of 102 mg/dL or greater and IgG4 levels of 20 mg/dL or greater.

Deficiencies in IgG subclasses IgG2 and IgG4 after ABMT are associated with an increased susceptibility to pneumococcal infection. Immunoglobulin subclass deficiency is long-lasting and renders patients susceptible to recurrent respiratory infections.

▶ This paper is a lovely demonstration that deficiency of IgG subclasses 2 and 4, from whatever cause, predisposes patients to pyogenic infections attributable to *S. pneumoniae* or *Hemophilus influenzae*. These 2 subclasses are the principal antipolysaccharide IgGs and are needed for opsonic activity; their levels were significantly lower in the group with infection compared to those without such complications. Also, IgG4 is locally made in the lung, and its role in lung defense has been speculated on. All 9 patients contracting late pyogenic infectious complications after allogeneic bone marrow transplantation had pneumonia, including 2 with 2 episodes and 1 with 3 episodes. Interestingly, 12 of the 15 IgG4 measurements in the infected group, before or after infection occurred, were less than 10 mg/dL, the lower value of the 95% confidence interval in the noninfected group. Because IgG2 and IgG4 levels declined post transplant in both groups, it is probably inevitable that the "uninfected" group would, with time, reach the threshold level for infection. Perhaps we need to develop a subclass product for prophylactic administration in these and other at-risk patients. The subject of intravenous immunoglobulin (IVIG) has recently been reviewed (1). In the same issue of the journal, cost-effectiveness analysis of the use of IVIG in chronic lymphatic leukemia concludes the gain is not worth the pain (or the cost).—G.T. Keusch, M.D.

Reference

1. Buckley RH, Schiff RI: *N Engl J Med* 325:110, 1991.

8 HIV Infection

Epidemiology

Transmission of HIV-1 Infections From Mothers to Infants in Haiti: Impact on Childhood Mortality and Malnutrition
Halsey NA, Boulos R, Holt E, Ruff A, Brutus J-R, Kissinger P, Quinn TC, Coberly JS, Adrien M, Boulos C, The CDS/JHU AIDS Project Team (Johns Hopkins Univ; Complexe Medico Sociale de la Cité Soleil, Port-au-Prince, Haiti)
JAMA 264:2088–2092, 1990 8–1

The impact of maternal infection with HIV type 1 (HIV-1) on childhood mortality and malnutrition was studied in a high-risk Haitian population. In addition, mother-to-infant HIV-1 transmission rates were compared to those reported in developed countries.

Of the 4,588 pregnant women seen for prenatal care, 443 (9.7%) were seropositive for HIV-1. Infants born to mothers who were HIV-1 seropositive were significantly more likely to be premature, of low birth weight, and malnourished at 3 months and 6 months of age than infants born to seronegative mothers. Furthermore, infants born to seropositive women had significantly lower survival rates (table). Mortality rates were 23.4% for infants born to women who were seropositive compared to 10.8% for infants born to women who were seronegative. Maternal HIV-1 infections resulted in an 11.7% increase in the overall infant mortality rate. Mother-to-infant transmission rates in these breast-fed infants were estimated at 25% by 2 different methods of data analysis. Similar rates have been reported for non–breast-fed populations in developing countries.

These data demonstrate the negative impact of maternal HIV-1 infections on birth weight, infant survival, and nutritional status in a high-risk population free of the confounding effects of drug abuse. The data also

Impact of Maternal HIV-1 Infection on Survival of Offspring in the First 2 Years of Life

		First Year		Birth-2 Years	
Maternal HIV-1 Status	**No. of Births**	**No. of Deaths**	**Mortality Rate†**	**No. of Deaths**	**Mortality Rate ***
Positive	100	23.4	234	31.3	313
Negative	900	97.2	108	127.8	142
Total	**1000**	**120.6**	121	**159.1**	159

*Number is per 1,000 live births; data from survival analysis.
(Courtesy of Halsey NA, Boulos R, Holt E, et al: *JAMA* 264:2088–2092, 1990).

show that the HIV-1 epidemic in this population has resulted in a significant increase in infant mortality.

▶ The studies from Haiti are consistent with what has been described in Zaire and Rawanda (1). The estimates of mother-to-infant transmission have also been confirmed in several other studies including Haitian mothers in the United States. It appears that breast-feeding did not have an impact on HIV transmission rates; therefore, breast-feeding can be continued with these infants in accord with current WHO recommendations. It may be that absence of highly avid gp120 antibodies will prove to be the major correlate of maternal-infant transmission of HIV (see Abstract 8–2).—D.R. Snydman, M.D.

Reference

1. 1991 Year Book of Infectious Diseases, pp 214–216.

Vertical Transmission of Human Immunodeficiency Virus Is Correlated With the Absence of High-Affinity/Avidity Maternal Antibodies to the gp120 Principal Neutralizing Domain

Devash Y, Calvelli TA, Wood DG, Reagan KJ, Rubinstein A (EI du Pont de Nemours, Glasgow, Del; Albert Einstein College of Medicine, Bronx)
Proc Natl Acad Sci USA 87:3445–3449, 1990 8–2

Although the majority of infants infected with HIV are born to HIV-infected mothers, not all pregnancies in HIV-infected mothers result in an infected infant. The factors that facilitate HIV transmission to the fetus are still not clear. A retrospective analysis of 15 pairs of maternal and neonatal serum samples was conducted with an enzyme-linked immunosorbent assay (ELISA) that preferentially detects high-affinity/avidity antibodies toward the principal neutralizing domain (PND). Mothers with high-affinity/avidity antibodies directed toward the PND of gp120 are less likely to transmit HIV to their children.

The assay correctly identified all 4 uninfected and 11 HIV-infected infants. All 11 HIV-infected infants and their mothers demonstrated only weak reactivity in the ELISA, whereas the sera of the 4 uninfected infants and 3 of 4 of their mothers showed strong reactivity. Other clinical and laboratory parameters, including p24 antigen, phytohemagglutinin mitogenic index, and absolute surface antigen $T4^+$ cell counts, were not predictive of HIV infection in the fetus.

These data show that vertical transmission of HIV is correlated with the absence of high-affinity/avidity maternal antibodies to the PND. This study also provides in vivo evidence that protective antibodies may prevent infection by HIV. The antigen-limited PND ELISA is a promising diagnostic tool.

▶ ↓ Studies from the same patient population, in fact the same sera set, previously demonstrated the extraordinarily high rate of HIV infection among patients seen in the emergency room in Baltimore (1). This report documents a high rate of human T cell lymphotropic virus I–II infection and the marked difference in epidemiologic characteristics in this group compared to HIV-infected emergency room patients.—D.R. Snydman, M.D.

Reference

1. 1990 Year Book of Infectious Diseases, pp 187–189.

Human T-Lymphotropic Virus (HTLV I–II) Infection Among Patients in an Inner-City Emergency Department

Kelen GD, DiGiovanna TA, Lofy L, Junkins E, Stein A, Sivertson KT, Lairmore M, Quinn TC (Johns Hopkins Univ; Ctrs for Disease Control, Atlanta; Natl Inst of Allergy and Infectious Disease, Bethesda, Md)

Ann Intern Med 113:368–372, 1990 8–3

Human T lymphotropic virus type II (HTLV-II) is a retrovirus closely related to HTLV-I that was recently documented in intravenous drug users. Although HTLV-II has not been associated specifically with any disease, co-infection with HIV-1 has been reported. Serologic surveys for HTLV-I or HTLV-II most accurately reflect the seroprevalence of HTLV I–II.

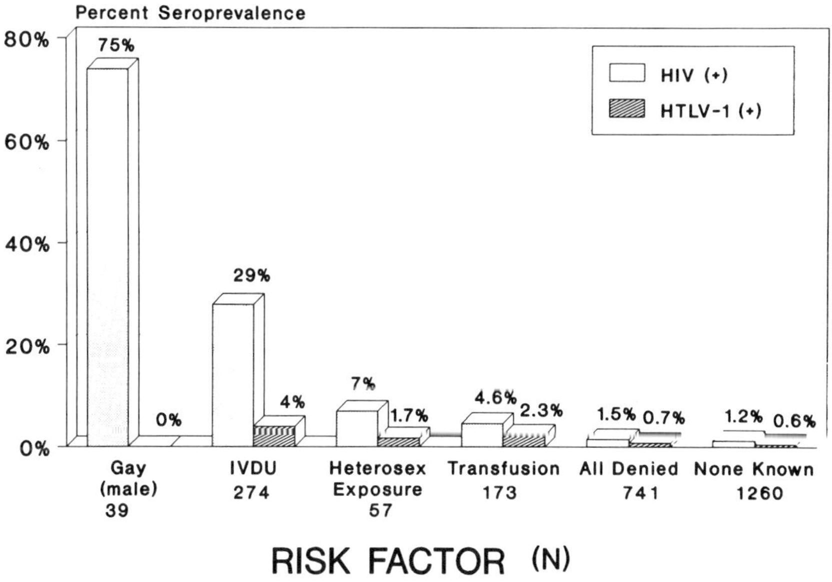

Fig 8–1.—Seroprevalence of HTLV I–II and HIV-1 by risk factors. *Black bars* indicate HIV-1. *Gray bars* indicate HTLV I–II. Risk factors were hierarchically ordered as follows: homosexual or bisexual, intravenous drug user *(IVDU)*, high-risk heterosexual partner, and transfusion or blood products recipient. *All denied* indicates that all risk factors were assessed and that all were denied. *None known* indicates that some risk factors may have been denied, but not all risk factors could be assessed. (Courtesy of Kelen GD, DiGiovanna TA, Lofy L, et al: *Ann Intern Med* 113:368–372, 1990.)

The seroprevalence and epidemiologic features of HTLV I–II among 2,544 adult emergency department patients with a high rate of HIV-1 infection were determined by identity-unlinked serum sampling. Of the 28 patients (1.1%) whose serum samples were seropositive for HTLV I–II, only 16 had identified risk factors (Fig 8–1). The 152 (6%) HIV-1 positive patients were concentrated among younger age groups. Of 39 identified homosexual men, 29 were HIV-1 seropositive, but none was positive for HTLV I–II antibodies.

The relatively high rate of HTLV I–II infection in the general emergency department population indicates a higher than expected prevalence of HTLV I–II having a different demographic distribution than HIV-1 infection. Bloodborne routes (e.g., via transfusion or intravenous drug use) are a risk factor that may represent nosocomial-related transmission. Adherence to universal precautions among health providers should minimize the risk of occupational transmission, which is probably less than that for hepatitis B virus or HIV-1.

Prevalence of Human Immunodeficiency Virus Type 1 p24 Antigen in U.S. Blood Donors—An Assessment of the Efficacy of Testing in Donor Screening

Alter HJ, Epstein JS, Swenson SG, VanRaden MJ, Ward JW, Kaslow RA, Menitove JE, Klein HG, Sandler SG, Sayers MH, Hewlett IK, Chernoff AI, and the HIV-Antigen Study Group (Natl Insts of Health, Bethesda, Md; Food and Drug Administration, Bethesda; Blood Systems Central Lab, Scottsdale, Ariz; Ctrs for Disease Control, Atlanta; Milwaukee Blood Ctr, et al)

N Engl J Med 323:1312–1317, 1990 8–4

Although the incidence of infection with HIV-I through transfusions has been reduced considerably, a residual risk does exist. There is a prolonged interval between infection and seroconversion, and some donors may not report recent infections or high-risk behavior. A multicenter study was undertaken to assess the value of screening donors for HIV-1 p24 antigen, which may appear in the blood before HIV-1 antibody (anti-HIV-1).

During a 6-month period, samples were obtained from 13 blood centers representing areas of both high and low prevalence of HIV-1. Of the 515, 494 donations initially screened for p24 antigen, 225 were repeatedly reactive on enzyme immunoassay. All but 5 of these repeatedly reactive samples were negative for anti-HIV-1 and failed to neutralize in the neutralization assay for p24 antigen. The 5 donors positive for p24 antigen (.001% of all donations tested) were also positive for anti-HIV-1 and HIV-1 by polymerase chain reaction.

All 5 donors with confirmed p24 antigen were men. Four were younger than age 30 and 3 had other markers of infections that would have resulted in their exclusion as donors. Three men had identified risk factors for HIV-1 infection, which should have led to their self-exclusion.

The findings of this study do not support routine testing for p24 antigens in blood donations. In this and other large field studies, no donor was both positive for p24 antigen and negative for anti-HIV-1. The period during which the antigen could be detected is generally less than 2 weeks, lessening the likelihood of positive results. Methods of improving the process of self-exclusion may be as efficient as additional testing.

▶ This carefully performed study clearly demonstrates that screening the blood supply for p24 antigen does not improve safety, as compared to testing for HIV-1 antibody.—S.M. Wolff, M.D.

Diagnostic Tests and Markers

Predicting Progression to AIDS: Combined Usefulness of CD4 Lymphocyte Counts and p24 Antigenemia

MacDonell KB, Chmiel JS, Poggensee L, Wu S, Phair JP (Northwestern Univ)
Am J Med 89:706–712, 1990 8–5

It has been estimated that up to 10 million persons worldwide are infected with HIV-1. Most will remain asymptomatic for years. Many markers have been recognized as predictors of progression to AIDS. Two markers, p24 core antigen and CD4 lymphocyte counts, were assessed prospectively for their usefulness as predictors of subsequent clinical disease in 924 homosexual and bisexual men without AIDS and with unknown HIV-1 serostatus. All were enrolled in the Multicenter AIDS Co-

Progression to AIDS Based on CD4 Lymphocyte Counts and P24 Antigen Status

			Estimated % of Men Developing AIDS Within			
CD4 †	**Pattern of Antigenemia†**	**Number of Men**	**1 Year**	**2 Years**	**3 Years**	**4 Years**
<200		20	36	59	65	86
	Ag–	5	20	20	47	47
	Ag– to Ag+	0	—	—	—	—
	Ag+	15	42	64	71	100
200–399		63	25	39	42	63
	Ag–	33	0	5	14	20
	Ag– to Ag+	6	0	17	38	38
	Ag+	24	17	57	68	81
≥400		421	0	6	12	21
	Ag–	333	0	3	7	14
	Ag– to Ag+	50	0	7	14	31
	Ag+	38	0	23	48	58

Abbreviations: Ag–, persistently antigen negative during 48 months of follow-up; *Ag– to Ag+*, antigen negative at entry but positive antigen status developed during 48 months of follow-up; *Ag+*, antigen positive at time of entry into study.

*Cd4 cells per microliter at entry.

†Kaplan-Meier estimates ($P < .0001$ for comparison of antigen groups stratified by CD4 number less than 400 and 400 or more cells/μL).

(Courtesy of MacDonell KB, Chmiel JS, Poggensee L, et al: *Am J Med* 89:706–712, 1990.)

hort Study in Chicago. Their CD4 lymphocyte counts, HIV-1 p24 antigen status, and clinical status were evaluated every 6 months during a 4-year period.

Of the 518 men found to be seropositive, 26% had detectable p24 antigen at some time during the study. Men with p24 antigenemia had significantly more rapid declines in CD4 lymphocyte counts than those without antigenemia. Antigenemia was detected in 61% of men who progressed to AIDS and in only 17% of those who did not. When the seropositive cohort was stratified by entry CD4 cell count and antigenemia status, Kaplan-Meier estimates showed that low CD4 cell counts at entry were associated with rapid progression to AIDS. In addition, within each CD4 stratum the presence of antigenemia was associated with significantly higher risk of AIDS developing within 4 years (table).

This study confirms the findings of previous smaller studies indicating that CD4 counts and p24 antigen are significant independent predictors of disease progression. The data also suggest that p24 antigenemia is a marker that can identify primarily asymptomatic individuals with moderate CD4 cell depletion who are at greater risk of disease progression. However, as a single marker of disease before the diagnosis of AIDS, the use of p24 antigen has major limitations.

▶ These data support smaller studies that have identified CD4 and p24 antigen as significant independent predictors of HIV-associated disease progression. Moreover, detection of p24 antigen is associated with a more rapid reduction in CD4 lymphocytes.—D.R. Snydman, M.D.

Increasing Viral Burden in CD4+ T Cells From Patients With Human Immunodeficiency Virus (HIV) Infection Reflects Rapidly Progressive Immunosuppression and Clinical Disease

Schnittman SM, Greenhouse JJ, Psallidopoulos MC, Baseler M, Salzman NP, Fauci AS, Lane HC (Natl Insts of Health, Bethesda, Md; Georgetown Univ; Frederick Cancer Research Facility, Frederick, Md)

Ann Intern Med 113:438–443, 1990 8–6

Although there is clearly an association of HIV-1 infection with AIDS, controversy continues over the role of HIV-1 in the pathogenesis of an immunodeficient state. A study was undertaken to examine the relationship between viral burden and immunologic status in 12 initially healthy HIV-1-seropositive patients followed for 14 months. In 6, rapidly progressive disease developed. In a second cohort of 15 healthy seropositive patients from the Multicenter AIDS Cohort Study, followed for an average of 32 months, rapidly progressive disease developed in 7. The viral burden of CD4+ T cells was estimated using the quantitative polymerase chain reaction.

Counts of HIV-infected CD4+ T cells were low in the patients who remained asymptomatic and did not increase above 1/1,000. In those who became symptomatic, in contrast, the frequency of infected T cells exceeded 1/1,000 at entry and usually rose above 1/100 within 3 months of the appearance of progressive disease. At the same time, the proportion of T4 cells fell from 31% to 16%. The proportion did not change in those who remained well. An increasing viral burden in peripheral blood CD4+ T cells is directly related to a progressive decrease in the CD4+ T cell count and a declining clinical course in HIV-infected patients.

▶ Other factors (such as autoimmunity) may play a role, but these studies increasingly show that infection of CD4+ and T cells is the major cause of immunosuppression in HIV-infected humans.—S.M. Wolff, M.D.

Tuftsin Deficiency in AIDS

Corazza GR, Zoli G, Ginaldi L, Cancellieri C, Profeta V, Gasbarrini G, Quaglino D (Univ of L'Aquila; Univ of Bologna; "GB Morgagni" Hosp, Forli, Italy)
Lancet 337:12–13, 1991 8–7

Tuftsin is an endogenous tetrapeptide that stimulates phagocytosis and is released from the Fc fragment of immunoglobulin G by a splenic en-

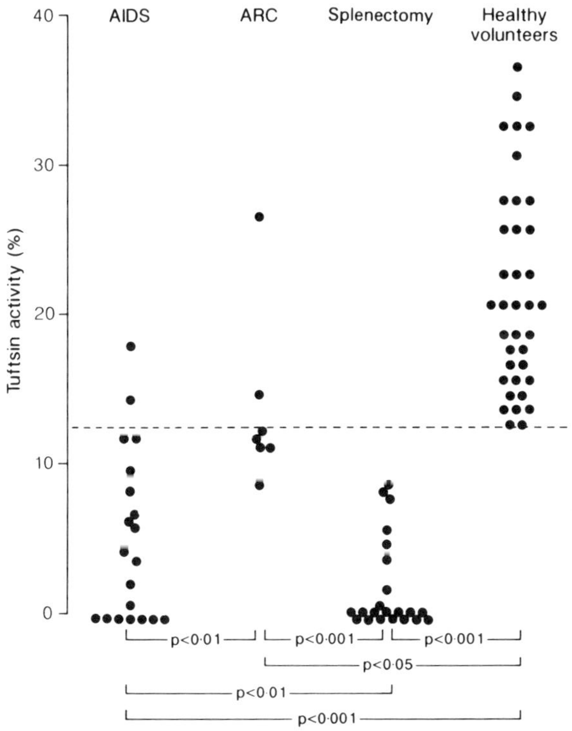

Serum tuftsin activity in study groups.

Fig 8–2.—Serum tuftsin activity was reduced significantly in the AIDS, ARC, and splenectomy groups. (Courtesy of Corazza GR, Zoli G, Ginaldi L, et al: *Lancet* 337:12–13, 1991.)

docarboxypeptidase. Because splenomegaly is common in AIDS that may be associated with functional asplenia, a study was designed to determine whether a deficiency in tuftsin activity may be another risk factor for infection in patients with AIDS.

Serum tuftsin activity and splenic function were measured in 21 patients with AIDS, 7 patients with AIDS-related complex (ARC), 22 patients who had splenectomy, and 37 healthy volunteers. Serum tuftsin activity was assayed by measuring its ability to stimulate phagocytosis of opsonized *Staphylococcus aureus* by neutrophilic granulocytes.

Serum tuftsin activity was significantly reduced in patients with AIDS (5.7%) and ARC (14.1%), and in the splenectomy group (2%), compared with healthy volunteers (21.6%) (Fig 8–2). Splenic function, as measured by pitted red blood cell counts, in patients with AIDS was significantly higher than in healthy volunteers, but significantly lower than in the splenectomized group. There was a significant inverse correlation between tuftsin activity and splenic function in all patients. There was no correlation between tuftsin activity and CD4 cell counts in patients with AIDS and ARC. These data suggest that tuftsin deficiency may contribute to the risk of bacterial infection in patients with HIV infection.

▶ I guess it's no surprise why I'm partial to studies describing the clinical relevance of tuftsin deficiency. But the recent demonstration that intravenous gammaglobulin reduces the incidence of bacterial infections in children with AIDS suggests that this may be a significant humoral immune deficiency in adults as well.—M.S. Klempner, M.D.

Impairment of Neutrophil Chemotactic and Bactericidal Function in Children Infected With Human Immunodeficiency Virus Type 1 and Partial Reversal After In Vitro Exposure to Granulocyte-Macrophage Colony-Stimulating Factor

Roilides E, Mertins S, Eddy J, Walsh TJ, Pizzo PA, Rubin M (Natl Cancer Inst, Bethesda, Md)

J Pediatr 117:531–540, 1990 8–8

The role of polymorphonuclear neutrophils (PMNs) in the host defense against bacteria has been examined more thoroughly in adults infected with HIV-1 than in HIV-1-infected children. Baseline PMN function in 25 such children was evaluated to determine whether this function is altered by granulocyte-macrophage colony-stimulating factor (GM-CSF), an agent likely to be used in children with AIDS.

Of the children, 12 had symptoms and 13 were symptom free at the time of the tests (table); a control group included 13 healthy HIV-1-seronegative young adults. The PMN functions assessed were chemotaxis, bacterial phagocytosis, superoxide generation, and bactericidal activity.

Although chemotaxis in symptom-free affected patients was significantly decreased compared with normal control values, the PMNs from patients with symptoms showed enhanced chemotaxis (Fig 8–3). The

Clinical and Laboratory Characteristics of Children With Asymptomatic and Those With Symptomatic HIV Infection

Clinical/ laboratory characteristic	Asymptomatic infection	Symptomatic infection
Gender (M/F)	7/6	8/4
Age (yr)		
Mean	6.4	5.3
Range	2-13	0.5-14
History of infections		
Oppórtunistic		8*/12
Bacterial		9†/12
Fungal		8‡/12
Leukocytes (cells/μl)		
Mean ± SD	5800 ± 2039	4360 ± 2274
Range	3300-9500	1700-8000
ANC (cells/μl)		
Mean	2043 ± 508	2037 ± 870
Range	1452-2812	255-2856
ANC <1500/μl	1/12	1/10
$CD4^+$ (cells/μl)		
Mean	771 ± 599	536 ± 557
Range	0-2134	1-1358
$CD4^+/CD8^+$ ratio		
Mean	0.82 ± 0.70	0.45 ± 0.49
Range	<0.01-2.4	0.02-1.35
$CD4^+$ <200/μl	3/13 (23%)	4/9 (44%)
Hypergammaglobulinemia§		
Hyper-IgG	7/12	6/8
Hyper-IgA	4/12	4/8
Hyper-IgM	0/12	2/8
p24 antigen‖ (pg/ml)	266.2 ± 250.0	568.8 ± 733.3

Abbreviation: ANC, absolute neutrophil count.

*Four children with *Pneumocystis carinii* pneumonia, 2 with toxoplasmosis, 2 with cytomegalovirus retinitis.

†One child with group A streptococcal bacteremia, 2 with pneumonia, 2 with sinusitis, 1 with osteomyelitis, 1 with epiglottis *(Hemophilus parainfluenzae)*, 1 with recurrent otitis media.

‡Six children with recurrent *Candida* stomatitis, 1 with *Candida* esophagitis, 1 with chronic fungal nail infection.

§Compared with age-matched normal values.

‖Tested at the same time with PMN function (or within 1 week); values are expressed as mean ± SD.

(Courtesy of Roilides E, Mertins S, Eddy J, et al: *J Pediatr* 117:531–540, 1990.)

bactericidal activity of the neutrophils against *Staphylococcus aureus* was defective in 8 of 12 asymptomatic children and in 8 of 9 symptomatic children (Fig 8–4). The PMNs from both patient groups and from normal controls released approximately equal amounts of superoxide anion. The bactericidal activity of PMNs in patients showed significant impairment. This activity was enhanced in vitro by GM-CSF.

Surprisingly, the significant defect in chemotaxis was evident only in

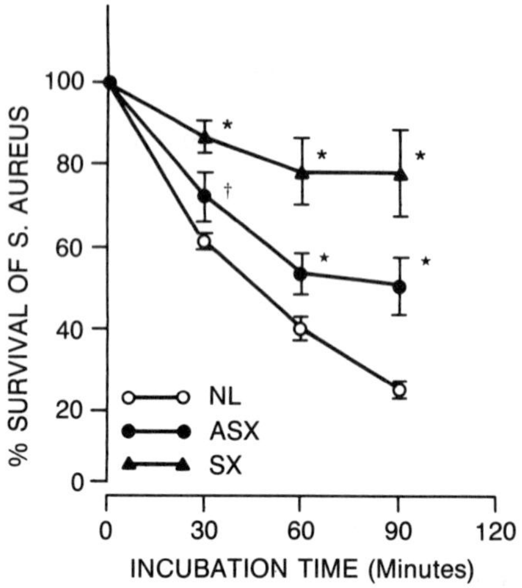

Fig 8–3.—Bactericidal activity of neutrophils from normal controls *(NL, open circles)* and children with asymptomatic *(ASX, closed circles)* and those with symptomatic *(SX; triangles)* HIV infection. *Staphylococcus aureus* was used as a target. *Vertical bars* denote SEM; *asterisk, P* < .00001; *star, P* < .02; dagger, *P* NS (differences between ASX or SX and NL children). (Courtesy of Roilides E, Mertins S, Eddy J, et al: *J Pediatr* 117:531–540, 1990.)

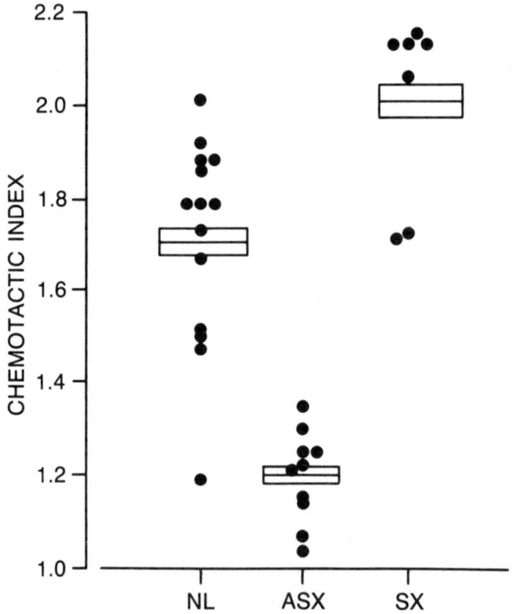

Fig 8–4.—Chemotactic response of neutrophils from normal controls *(NL)* and from children with asymptomatic *(ASX)* and those with symptomatic *(SX)* HIV infection. Results are expressed as chemotactic index: ratio of number of cells with directed migration divided by randomly migrating cells. *Horizontal bars* denote means; *open boxes* denote SEM. (Courtesy of Roilides E, Mertins S, Eddy J, et al: *J Pediatr* 117:531–540, 1990.)

the children with asymptomatic HIV-1 infection. This contrast between the 2 groups of children may relate to the differential release of cytokines at various stages of AIDS. These findings suggest that both cellular and humoral defects can be found in HIV-1-infected children and may contribute to the increased incidence of bacterial infection in such children. Treatment with GM-CSF appears to partially reverse this cellular defect.

▶ As someone with a longstanding interest in neutrophil function, I have been closely following the literature on abnormal neutrophil function in patients with AIDS. There is clear documentation of abnormal neutrophil migration and perhaps abnormal bactericidal activity in both children and adults. That this is functionally important is brought home to me by the increasing incidence of bacterial infections, especially those caused by *Staphylococcus aureus*. Infection with this particular organism is one of the hallmarks of a relevant neutrophil defect because complement, immunoglobulins, and T cells have a relatively small role in host defense against this bacteria. It will be interesting to see whether in vivo treatment with CSFs, which is being done in some patients with AIDS now, will also reverse the chemotactic defect as it did in vitro here.—M.S. Klempner, M.D.

Frequency of Indeterminate Western Blot Tests in Healthy Adults at Low Risk for Human Immunodeficiency Virus Infection

Midthun K, Garrison L, Clements ML, Farzadegan H, Fernie B, Quinn T, and the NIAID AIDS Vaccine Clinical Trials Network (Johns Hopkins Univ; Georgetown Univ, Rockville, Md)

J Infect Dis 162:1379–1382, 1990 8–9

Indeterminate Western blot (WB) test results have been described in early and advanced infection with HIV-1 and in the absence of infection. As part of a phase 1 trial of a candidate vaccine for AIDS, 168 healthy adult volunteers at minimal or no risk of acquiring HIV-1 infection were screened. Blood specimens from these volunteers were tested by enzyme immunoassay (EIA), the Biotech/Du Pont WB, culture, and polymerase chain reaction assay.

None of the volunteers tested positive for any of the assays, but in 53 (32%) the WB results were indeterminate. Most of the indeterminate WB tests (85%) demonstrated a single band of low intensity. Bands corresponding to p24, p55, and p66 occurred most frequently, whereas envelope bands were unusual. Within 2–11 months, 33 volunteers with indeterminate WB tests were retested. None progressed to a positive WB, EIA, or p24 antigen test, and none was positive for antibodies to HIV-2 or human T cell lymphotropic virus type I. Analysis of the lot-to-lot variability as a contributory factor to the variation in the frequency of indeterminate WB tests showed a 91% agreement in test results of the first and second serum samples when the same lot of WB kit was used but only 39% agreement when different lots were used. These data show that the Biotech/Du Pont WB kit frequently yields indeterminate test results in the absence of HIV-1 infection, and that the reproducibility of WB may be subject to lot-to-lot variability.

▶ Clinicians should realize that Western blots can vary from lot to lot. Although this was a select group of subjects with indeterminate Western blots, the intensity of bands varied greatly. The experience reported here and that of others reviewed previously confirm the absence of HIV infection in those patients with repeatedly indeterminate Western blots (1).—D.R. Snydman, M.D.

Reference

1. 1991 Year Book of Infectious Diseases, pp 230–233.

Opportunistic Infections

The Radiographic Appearance of Pulmonary Nocardiosis Associated With AIDS

Kramer MR, Uttamchandani RB (Univ of Miami)
Chest 98:382–385, 1990 8–10

Nocardia asteroides is the most common pathogen in the 500–1,000 patients with nocardiosis identified each year in the United States. Be-

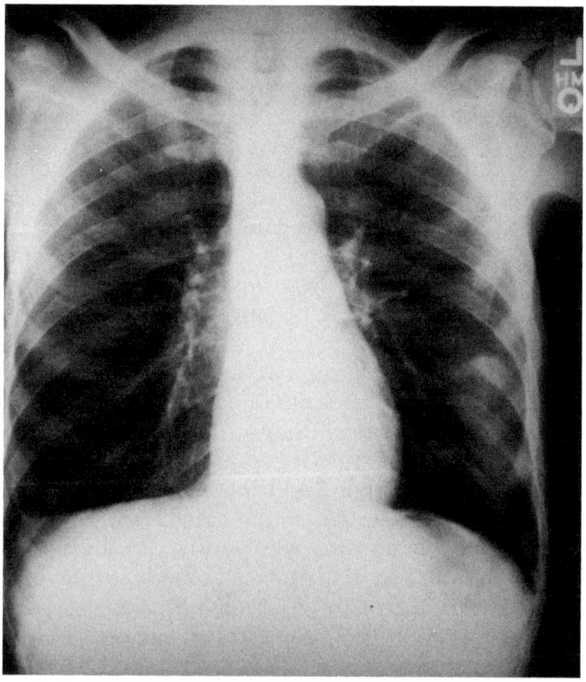

Fig 8–5.—Left lower lobe; rounded, well-defined soft mass. (Courtesy of Kramer MR, Uttamchandani RB: *Chest* 98:382–385, 1990.)

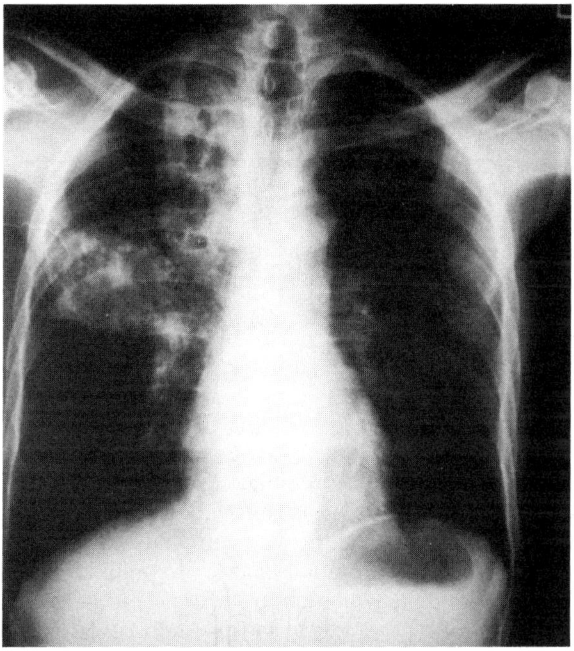

Fig 8–6.—Right upper lobe cavitary infiltrate. (Courtesy of Kramer MR, Uttamchandani RB: *Chest* 98:382–385, 1990.)

cause cell-mediated immunity defends the host from infection, this opportunistic infection occurs significantly in immunocompromised patients, e.g., posttransplant patients. The radiographic findings in 21 patients with pulmonary nocardiosis associated with HIV infection were reviewed.

Although the radiographic appearances were variable among patients with AIDS-associated nocardiosis, the patterns were not significantly different from those in patients without AIDS. Lobar or multilobar consolidation was evident in 11 of 21 patients. Solitary masses appeared in 5 patients (24%). Reticulonodular infiltrates and pleural effusion each appeared in 7 (33%) patients. Cavitary lesions were common and were observed in 13 patients (62%). Upper lobes were more commonly involved (71%) (Figs 8–5 and 8–6).

Nocardiosis should be suspected in HIV-positive patients with subacute pulmonary disease and an unexplained lung mass or cavitary lesions. The final diagnosis should be based on a positive sputum culture or bronchoscopic findings.

▶ Pulmonary nocardiosis can have virtually any radiographic appearance. However, the most suggestive presentations in immunosuppressed patients are a solitary rounded mass (with or without cavitation) and an upper lobe cavitary lesion. The presence of extrapulmonary lesions, especially soft tissue and cerebral lesions, is another suggestive clue.—M.J. Barza, M.D.

Microsporidial Keratoconjunctivitis in Acquired Immunodeficiency Syndrome

Friedberg DN, Stenson SM, Orenstein JM, Tierno PM, Charles NC (New York Univ Med Ctr; George Washington Univ)

Arch Ophthalmol 108:504–508, 1990 8–11

Microsporida are small obligate intracellular parasites found throughout the animal kingdom. The incidence of human microsporidiosis among patients with AIDS has been increasing. Data were reviewed on patients with AIDS in whom a recalcitrant bilateral epithelial keratitis developed.

In 2 patients, microsporidial keratoconjunctivitis was diagnosed on the basis of typical findings on light and electron microscopy. All 3 patients had exposure to household pets. The appearance of the keratitis was similar in all 3 patients, with disease confined to the superficial corneal epithelium and only minimal clinical involvement of the conjunctiva (Fig 8–7). Symptoms included photophobia, foreign-body sensation, blurred vision, and dryness. The frequent use of ocular lubricants provided symptomatic relief, but no clinical improvement occurred. Despite the extent of the keratitis, there was a minimal degree of conjunctival inflammation in all 3 patients. Scraping, which showed numerous protozoans, proved to be a simple, benign way to establish the diagnosis of microsporida infection (Fig 8–8).

Household pets (e.g., cats, dogs, and birds) acquire and harbor *Enceph-*

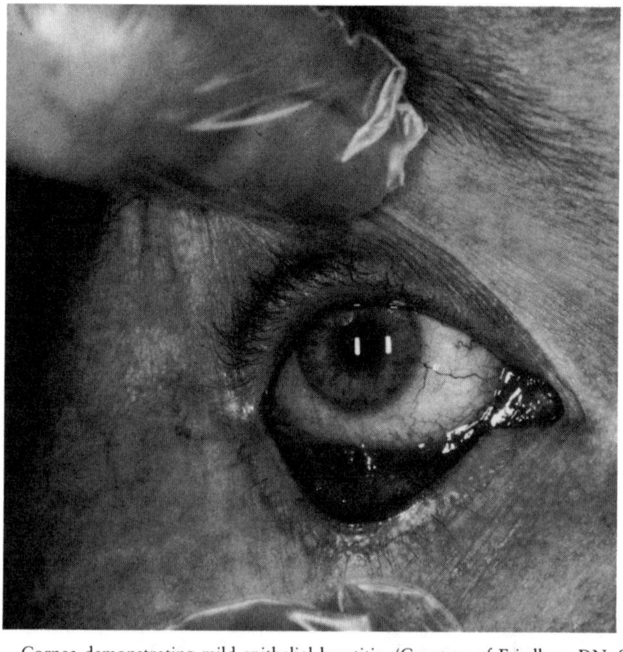

Fig 8–7.—Cornea demonstrating mild epithelial keratitis. (Courtesy of Friedberg DN, Stenson SM, Orenstein JM, et al: *Arch Ophthalmol* 108:504–508, 1990.)

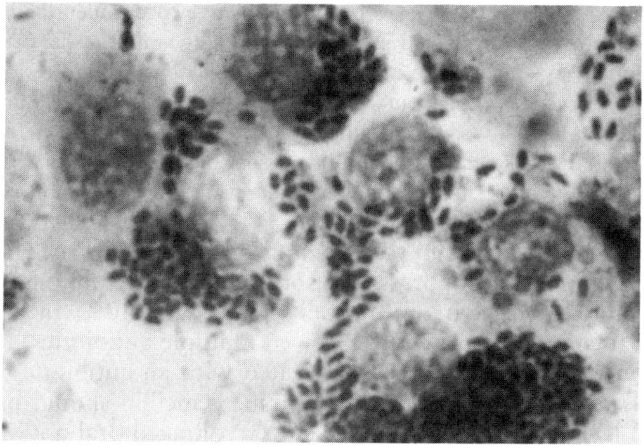

Fig 8–8.—Conjunctival scraping shows numerous large gram-positive ovoid organisms within conjunctival epithelial cells (Gram's stain; original magnification, ×500). (Courtesy of Friedberg DN, Stenson SM, Orenstein JM, et al: *Arch Ophthalmol* 108:504–508, 1990.)

alitozoon cuniculi organisms that may have been the source of the topical infection in these 3 patients. There is no known effective treatment for microsporidia in human beings. Sulfa drugs reportedly have some effect. The cytologic appearance of the organisms, coupled with the distinctive superficial keratitis, enables the diagnosis of microsporidial infection.

▶ Just when I was learning to pronounce the new species of microsporida that causes diarrhea and malabsorption in patients with AIDS *(Enterocytozoon bieneusi),* along comes this report of a different species that can cause keratoconjunctivitis. This is a different species *(Encephalitozoon cuniculi)* and appears to have a different pathogenesis than the enteric infection. It is inoculated topically and is probably associated with exposure to pets.—M.S. Klempner, M.D.

Rhodococcus equi **Infection in Patients With and Without Human Immunodeficiency Virus Infection**

Harvey RL, Sunstrum JC (Wayne State Univ, Detroit; VA Med Ctr, Allen Park, Mich)

Rev Infect Dis 13:139–145, 1991 8–12

Rhodococcus equi (formerly *Corynebacterium equi*) is a pathogen of farm animals that can cause cavitary pneumonia in immunosuppressed human contacts. Ten infections have been described in patients with AIDS. Another such patient was encountered.

Man, 30, an abuser of alcohol and intravenous drugs, had a sharp retrosternal pain and a right lower lobe infiltrate associated with a chronic nonproductive cough. He had a history of multiple episodes of pneumonia as well as upper gastrointestinal bleeding. Generalized adenopathy was noted, as was oral candidiasis. Anergy was demonstrated and the T cell ratio in peripheral blood was reversed. Blood culture yielded an aerobic gram-positive coccus identified as *R. equi*. The organism grew from resected lung tissue including a hilar node. *Candida albicans* fungemia also was present, as was possible mycobacterial infection. The patient was given erythromycin, isoniazid, rifampin, and ketoconazole. Subsequently, cavitary pneumonia involved the left upper lobe, and cultures again yielded *R. equi*. Infection with HIV was confirmed, and the patient died of respiratory insufficiency 2 months later. *Pneumocystis carinii* pneumonia was confirmed at autopsy.

Most *R. equi* infections in patients not infected by HIV occurred in association with immunosuppressive disorders such as lymphoma and renal transplantation. The overall mortality rate was 20% in non–HIV-infected patients, most of whom received multiple antibiotics.

Infection with *R. equi* should be treated with an antibiotic that penetrates cells, e.g., erythromycin or rifampin. Penicillin should be avoided because β-lactam resistance may develop. Prolonged oral antibiotic therapy after intravenous treatment has been proposed.

Treatment of Tuberculosis in Patients With Advanced Human Immunodeficiency Virus Infection

Small PM, Schecter GF, Goodman PC, Sande MA, Chaisson RE, Hopewell PC (San Francisco Gen Hosp; Dept. of Public Health, City and County of San Francisco; Univ of California, San Francisco)

N Engl J Med 324:289–294, 1991 8–13

Infection with HIV increases the risk of tuberculosis and may also decrease the effectiveness of antituberculous treatment. The American Thoracic Society and the Centers for Disease Control have recommended that antituberculous chemotherapy for patients infected with HIV be administered for a minimum of 9 months, or for at least 6 months after organisms have been cleared from the sputum. In a retrospective study the clinical course of all 132 patients with both AIDS and tuberculosis was reviewed.

When tuberculosis was diagnosed, 78 patients (59%) did not yet have a diagnosis of AIDS (group 1), 18 patients (14%) were given a concomitant diagnosis of AIDS (group 2), and 36 patients (27%) already had AIDS (group 3). The treatment regimen was isoniazid and rifampin sup-

Vital Status and Outcome in Treated Patients as of August 31, 1990

Group No.	No. of Patients	Alive	Dead	Death from TB	Adverse Reaction	Treatment Failure	Relapse
				number (percent)			
1	77	19 (25)	58 (75)	1 (1)	14 (18)	1 (1)	3 (4)
2	17	4 (24)	13 (76)	4 (24)	2 (12)	0	0
3	31	6 (19)	25 (81)	3 (10)	7 (38)	0	0
Total	125	29 (23)	96 (77)	8 (6)	23 (18)	1 (1)	3 (2)

Abbreviation: TB, tuberculosis.
(Courtesy of Small PM, Schecter GF, Goodman PC, et al: *N Engl J Med* 324:289–294, 1991.)

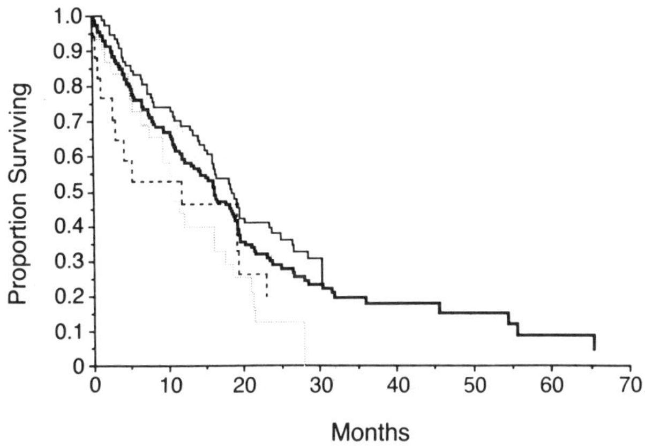

Fig 8–9.—Kaplan-Meier life table for survival after diagnosis of tuberculosis in patients with tuberculosis and AIDS. *Heavy solid line* denotes all patients, *light solid line* depicts group 1, *dashed line* depicts group 2, and *dotted line* depicts group 3. Lines for all patients and for group 1 are superimposed beyond 30 months. (Courtesy of Small PM, Schecter GF, Goodman PC, et al: *N Engl J Med* 324:289–294, 1991.)

plemented by ethambutol for the first 2 months in 52 patients, isoniazid and rifampin supplemented by pyrazinamide and ethambutol for the first 2 months in 39 patients, isoniazid and rifampin in 13 patients, isoniazid and rifampin supplemented by pyrazinamide for the first 2 months in 4 patients, and other drug regimens in 17 patients. The intended duration of treatment was 6 months when the regimen included pyrazinamide and 9 months when the regimen did not include pyrazinamide.

The vital status and outcome in treated patients as of August 31, 1990, are shown in the table. Seven patients died before tuberculosis was diagnosed, and therapy failed in 1 noncompliant patient. The median survival of the 125 treated patients was 16 months after the diagnosis of tuberculosis (Fig 8–9).

Patient noncompliance is the most serious barrier to successful therapy for tuberculosis. In compliant patients conventional therapy results in sterilization of sputum (within 10 weeks in this study), radiographic improvement, and low rates of relapse.

▶ The clinical presentation of tuberculosis in this HIV-infected cohort was atypical, consistent with previous studies. The response to chemotherapy was surprisingly good and comparable to previous reports from this same group. However, the rate of adverse drug reactions was higher than that seen in non–HIV-infected groups. Although reactions were generally mild and early (rash and hepatitis), 1 anaphylactic reaction occurred.—D.R. Snydman, M.D.

Spontaneous Pneumothorax in Patients With Acquired Immunodeficiency Syndrome Treated With Prophylactic Aerosolized Pentamidine

Newsome GS, Ward DJ, Pierce PF (Georgetown Univ)

Arch Intern Med 150:2167–2168, 1990 8–14

Characteristics of Patients With AIDS With Spontaneous Pneumothorax During Aerosolized Pentamidine Prophylaxis

Case	Age, y/ Race/ Sex	Risk Factor	Duration of AIDS Diagnosis, mo	Previous Episodes of PCP	Duration of Aerosolized Prophylaxis, mo	Location of Pneumothorax	Treatment	Outcome
1	31/B/M	Homosexual	30	3	13	Bilateral	Chest tube	Recovered
2	38/W/M	Homosexual	21	1	9	Left	Chest tube	Died
3	33/W/M	Homosexual	15	2	7	Left	Observation	Recovered
4	35/W/M	Homosexual	16	1	12	Right	Chest tube	Reexpansion, died (disseminated *Pneumocystis carinii*)
5	34/W/M	Homosexual	9	1	8	Bilateral	Chest tube	Recovered
6	43/W/M	Homosexual	19	2	5	Bilateral	Chest tube	Recovered, later developed emphysema, died
7	47/W/M	Homosexual	18	2	6	Right	Chest tube	Died
8	33/W/M	Homosexual	17	2	3	Bilateral	Observation	Recovered
9	40/W/M	Homosexual	7	1	6	Bilateral	Chest tube	Died
10	35/B/M	Homosexual	24	2	?	Bilateral	Chest tube	Died
11	31/W/M	Homosexual	19	1	16	Left	Chest tube	Recovered
12	31/W/M	Homosexual	15	1	12	Right	Chest tube	Left pneumothorax; refused further treatment

Abbreviations: B, black; *W,* white; *M,* male.
(Courtesy of Newsome GS, Ward DJ, Pierce PF: *Arch Intern Med* 150:2167–2168, 1990.)

Some spontaneous pneumothoraces in patients with AIDS who have *Pneumocystis carinii* pneumonia (PCP) have been associated with prophylactic aerosolized pentamidine. Data were reviewed on 327 outpatients who were HIV positive and had at least 1 past episode of PCP. The patients were given pentamidine, 100 mg weekly for 4 weeks, followed by 100 mg on alternate weeks by inhalation.

During the study, there were 12 spontaneous pneumothoraces (table). None of the patients had a history of pneumothorax, and no iatrogenic cause was identified. The episodes occurred after a mean of 9 months of aerosolized pentamidine. Most of these affected patients had active PCP and roentgenographic evidence of fibrocystic lung changes. Half of the patients died of progressive respiratory failure.

Spontaneous pneumothorax in patients given aerosolized pentamidine is associated primarily with concurrent acute pulmonary infection. The risk of pneumothorax may well be greater when prophylaxis fails to prevent recurrent PCP.

▶ This retrospective analysis is in accord with a recently published prospective study documenting the risk of pneumothorax in patients receiving aerosolized pentamidine.

Presumably, there are areas of the lung in which *P. carinii* is not being adequately controlled with aerosolized pentamidine therapy. Fibrosis and dissection into the pleural cavity or mediastinum may occur, leading to a bronchopleural fistula.—D.R. Snydman, M.D.

▶ ↓ Extrapulmonary *Pneumocystis carinii* infection has become more commonplace. This review is one of several that document some of the clinical findings.—D.R. Snydman, M.D.

Extrapulmonary Pneumocystosis: The First 50 Cases

Raviglione MC (Cabrini Med Ctr, New York)

Rev Infect Dis 12:1127–1138, 1990 8–15

Despite the increasing frequency of pneumonia caused by *Pneumocystis carinii* (PCP) in patients with AIDS, extrapulmonary infection with *P. carinii* remains uncommon. In 31 months, 5 cases of extrapulmonary pneumocystosis were diagnosed at the Cabrini Medical Center compared to 940 cases with pulmonary PCP. There appears to be an increasing frequency of extrapulmonary pneumocystosis in patients with AIDS, particularly those given aerosolized pentamidine for prophylaxis of PCP. The records of 50 patients with extrapulmonary pneumocystosis reported in the literature since 1954 were reviewed. Characteristics and effects of this infection were compared for patients with and without HIV infection.

Extrapulmonary pneumocystosis occurred in 16 patients with diseases other than AIDS and in 34 patients with AIDS. Of the latter infections, 33 occurred during the last 3 years, and all but 3 occurred in the United States. Concomitant PCP was diagnosed in 14 patients (87%) without AIDS and in only 16 (47%) of those with AIDS. Several organs or tissues were involved, but the most common sites were lymph nodes, spleen, liver, and bone marrow (table). Both lymphatic and hematogenous routes were involved in the extrapulmonary spread of *P. carinii* infection. Half of the patients had a single site of extrapulmonary involvement. All pa-

Extrapulmonary Sites of Infection With *P. carinii* in 50 Patients

Site of infection	No. of patients with infected site (%)	No. of HIV-infected patients (n = 34) with site of infection	No. of patients who had other conditions (n = 16) with site of infection	No. of patients with concomitant PCP
Lymph nodes	23 (46)	12	11	19
Spleen	18 (36)	12	6	14
Liver	16 (32)	12	4	12
Bone marrow	13 (26)	8	5	11
Gastrointestinal tract	9 (18)	8	1	7
Eyes	9 (18)	9	...	5
Thyroid gland	8 (16)	7	1	6
Adrenal glands	8 (16)	6	2	8
Kidneys	7 (14)	4	3	6
Vessels	6 (12)	4	2	5
Heart	5 (10)	5	...	5
Pancreas	4 (8)	3	1	4
External auditory canal	3 (6)	3	...	1
Pleurae	2 (4)	2	...	2
Brain	2 (4)	1	1	2
Thymus gland	2 (4)	...	2	2
Ureters	1 (2)	1	...	1
Virchow-Robin spaces	1 (2)	1	...	1
Diaphragm	1 (2)	1	...	1
Middle ear/mastoid	1 (2)	1	...	...
Pericardium	1 (2)	...	1	1
Retroperitoneal tissue	1 (2)	...	1	1
Hard palate	1 (2)	...	1	1

(Courtesy of Raviglione MC: *Rev Infect Dis* 12:1127–1138, 1990.)

tients who did not have AIDS and had a single site of extrapulmonary infection died shortly after diagnosis, but 11 of 17 patients with AIDs survived. Overall, 15 of 16 patients who did not have AIDS died, whereas 15 (44%) of 34 patients with AIDS survived. In the latter group, the absence of concomitant PCP and single-organ involvement were associated with survival.

There is an increasing frequency of extrapulmonary and truly disseminated pneumocystosis, particularly among patients with AIDS. The widespread use of aerosolized pentamidine as prophylaxis for PCP may play a role in the increase among AIDS patients because of its inadequate systemic absorption. Longer survival of these patients in immunocompromised states and the frequent presence of dysgammaglobulinemia may also be factors. Because of the increasing frequency of this condition in patients who do not have pneumonia caused by *P. carinii*, extrapulmonary pneumocystosis should be included among the AIDS-defining criteria.

A Controlled Trial of Early Adjunctive Treatment With Corticosteroids for *Pneumocystis carinii* Pneumonia in the Acquired Immunodeficiency Syndrome

Bozzette SA, Sattler FR, Chiu J, Wu AW, Gluckstein D, Kemper C, Bartok A, Niosi J, Abramson I, Coffman J, Hughlett C, Loya R, Cassens B, Akil B, Meng T-C, Boylen CT, Nielsen D, Richman DD, Tilles JG, Leedom J, McCutchan JA and the California Collaborative Treatment Group (Univ of California, San Diego; Univ of Southern California; Los Angeles County Hosp; Univ of California, Irvine; Kaiser Permanente Med Ctr, Los Angeles; et al)
N Engl J Med 323:1451–1457, 1990 8–16

Reports of clinical improvement in *Pneumocystis carinii* pneumonia (PCP) from adjunctive steroid therapy prompted a prospective multicenter trial in 333 AIDs patients with PCP. The patients, all receiving standard tratment, were assigned to receive steroid therapy in an equivalent of 40 mg of prednisone twice daily or no additional treatment. A total of 251 patients with confirmed or presumed disease were evaluated.

the risk of respiratory failure in steroid-treated patients was less than half that in the control group. Mortality was twice as great in controls. Dose-limiting toxicity from standard drugs was comparably frequent in the steroid-treated and control patients. Patients with mild disease, as assessed from the degree of hypoxemia, did not benefit clinically from receiving steroid. Herpetic lesions were more frequent in steroid recipients.

Adjunctive steroid therapy can lower mortality from PCP in patients having moderate to severe disease. It is important to confirm the diagnosis so that adverse effects from unsuspected infections such as tuberculosis or cryptococcosis can be avoided.

Corticosteroids as Adjunctive Therapy for Severe *Pneumocystis carinii* Pneumonia in the Acquired Immunodeficiency Syndrome: A Double-Blind, Placebo-Controlled Trial
Gagnon S, Boota AM, Fischl MA, Baier H, Kirksey OW, La Voie L (Univ of Miami; Jackson Med Med Ctr, Miami)
N Engl J Med 323:1444–1450, 1990 8–17

Pneumocystis carinii pneumonia (PCP) is the most common opportu nistic infection in AIDS and causes mortality approaching 25%. Several reports suggest that adjunctive steroid therapy may be helpful if instituted before respiratory failure develops. Accordingly, a double-blind study of methylprednisolone therapy was carried out in 23 patients with severe PCP who had received antibiotics for less than 72 hours.

Twelve patients were randomized to receive methylprednisolone intravenously in a dose of 40 mg every 6 hours for 1 week. Eleven others were assigned to placebo treatment. Trimethoprim-sulfamethoxazole was given to all patients for 3 weeks.

Three steroid-treated patients and 9 placebo recipients had respiratory failure. Steroid recipients spent more time in the hospital on average, but they defervesced more rapidly and had a better arterial blood gas pattern. One patient in each group required transfusion because of gastrointestinal bleeding. Four patients deteriorated after steroid withdrawal and required reinstitution and tapering of the treatment.

Adjunctive corticosteroid treatment tends to prevent respiratory failure when given at an early stage to patients with PCP. Nine of 12 steroid-treated patients in this study survived to be discharged, compared with 2 of 11 placebo recipients. Treatment for at least a week is recommended, followed by tapering of the dosage.

▶ The risk of corticosteroid therapy in AIDS patients seemed enormous. No doubt, long-term use would lead to deleterious consequences, but Abstracts 8–16 and 8–17 studies clearly demonstrate the benefits of the use of corticosteroids in AIDS patients with PCP.—S.M. Wolff, M.D.

Corticosteroids Prevent Early Deterioration in Patients With Moderately Severe *Pneumocystis carinii* Pneumonia and the Acquired Immunodeficiency Syndrome (AIDS)

Montaner JSG, Lawson LM, Levitt N, Belzberg A, Schechter MT, Ruedy J (St Paul's Hosp, Vancouver; Univ of British Columbia, Vancouver)

Ann Intern Med 113:14–20, 1990 8–18

The efficacy of systemic corticosteroid therapy in preventing deterioration in patients with AIDS-related *Pneumocystis carinii* pneumonia (PCP) was investigated in a double-blind, placebo-controlled, randomized study of 37 patients in their first episode of PCP. The patients were within 24 hours of microbiologic confirmation of the diagnosis and within 48 hours of starting antimicrobials specific for *P. carinii* pneumonia. All had oxygen saturation of 85% or more and less than 90% at rest, or a 5% decrease in baseline oxygen saturation with exercise (Fig 8–10). They were randomly assigned to receive either placebo or orally administered prednisone, beginning with a 60-mg dose for 7 days followed by a progressive tapering over 14 days. Early deterioration, defined as a 10% decrease in baseline oxygen saturation at rest occurring not before day 3, was the major end point of the study.

Early deterioration developed in 8 of 19 placebo-treated patients compared with 1 of 18 corticosteroid-treated patients. The adjusted point estimates for the probabilities of early deterioration were 43% in the placebo group and 12% in the treated group. The only treated patient in whom deterioration developed died on day 6 of overwhelming *P. carinii* pneumonia. The 8 patients with early deterioration in the placebo-treated group responded satisfactorily with the addition of corticosteroid treatment. The corticosteroid-treated group also had an increased exercise tolerance on day 7 that persisted at day 30 (Fig 8–11). Oral corticosteroid treatment prevents early deterioration and increases exercise tolerance in patients with AIDS with moderately severe *P. carinii* pneumonia, and is useful adjunctive therapy, particularly when administered early after the diagnosis of *P. carinii* pneumonia.

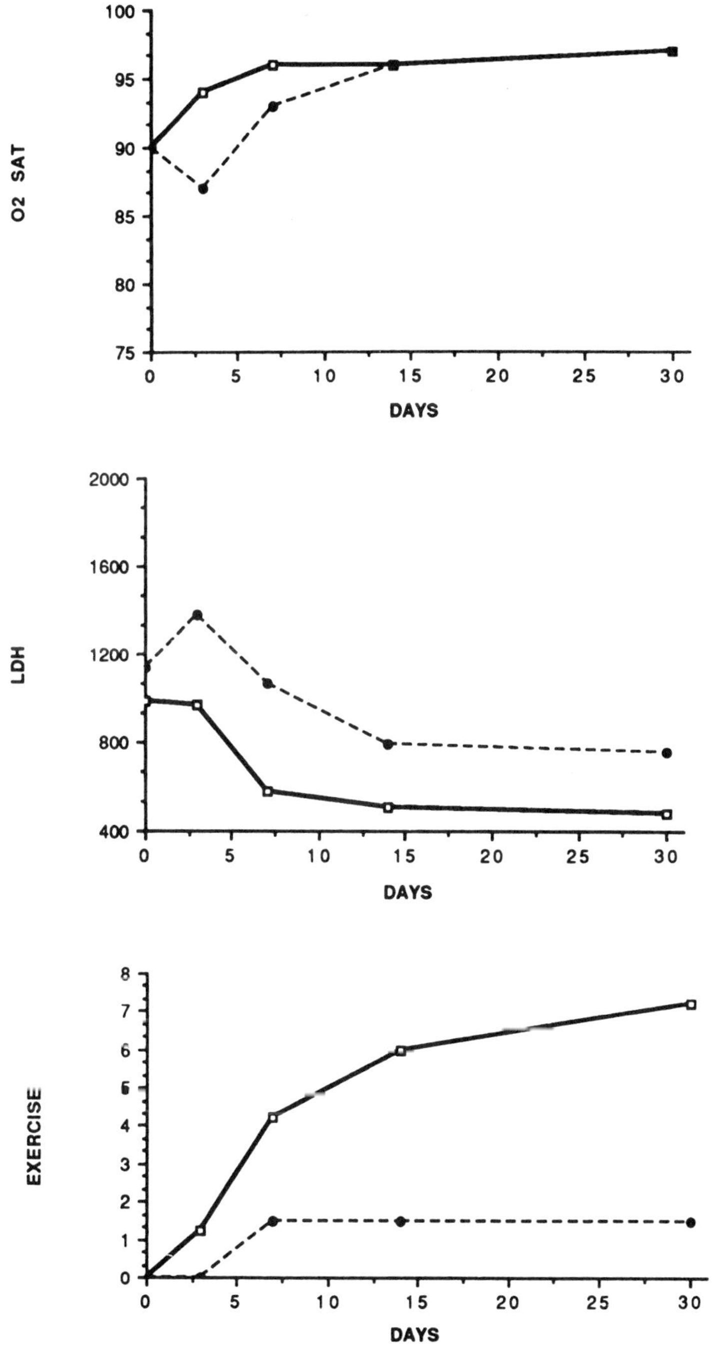

Fig 8–10.—Median oxygen saturation at rest (*O2 SAT,* as a percentage), median lactic dehydrogenase (*LDH,* in units per liter), and median exercise tolerance (*EXERCISE,* in minutes) in patients randomly assigned to receive corticosteroids *(squares)* and placebo *(circles).* (Courtesy of Montaner JSG, Lawson LM, Levitt N, et al: *Ann Intern Med* 113:14–20, 1990.)

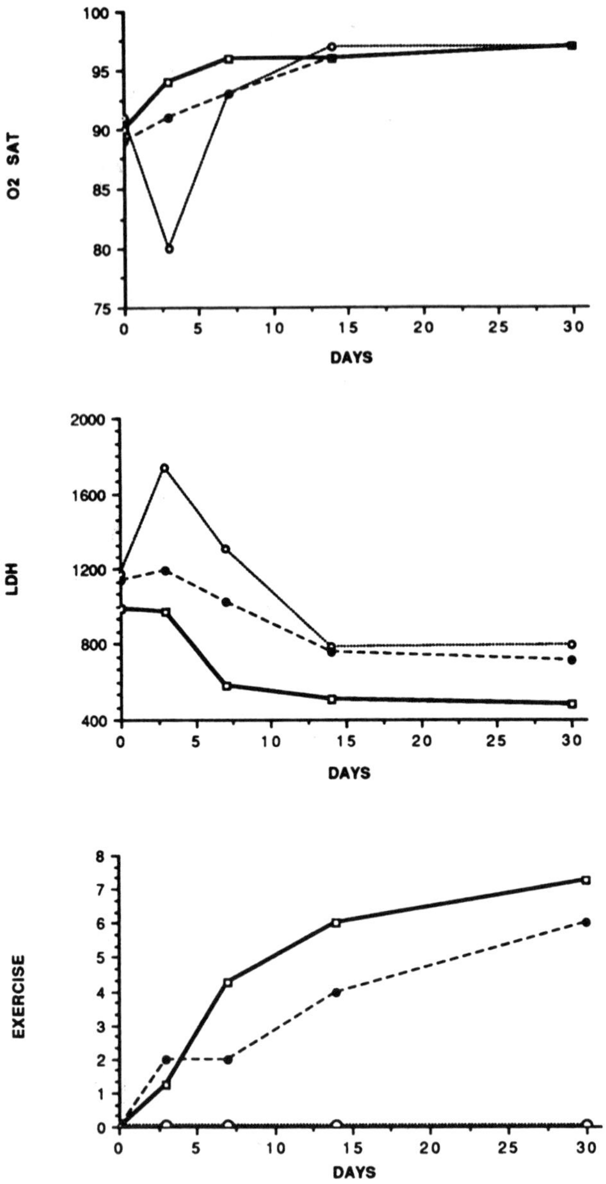

Fig 8–11.—Median oxygen saturation at rest (*o2 SAT,* as a percentage), median lactic dehydrogenase (*LDH,* in units per liter), and median exercise tolerance (*EXERCISE,* in minutes), according to treatment received. Patients initially randomly assigned to corticosteroids *(squares),* patients initially randomly assigned to placebo in whom early deterioration developed and were treated with corticosteroids after day 4 *(open circles),* and patients initially randomly assigned to placebo in whom early deterioration did not develop *(closed circles).* (Courtesy of Montaner JSG, Lawson LM, Levitt N, et al: *Ann Intern Med* 113:14–20, 1990.)

Inhaled or Intravenous Pentamidine Therapy for *Pneumocystis carinii* Pneumonia in AIDS: A Randomized Trial

Soo Hoo GW, Mohsenifar Z, Meyer RD (Cedars-Sinai Med Ctr, Los Angeles; Univ of California, Los Angeles)

Ann Intern Med 113:195–202, 1990 8–19

The standard treatments for *Pneumocystis carinii* pneumonia—trimethoprim-sulfamethoxazole and parenteral pentamidine—frequently cause adverse reactions. Inhaled pentamidine has had some success as an alternative therapy for patients with AIDS and *Pneumocystis* pneumonia, but results of these trials have been mixed. In a prospective randomized trial, inhaled and intravenous pentamidine therapies were compared in 21 men with *Pneumocystis* pneumonia.

Eligible patients were stratified into groups according to room air oxygen pressure less than 8 kPa or at least 8 kPa and the episode of *Pneumocystis* pneumonia (initial or recurrent). They were then randomly assigned to treatment with inhaled pentamidine (11 patients) or intravenous pentamidine (10 patients) given daily for 21 days. Follow-up continued for at least 3 months.

Intravenous pentamidine resulted in a 100% response compared with a 55% response in patients who inhaled the drug. Of the 5 patients who failed to respond, 3 were treated successfully with trimethoprim-sulfamethoxazole. The deaths of the other 2 patients resulted in an 18% mortality rate in the inhaled pentamadine group. Because of this low response rate, the study was terminated before its scheduled completion.

Patients who failed to respond to inhaled pentamidine appeared to have a greater severity of illness at study entry. Compared with respond-

Toxicity Associated With Pentamidine Therapy

Toxicity	Intravenous Pentamidine (n = 10)	Inhaled Pentamidine (n = 11)	P Value*
	n (%)		
Clinical			
Hypotention	4 (40)	0 (0)	0.04
Nausea or emesis	6 (60)	2 (18)	0.06
Rash	1 (10)	0 (0)	0.48
Drug fever	2 (20)	0 (0)	0.21
Dysgeusia	5 (50)	0 (0)	0.01
Cough or wheezing	0 (0)	9 (82)	0.002
Laboratory			
Neutropenia	5 (50)	0 (0)	0.01
Thrombocytopenia	1 (10)	0 (0)	0.48
Azotemia	3 (30)	0 (0)	0.09
Dysglycemia	5 (50)	3 (27)	0.27
Hypoglycemia	3 (30)	3 (27)	0.63
Hyperglycemia	2 (20)	0 (0)	0.21

**P* value from the Fisher exact test.

(Courtesy of Soo Hoo GW, Mohsenifar Z, Meyer RD: *Ann Intern Med* 113:195–202, 1990.)

ers, nonresponders had a lower mean arterial oxygen pressure and a higher arterial-alveolar gradient in PO_2. Those with milder disease clearly improved with inhaled pentamidine, but this form of therapy should not be used in patients with moderate or severe disease. Although intravenous therapy produced a higher response rate, it also caused substantially greater adverse systemic effects (table).

▶ This study, which was prematurely discontinued because of the poor response to aerosolized pentamidine, constitutes another blow to the popularity of inhaled pentamidine, which had already been falling into disfavor for prophylaxis. The results were particularly poor among patients with more severe disease. The authors attribute this result to the observation that sicker patients breathe more rapidly and shallowly than less sick ones, reducing alveolar ventilation and drug delivery. Moreover, the most heavily infected areas of the lung tend also to be poorly ventilated, further reducing drug delivery to important sites. As would be expected, the patients given pentamidine intravenously had a much higher rate of drug toxicity than those given the drug by aerosol, and the intravenous treatment had to be discontinued in 4 of 10 patients. Surprisingly, 3 of 10 patients given aerosolized pentamidine had hypoglycemia. Based on the accumulating data, it seems likely that aerosolized pentamidine will be relegated to a minor role for the prophylaxis and treatment of patients with HIV infection.—M. Barza, M.D.

Intravenous or Inhaled Pentamidine for Treating *Pneumocystis carinii* Pneumonia in AIDS: A Randomized Trial

Conte JE Jr, Chernoff D, Feigal DW Jr, Joseph P, McDonald C, Golden JA (Univ of California, San Francisco; Pacific Presbyterian Med Ctr, San Francisco; Peralta Hosp, Oakland, Calif)

Ann Intern Med 113:203–209, 1990 8–20

The value of aerosolized pentamidine was compared with that of reduced-dose intravenous treatment in treating mild to moderate *Pneumocystis carinii* pneumonia (PCP) in 45 patients with AIDS. In the initial episode of PCP, the arterial oxygen pressure was 55 mm Hg or greater. Pentamidine isethionate, 600 mg, was administered to 23 patients using a Respigard II nebulizer, and pentamidine, 3 mg/kg, was administered intravenously daily for 2–3 weeks in 22 patients.

Aerosol therapy failed in 12% of patients and intravenous treatment failed in 19%. The respective rates of early recrudescence was 35% and 0. Relapse occurred in 24% of aerosol-treated patients, but in none of those given pentamidine intravenously. Major toxicity occurred in 10% of patients given intravenous treatment. Much greater concentrations of drug were present in the bronchoalveolar lavage fluid in patients given aerosolized treatment. The mean trough plasma drug level after 3 weeks of intravenous therapy was 61 ng/mL.

A comparatively low dose of intravenously administered pentamidine was more effective than aerosolized pentamidine in treating mild to moderate PCP in these patients. Whether adjunctive measures can prevent early recrudescence of symptoms or relapse warrants further investigation.

▶ There have been several trials comparing inhaled pentamidine with reduced-dose intravenous pentamidine. The rate of early relapse in the group given the inhaled form precludes this approach, in my view.—D.R. Snydman, M.D.

Aerosolized Pentamidine for Prophylaxis Against *Pneumocystis carinii* Pneumonia: The San Francisco Community Prophylaxis Trial

Leoung GS, Feigal DW Jr, Montgomery AB, Corkery K, Wardlaw L, Adams M, Busch D, Gordon S, Jacobson MA, Volberding PA, Abrams D and the San Francisco County Community Consortium (San Francisco Gen Hosp; Univ of California, San Francisco; Children's Hosp, San Francisco; Pacific Med Ctr, San Francisco; State Univ of New York, Stony Brook; et al)

N Engl J Med 323:769–775, 1990 8–21

Pneumocystis carinii pneumonia (PCP) remains the most frequent life-threatening opportunistic infection leading to the diagnosis of AIDS and the most common cause of death from HIV infection. A controlled trial of aerosolized pentamidine, which is becoming standard community practice, was undertaken in a prospective series of 441 patients seen in an 18-month period at 12 treatment centers in the San Francisco area. Study patients received 30 mg of aerosolized pentamidine isethionate every 2 weeks, 150 mg every 2 weeks, or 300 mg every 4 weeks.

Episodes of PCP were least frequent with 300 mg of pentamidine. The 150-mg dose was consistently less effective than the higher dose. Zidovudine therapy independently lowered the risk of PCP by a factor of 2. Mortality did not differ significantly among any of the groups. During the study period, PCP caused 12% of deaths. About 6% of participants discontinued taking aerosolized pentamidine because of adverse effects, but in only 2% were those associated directly with treatment.

Aerosolized pentamidine is an effective means of preventing PCP in HIV-infected patients at high risk. Adverse effects are less frequent and less severe than with systemic treatment. A combination of prophylaxis with antiretroviral treatment may prevent most episodes of PCP in HIV-infected persons.

▶ This well-done study clearly demonstrates the beneficial effects of aerosolized pentamidine as prophylaxis against PCP. I look forward to the time when we can correct the underlying immune deficit in AIDS patients and can avoid the necessity for treating the opportunistic infections.—S.M. Wolff, M.D.

Oral Therapy for *Pneumocystis carinii* Pneumonia in the Acquired Immunodeficiency Syndrome: A Controlled Trial of Trimethoprim-Sulfamethoxazole versus Trimethoprim-Dapsone

Medina I, Mills J, Leoung G, Hopewell PC, Lee B, Modin G, Benowitz N, Wofsy CB (Univ of California, San Francisco)

N Engl J Med 323:776–782, 1990 8–22

Patients with AIDS require orally active antimicrobials for use in treating *Pneumocystis carinii* pneumonia (PCP). There is some evidence that dapsone combined with trimethoprim may be an effective alternative to trimethoprim-sulfamethoxazole (TMP-SMX), which often has toxic effects.

In a double-blind trial, 60 AIDS patients with a first episode of PCP who were mildly to moderately ill were assigned to receive 1 of 2 regimens for 3 weeks. Some patients received TMP-SMX in respective daily doses of 10 mg/kg and 100 mg/kg, whereas others received 20 mg of trimethoprim per kg combined with 100 mg of dapsone daily.

Five patients deteriorated markedly early in the course of treatment and were given pentamidine intravenously; 1 of them died. Hepatitis and neutropenia were more frequent in patients given TMP-SMX therapy. Most clinical features failed to distinguish between the 2 treatment groups. Overall survival and relapse rates also were comparable in the 2 groups.

The oral administration of trimethoprim and dapsone is a reasonable approach to AIDS patients with mild to moderately severe PCP. Further experience with this treatment is needed, however, to assess the importance of such complications as methemoglobinemia and hyperkalemia.

▶ Important support for the use of trimethoprim-dapsone rather than TMP-SMX. However I am afraid the latter is so commonly used that change will be slow, if at all.—S.M. Wolff, M.D.

Treatment of Disseminated *Mycobacterium avium* Complex Infection in AIDS With Amikacin, Ethambutol, Rifampin, and Ciprofloxacin

Chiu J, Nussbaum J, Bozzette S, Tilles JG, Young LS, Leedom J, Heseltine PNR, McCutchan JA, and the California Collaborative Treatment Group (Univ of California, Irvine; Los Angeles County-Univ of Southern California Med Ctr; Univ of California, San Diego; Kuzell Inst for Arthritis and Infectious Diseases, San Francisco)

Ann Intern Med 113:358–361, 1990 8–23

The treatment of *Mycobacterium avium* complex infection in the immunocompromised patient has been frustrating. In a prospective nonrandomized study the efficacy of combination drug therapy with amikacin, ethambutol, rifampin, and ciprofloxacin in treating disseminated *M. avium* complex infection was evaluated in patients with AIDS.

Fifteen of the 17 patients with at least 2 consecutive blood cultures positive for *M. avium* complex who had not been treated previously with antituberculous drugs completed at least 4 weeks of treatment. These patients received daily intravenous injections of amikacin, 7.5 mg/kg, for the first 4 weeks plus the following oral medications for at least 12 weeks: ciprofloxacin, 750 mg twice daily; ethambutol, 1,000 mg daily; and rifampin, 600 mg daily.

Effect of Length of Therapy on Symptoms Associated With *Mycobacterium avium* Complex and on Colony Count

Variable	Weeks of Therapy				
	0	4	8	12	More Than 12
Patients, *n*	15	15	11	10	8
Weight†, *kg*	57.4 ± 10.5	57.5 ± 9.0	55.3 ± 9.3	56.9 ± 9.0	51.0 ± 5.5
Patients reporting symptoms, *n(%)*					
Fever	14 (93)	4 (27)‡	4 (36)	3 (30)	5 (63)
Night sweats	13 (87)	6 (40)‡	2 (18)	1 (10)	2 (25)
Diarrhea	6 (40)	4 (27)§	2 (18)	4 (40)	4 (50)
M. avium bacteremia, *CFU/mL**					
Geometric mean	537	14‖	28‖	15‖	1‖
Log mean ± SE	2.7 ± 0.4	1.2 ± 0.3	1.4 ± 0.4	1.2 ± 0.5	0.1 ± 0.3
Range	5–100 000	0–1000	0–12 800	0–24 160	0–10

*CFU, colony-forming unit.
†Mean ± standard deviation.
‡$P < .05$ compared with week 0 using chi-square analysis.
§$P = .698$ compared with week 0 using chi-square analysis.
‖$P < .05$ compared with week 0 using 2-tailed t test.
(Courtesy of Chiu J, Nussbaum J, Bozzette S, et al: *Ann Intern Med* 113:358–361, 1990.)

The geometric mean colony count from blood cultures fell from 537/mL at baseline to 14/mL after 4 weeks of therapy (table). This microbiologic suppression was sustained during treatment and was accompanied by significant improvement of systemic symptoms. Of the 10 patients who completed 12 weeks of therapy, bacteremia was terminated in 3, reduced in 5, and increased only in 2. Clinical and microbiologic improvement occurred early and rapidly in most patients, and none acquired concomitant infections before 12 weeks.

Symptoms recurred after 12 weeks of therapy in 7 patients, often because of new opportunistic infections. All isolates were sensitive to amikacin, but no isolate was sensitive to all 3 oral agents. Treatment was discontinued prematurely in 7 patients because of gastrointestinal intolerance and hepatic toxicity.

Combination therapy with amikacin, ethambutol, rifampin, and ciprofloxacin is the first drug regimen to show symptomatic relief and reduction of bacteremia prospectively in patients with AIDS and disseminated *M. avium* complex infection. The morbidity associated with *M. avium* complex infection may be related to mycobacterial load and can be reduced with appropriate regimens that suppress mycobacterial growth.

Quadruple-Drug Therapy for *Mycobacterium avium-intracellulare* Bacteremia in AIDS Patients

Hoy J, Mijch A, Sandland M, Grayson L, Lucas R, Dwyer B (Fairfield Infectious Diseases Hosp, Melbourne)
J Infect Dis 161:801–805, 1990

8–24

TABLE 1.—Symptoms and Signs of Patients With AIDS on Presentation With Disseminated MAC and Subsequent Clinical Response

Symptom/sign	No. at presentation	No. resolved after 3 months treatment
Sweats	22	21
Fever	21	20
Lethargy	11	7
Cough	6	3
Myalgia	5	5
Abdominal pain	5	3
Headache	4	4
Acute brain syndrome	2	2
Lymphadenopathy		
Cervical/inguinal	6	5
Mediastinal/hilar	2	0
Mesenteric/paraaortic	2	1

(Courtesy of Hoy J, Mijch A, Sandland M, et al: *J Infect Dis* 161:801–805, 1990.)

TABLE 2.—Effect of Quadruple Drug Regimen on MAC Bacteremia in Patients With AIDS

Patient	No., type of pretherapy cultures positive for MAC	Weeks of quadruple-drug therapy (to May '89)	Rifabutin daily dose (mg)	Blood cultures by week of therapy: Positive	Blood cultures by week of therapy: Negative
1	2, B	50	300	None	4, 10, 14, 18, 22, 32, 34, 38, 42, 44, 46, 50, 52, 56, 62
2	2, B, brain biopsy	39	300	4	9, 14, 16, 24
3	2, B, bone marrow; bronchial lavage	52	300	6	4, 10, 16, 18, 20, 24, 30, 36, 40, 50
4	B, bone marrow, lymph node	74	450	None	2, 4, 6, 10, 12, 16, 18, 26, 40, 46, 52, 60, 64, 72
5	2, B; F, urine; bronchial lavage	35	300	2, 25, 28	4, 8, 10, 12, 14, 16, 18
6	4, B; urine, F	26	300	11, 15, 22, 30	2, 28
7	3, B; F	59	600	None	4, 6, 8, 10, 12, 14, 16, 20, 24, 30, 33, 37, 56
8	2, B; F	8	300	6, 8	2, 4, 7
9	Sputum, B, F	17	300	4, 8, 11	None
10	B, F	26	450	None	2, 4, 6, 8, 11, 18
11	2, B; F	34	300	1	3, 6, 8, 10, 14, 26
12	3, B	22	450	2	4, 11, 14
13	3, B; sputum	52	600	None	10, 15, 20, 25, 29, 35, 44
14	4, B; bronchial lavage	52	300	5	8, 16, 18, 23, 25, 29, 32, 36, 39
15	3, B	44	600	6, 12	2, 4, 16, 19, 20, 24, 27, 30, 33, 40
16	3, B	45	450	2, 11, 14, 19, 21, 27, 31, 34, 37, 40	None
17	4, B	45	300	1, 4, 38, 40	10, 12, 21, 24, 28, 33
18	B, lymph node, F	54	300	17	6, 12, 21, 26, 39
19*	B, F	21	600	45, 47, 50, 52	23, 27, 34, 38, 65
20	2, B; F	40	600	0	5, 6, 8, 10, 13, 15, 18, 22, 31
21	3, B; sputum	35	450	1	9, 12, 13, 15, 19, 23, 25
22	4, B; sputum; 3, F; urine	38	450	1	7, 9, 11, 14, 16, 19
23	3, B	39	450	2	8, 12, 16
24	2, B	24	450	1, 4	3, 5, 15, 16
25	4, B; F; sputum	24	450	None	7, 9, 14, 20

Abbreviations: B, blood; *F*, feces.
*Treated initially for 6 weeks; resumed treatment 40 weeks after cessation.
(Courtesy of Hoy J, Mijch A, Sandland M, et al: *J Infect Dis* 161:801–805, 1990.)

Mycobacterium avium-intracellulare complex (MAC) is a frequent opportunistic pathogen in AIDS patients. The value of quadruple-drug therapy was examined in 25 patients with AIDS who had MAC cultured from the blood on multiple occasions, or from the blood and another source. All had an illness consistent with MAC infection. The drugs administered were rifabutin, clofazimine, ethambutol, and isoniazid. Treatment usually was continued indefinitely.

Signs and symptoms of patients with AIDS on presentation with MAC and subsequent clinical responses are shown in Table 1. All but 3 of the 25 patients had negative blood cultures after starting treatment, but MAC bacteremia recurred in 6 patients, transiently in 2 of them. Mycobacteremia cleared in 13 of 16 patients harboring rifabutin-resistant MAC and in all 8 whose strains were susceptible to this drug. Symptoms resolved completely in 18 patients. Fourteen patients died, none of disseminated MAC infection. Quadruple therapy including rifabutin in a daily dose of 300–600 mg (Table 2) appears to clear mycobacteremia and to combat symptoms effectively in patients with AIDS who have MAC bacteremia.

▶ In a recent review of MAC infections in AIDS patients, Horsburgh (1) argues strongly in favor of multidrug treatment. The more favorable results of recent studies, including those reported in Abstract 8–23 and 8–24, may in part relate to the use of combined antimicrobial therapy started early in the course of the patient's symptoms. In previous studies, therapy was usually delayed until patients were almost terminal. The oral combination of ciprofloxacin, clofazamine, ethambutol, and rifampin provides a good starting point with agents that are currently available and are usually well tolerated in this patient population. If the patient does not respond after 4–6 weeks, the addition of amikacin is reasonable. Studies in progress include trials of the macrolides, clarithromycin, and azithromycin, and I'm sure we'll see changes in the recommended regimens in the coming year. However, I favor early treatment of symptomatic MAC infections in patients with AIDS.—M.S. Klempner, M.D.

Reference

1. Horsburgh CR: *N Engl J Med* 324:1332, 1991.

Radiographic Distribution of *Pneumocystis carinii* Pneumonia in Patients With AIDS Treated With Prophylactic Inhaled Pentamidine

Chaffey MH, Klein JS, Gamsu G, Blanc P, Golden JA (Univ of California, San Francisco)

Radiology 175:715–719, 1990 8–25

The monthly administration of inhaled pentamidine has been shown to be an effective prophylaxis against *Pneumocystis carinii* in patients with AIDS. Recurrent *P. carinii* pneumonia is distributed in the upper lobes of the lungs of patients treated with inhaled pentamidine. To determine whether other factors might account for this finding, 64 patients with AIDS and *P. carinii* pneumonia were studied.

Twenty-three patients received 300 mg of aerosolized pentamidine monthly; the remaining 41 patients were not receiving this treatment. All but 1 of the 64 patients had parenchymal abnormalities. Fifty had radiographic opacities of a grade at least 1+ in the upper lung zones caused by *P. carinii* pneumonia.

Patients who received inhaled pentamidine were more likely than control patients to have disease isolated or predominant in the upper lobes (odds ratio = 3.9). Prophylaxis remained a significant risk factor independent of patient age and the duration of pentamidine therapy. Although previous *P. carinii* pneumonia may independently predispose the upper lobes of the lung to recurrent pneumonia, data did not suggest that prior *P. carinii* pneumonia accounted for the relationship of prophylaxis to upper lung disease.

The reason for a predisposition to isolated or dominant *P. carinii* pneumonia in the upper lobes among patients who receive prophylaxis remains unclear. The finding may be traced, however, to the pattern of deposition or retention of the aerosolized drug.

▶ Recurrent *Pneumocystis* infection remains a problem in AIDS patients receiving aerosolized pentamidine (AP) prophylaxis. Because drug resistance is not the reason, other possibilities need to be evaluated so that appropriate measures may be taken. This study shows a significant predilection for patients given AP to have either isolated or predominant disease in the upper lobes, although a similar percentage of non–AP-treated patients had some degree of upper lobe abnormalities. The proportion with upper lobe involvement did not differ among first-time and repeat *P. carinii* infections, thus it is not likely that the difference observed with AP was related to recurrence per se. It is suggested that mechanical factors relating to distribution of the inhaled drug may be the responsible factor. If so, then in-progress studies described by the investigators to determine the physical factors influencing regional pulmonary drug distribution may permit selection of more optimal conditions for AP administration.—G.T. Keusch, M.D.

Intestinal Microsporidiosis as a Cause of Diarrhea in Human Immunodeficiency Virus-Infected Patients: A Report of 20 Cases

Orenstein JM, Chiang J, Steinberg W, Smith PD, Rotterdam H, Kotler DP
(George Washington Univ; Natl Inst of Dental Research, Washington DC; New York Univ, St Luke's-Roosevelt Hosp, New York)

Hum Pathol 21:475–481, 1990 8–26

Chronic diarrhea accompanied by weight loss is a common, often debilitating problem in patients with HIV infection. *Enterocytozoon bieneusi,* a newly identified species of the protozoan phylum Microspora, has been associated with chronic diarrhea and wasting in a small number of AIDS patients in the United States, Europe, and Africa. Diagnosis was based solely on the ultrastructural identification of this small, intracellular parasite in bowel biopsy specimens. Another series was reviewed in which intestinal microsporidiosis was a cause of diarrhea in HIV-infected patients.

Seventy-one small bowel biopsies were done in 67 homosexual patients with AIDS and AIDS-related complex. The patients had chronic diarrhea, but no pathogens were identified by light microscopy on paraffin sections. The biopsy specimens were embedded in plastic and studied by light and transmission electron microscopy. *Enterocytozoon bieneusi* microsporidiosis was diagnosed by electron microscopy in 22 biopsy specimens obtained from 20 patients. More jejunal biopsies than duodenal biopsies were positive. Parasites and spores could be seen clearly at the light microscopic level in the semithin plastic sections from 17 and 21 of the specimens, respectively. Parasites could be identified retrospectively by light microscopy in standard hematoxylin- and eosin-stained paraffin sections. Infection was confined to enterocytes covering the villi, especially the tips. It was associated with villous atrophy and cell degeneration, necrosis, and sloughing. Spores were released into the bowel lumen. In 2 patients with small bowel microsporidiosis, colorectal biopsies were negative for microsporidia.

This study documents the association between infection of the small intestine by a species of Microspora and severe diarrhea in HIV infection. It stresses the need for doing more than simply stool examinations and light microscopic studies of endoscopic biopsy specimens, particularly if the patient is immunocompromised.

▶ Chronic diarrhea and wasting syndrome in AIDS patients remains a vexing problem, both from the lack of certainty as to etiology as well as the difficulty of management. This study shows the presence of *E. bieneusi* in the small bowel biopsy tissue of a large number of patients with chronic diarrhea of unknown cause. Unfortunately, the diagnosis is difficult by other than invasive methods and electron microscopy, although there are attempts to develop an enzyme-linked immunoassay or other methods to look for parasite markers in the stool. The real prevalence of this organism remains unknown, and without the ability to treat (and thus to collect data from therapeutic trial), or to fulfill Koch's third postulate by experimental infection of humans, its pathogenic potential cannot be fully assessed. If reinfection from the gut lumen is a part of the life cycle contributing to intestinal manifestations, as it is in cryptosporidiosis, then like *Cryptosporidium parvum, Microspora* infection may be amenable to passive immunotherapy using antibody derived from bovine colostrum from immunized cows. Assuming that nothing else will come along to treat the infection, and that subsequent studies will confirm the high prevalence of infection in AIDS patients with undiagnosed chronic diarrhea, it may be wise now to encourage applied research designed to develop an antibody product for clinical testing.—G.T. Keusch, M.D.

Disseminated Adenovirus Infection With Hepatic Necrosis in Patients With Human Immunodeficiency Virus Infection and Other Immunodeficiency States

Krilov LR, Rubin LG, Frogel M, Gloster E, Ni K, Kaplan M, Lipson SM (Schneider Children's Hosp, Long Island Jewish Med Ctr, New Hyde Park, NY; State Univ

of New York, Stony Brook; North Shore Univ Hosp, Manhasset, NY; Cornell Med College; Nassau County Med Ctr, East Meadow, NY)
Rev Infect Dis 12:303–307, 1990 8–27

Disseminated adenovirus infection with fatal hepatic necrosis has been described in immunodeficiency states. Three patients were seen with HIV infection who also had disseminated adenovirus infection with hepatic necrosis.

Sixteen cases of disseminated adenovirus infection with fatal hepatic necrosis have been described. All but 1 patient had an underlying immunodeficiency state (table). In the 3 patients examined in this report, the cause of the immunodeficiency state was infection with HIV. One patient had no antibody to HIV, but the presence of HIV core antigen plus thrush and failure to thrive indicated an HIV-related immunodeficiency state. The majority of the 16 patients were children, and the median age was 4.7 years. In addition to hepatitis, the clinical course was characterized by fever, coagulopathy, lower respiratory tract disease, and gastrointestinal hemorrhage. Signs of pulmonary involvement were absent in 6 patients. The most commonly recovered isolates were of the serotypes 1, 2, 3, 5, and 7 that accounted for 13 of the 15 isolates. One patient had serotype 4, and another had serotype 31.

Considering the high frequency of adenovirus infection in humans and

Data From Patients With Adenovirus Hepatic Necrosis

Underlying condition	Adenovirus type	Patient's age (y)	Reference
HIV infection	1	7	PR
HIV infection	2	0.5	PR
HIV infection, lymphoma	3	24	PR
SCID	2	0.83	1
SCID	2	0.17	2
SCID	31	0.5	3
SCID	7	0.46	4
SCID	5	0.10	5
ALL	5	19	6
Hodgkin's disease	ND	28	7
Bone marrow transplantation, AA	5	13	8
Bone marrow transplantation, AML	1	24	8
Bone marrow transplantation, XEBV	5	19	9
Liver transplantation	5	1.5	10
Liver transplantation	5	4	10
None	4	5.5	12

Abbreviations: PR, present report; *SCID,* severe combined immunodeficiency; *ALL,* acute lymphocytic leukemia; *ND,* not determined; *AA,* aplastic anemia; *AML,* acute myelogenous leukemia; *XEBV,* X-linked lymphoproliferative syndrome with Epstein-Barr virus infection.

(Courtesy of Krilov LR, Rubin LG, Frogel M, et al: *Rev Infect Dis* 12:303–307, 1990.)

the increasing prevalence of HIV infection in children, it appears that disseminated adenovirus infection will continue to be seen. Currently, there are no effective chemotherapeutic agents against adenoviruses.

▶ In this review of published cases of disseminated adenovirus infection, nearly all of the patients were immunosuppressed and two thirds were children with severe combined immunodeficiency disease or organ transplants as the underlying reason for the immunosuppression. This study adds 3 more patients with HIV infection, including a 24-year-old woman with AIDS and non-Hodgkin's lymphoma. This suggests that as the HIV epidemic progresses, we will see more systemic adenovirus infections. Treatment at present is rather limited. Ribavirin is the likely agent to try first, based on in vitro activity, but I wouldn't expect too much.—G.T. Keusch, M.D.

Life-Threatening Bacteraemia in HIV-1 Seropositive Adults Admitted to Hospital in Nairobi, Kenya

Gilks CF, Brindle RJ, Otieno LS, Simani PM, Newnham RS, Bhatt SM, Lule GN, Okelo GBA, Watkins WM, Waiyaki PG, Were JBO, Warrell DA (Kenya Med Research Inst, Nairobi; Univ of Nairobi; Oxford Univ, England)

Lancet 336:545–549, 1990 8–28

The risk of infection with nonopportunistic bacterial pathogens in patients infected with HIV type I is well recognized in the industrialized world, but this relationship has not been studied in Africa. A cross-sectional study was carried out to assess the prevalence of bacteremia and its relation to HIV status and outcome among adult emergency admissions to the main government hospital serving Nairobi.

The study population comprised 304 men and 202 women hospitalized during a 6-month study period. Laboratory evaluation included blood culture, HIV serology, and antimicrobial sensitivity. Of the 506 patients, 95 (19%) were seropositive and 411 were seronegative for HIV-1. Bacteremia was confirmed in 25 (26.3%) seropositive patients and in 26 (6.3%) seronegative patients (Table 1). The difference was statistically significant. *Streptococcus pneumoniae* and *Salmonella typhimurium* were the predominant organisms isolated from the seropositive patients. Mortality was higher in the seropositive than in the seronegative bacteremic patients, but the numbers were too small to be statistically significant (Table 2). As acute bacterial infections caused at least 25% of all HIV-related medical admissions to the largest hospital in East Africa, they are likely causing similar problems elsewhere.

▶ This is an extremely simple, but extraordinarily useful, study. The authors are to be congratulated and encouraged to continue with this sort of applied clinical research. I say, simple; however, I know very well how difficult it can be to carry out "simple" studies in resource-limiting environments in developing countries. Gilks et al. have shown that bacteremia is common in HIV-1 patients in Nairobi, and that the most common causes are common organisms, and not

TABLE 1.—Clinically Significant Blood Culture Isolates

Organism	HIV-1 antibody status: Positive *(%)* (n=95)	Negative *(%)* (n=411)	Odds-ratio (95% CI)
Enterobacteriaceae			
Salmonella typhimurium	10 *(11·1)*	1 *(0·3)*	48·2 (13–176)
Salmonella vitiki	0	1 *(0·3)*	*
Salmonella typhi	2 *(2·1)*	5 *(1·2)*	NS
Escherichia coli	2 *(2·1)*	1 *(0·3)*	*
Shigella flexneri	1 *(1·1)*	0	*
Enterobacter cloacae	0	1 *(0·3)*	*
Other gram-negative organisms			
Neisseria meningitidis	1 *(1·1)*	4 *(1·0)*	NS
Bacteroides fragilis	1 *(1·1)*	1 *(0·3)*	*
Pseudomonas aeruginosa	0	1 *(0·3)*	*
Aeromonas salmonicida	0	1 *(0·3)*	*
Gram-positive organisms			
Streptococcus pneumoniae	7 *(7·4)*	7 *(1·7)*	4·6 (1·5–14·0)
Streptococcus pyogenes	0	1 *(0·3)*	*
Staphylococcus aureus	1 *(1·1)*	2 *(0·5)*	*
Total bacteraemias	25 *(26·3)*	26 *(6·3)*	5·3 (3·0–9·4)
Yeast			
Cryptococcus neoformans	1 *(1·1)*	0	*

Abbreviations: CI, confidence interval; *NS,* not significant.
*Insufficient numbers for statistical comparison.
(Courtesy of Gilks CF, Brindle RJ, Otieno LS, et al: *Lancet* 336:545–549, 1990.)

exotic or rare opportunists. As such, these infections are eminently treatable using inexpensive and readily available antibiotics. These data can form the basis of a treatment algorithm in Kenya, and it would not be unreasonable to expect that a similar algorithm could be proposed for other African countries, with some local refinements as culture data became available. An algorithm would

TABLE 2.—Mortality in 24 HIV Seropositive and 25 Seronegative Patients Who Were Bacteremic on Admission

	No of deaths *(%)*: HIV-1-seropositive	HIV-1-seronegative
All Enterobacteriaceae	11/15 *(73)*	1/9 *(11)*‡
Salm typhimurium	8/10 *(80)*	0/1
Strep pneumoniae	2/7 *(29)*	3/7 *(43)*
Other bacteria	1/2* *(50)*	3/7† *(43)*
All bacteraemias	14/24* *(58)*	8/25† *(32)*

*One seropositive patient with *Staphylococcus* bacteremia absconded after 24 hours and is excluded.
†One seropositive patient with *Bacteroides fragilis* bacteremia absconded after 2 days and is excluded.
‡P = .0009, Fisher's exact 2-tail test.
(Courtesy of Gilks CF, Brindle RJ, Otieno LS, et al: *Lancet* 336:545–549, 1990.)

be preferable to existing practice and the sense of frustration among dedicated African clinicians working with large numbers of HIV-infected patients with little laboratory resources to help them determine etiology and direct therapy. Unfortunately, research related to patient-care issues, especially in adults, is not attractive to funding agencies. Nonetheless, attention to adult health in the Third World is a key to improved child survival. In the AIDS belt, diminished adult morbidity and delayed mortality will favorably affect the survival of the two thirds of their offspring who are HIV negative. Its not too late to remember that adults care for and nurture children, are the economically productive members of the family, and must be considered in health care programs.—G.T. Keusch, M.D.

Therapy

Zidovudine in Asymptomatic Human Immunodeficiency Virus Infection: A Controlled Trial in Persons With Fewer than 500 CD4-Positive Cells per Cubic Millimeter

Volberding PA, Lagakos SW, Koch MA, Pettinelli C, Myers MW, Booth DK, Balfour HH Jr, Reichman RC, Bartlett JA, Hirsch MS, Murphy RL, Hardy WD, Soeiro R, Fischl MA, Bartlett JG, Merigan TC, Hyslop NE, Richman DD, Valentine FT, Corey L, and the AIDS Clinical Trial Group of the National Institute of Allergy and Infectious Diseases (Univ of California, San Francisco; Harvard School of Public Health; Research Triangle Inst, Research Triangle Park, NC; Natl Inst of Allergy and Infectious Diseases, Bethesda, Md; Univ of Minnesota; et al)
N Engl J Med 322:941–949, 1990 8–29

The use of zidovudine in patients with advanced HIV infection has led to improvement in survival beyond 18 months of treatment; however, prolonged use of zidovudine has been associated with increased tolerance to the drug and a risk for myopathy. To provide further information, asymptomatic adults with HIV infection and initial CD4+ cell counts below 500/μL were entered into a study. Subjects (92% of whom were men) were randomized to receive either placebo; zidovudine, 500 mg/day; zidovudine, 1,500 mg/day. Patients were followed for a mean of 55 weeks.

In 33 of 428 subjects receiving placebo, AIDS developed during follow-up; AIDS developed in 11 of 453 receiving 500 mg of zidovudine and 14 of 457 receiving 1,500 mg of zidovudine. Rates of progression to either AIDS or advanced AIDS-related complex per 100 person-years were 7.6, 3.6, and 4.3 for the placebo-treated group, the 500-mg zidovudine group, and the 1,500-mg zidovudine group, respectively. Patients given zidovudine had significant increases in the number of CD4+ cells and significant declines in p24 antigen levels as compared to those given placebo. In the higher-dose zidovudine group, patients were more likely to have anemia or neutropenia. Nausea was the only side effect that was significantly more frequent in the 500-mg zidovudine group than in the placebo group.

Zidovudine is safe and effective in patients with asymptomatic HIV infection and fewer than 500 CD4+ cells/μL. It remains to be seen whether zidovudine treatment will improve survival in these patients.

▶ Although both the low dose (500 mg/day) and the commonly employed dose (1,500 mg/day) slowed progression to AIDS, the low dose offers major advances in decreasing toxicity and cost. As early trials are beginning to suggest, combination therapy with low-dose zidovudine and other agents such as ddI (see Abstract 8–30) will be the regimes of choice in the future.—S.M. Wolff, M.D.

A Randomized Controlled Trial of a Reduced Daily Dose of Zidovudine in Patients With the Acquired Immunodeficiency Syndrome

Fischl MA, Parker CB, Pettinelli C, Wulfsohn M, Hirsch MS, Collier AC, Antoniskis D, Ho M, Richman DD, Fuchs E, Merigan TC, Reichman RC, Gold J, Steigbigel N, Leoung GS, Rasheed S, Tsiatis A and the AIDS Clinical Trials Group (Univ of Miami; Research Triangle Inst, Research Triangle Park, NC; Natl Inst of Allergy and Infectious Diseases, Bethesda, Md; Harvard School of Public Health, Boston; Harvard Med School; et al)

N Engl J Med 323:1009–1014, 1990 8–30

Initially, a dose of 1,500 mg of zidovudine was used to treat patients with advanced HIV-1 disease. This dose is effective but produces substantial toxicity. The efficacy of lower doses was examined in 524 patients having a first episode of *Pneumocystis carinii* pneumonia (PCP). Patients took either 250 mg of zidovudine orally every 4 hours, or 200 mg every 4 hours for 4 weeks followed by 100 mg every 4 hours. The median follow-up was 26 months.

Survival rates at 18 months were 52% for patients given standard treatment and 63% for the low-dose group. At 2 years, 27% and 34%, respectively, were alive. About 80% of patients in both groups had further opportunistic infection at a similar interval. A fall in hemoglobin and neutropenia both were more prevalent in patients given standard treatment.

A reduced daily dose of zidovudine was at least as effective in treating advanced HIV disease as conventional dosing in this study and was less toxic. In particular, problems with severe anemia were less frequent when a lower dose was used.

▶ Both this paper and Abstract 8–25 make powerful arguments for the use of 500–600 mg of zidovudine per day.—S.M. Wolff, M.D.

The Safety and Efficacy of Zidovudine (AZT) in the Treatment of Subjects With Mildly Symptomatic Human Immunodeficiency Virus Type 1 (HIV) Infection: A Double-Blind, Placebo-Controlled Trial

Fischl MA, Richman DD, Hansen N, Collier AC, Carey JT, Para MF, Hardy WD, Dolin R, Powderly WG, Allan JD, Wong B, Merigan TC, McAuliffe VJ, Hyslop NE, Rhame FS, Balfour HH Jr, Spector SA, Volberding P, Pettinelli C, Anderson J; and the AIDS Clinical Trials Group (Univ of Miami; Univ of California, San Diego; Univ of Washington; Case Western Reserve Univ; Ohio State Univ; et al)

Ann Intern Med 112:727–737, 1990 8–31

Correlation of a First Critical Event With CD4 T-Lymphocyte Count Before Treatment, Status of Serum HIV Type I Antigen, and Number of Symptoms

Variable	Subjects with First Critical Events			
	Overall	Placebo Group	Zidovudine Group	*P* Value*
CD4 T-lymphocyte count before treatment				
Total subjects, *n*	711	351	360	
200-300 cells/mm³, *n/n*†	19/140	12/64	7/76	0.04
300-400 cells/mm³, *n/n*	15/209	12/101	3/108	0.01
400-500 cells/mm³, *n/n*	12/168	10/90	2/78	0.06
> 500 cells/mm³, *n/n*	5/194	2/96	3/98	0.63
HIV antigen status before treatment				
Total subjects, *n*	642	313	329	
HIV antigen positive, *n/n*	19/147	13/68	6/79	0.05
HIV antigen negative, *n/n*	28/495	20/245	8/250	0.01
Number of symptoms before treatment				
Total subjects, *n*	711	351	360	
One symptom, *n/n*	37/547	26/265	11/282	0.003
Two symptoms, *n/n*	14/164	10/86	4/78	0.20

*By log rank tests.
†Number of subjects with a first critical event/total number of subjects.
(Courtesy of Fischl MA, Richman DD, Hansen N, et al: *Ann Intern Med* 112:727–737, 1990.)

To determine the efficacy of zidovudine when given early in the course of HIV infection, double-blind, placebo-controlled trial stratified patients by baseline CD4 T lymphocyte count to assess the efficacy of zidovudine given orally in a dose of 200 mg every 4 hours. All subjects had initial CD4 counts of 200–800/mm³. The 360 zidovudine-treated patients were compared with 351 placebo recipients. The median follow-up was 11 months.

The relative risk of progressive HIV disease or death was 2.7 in the placebo-treated group. The first critical event was AIDS in 21 placebo recipients and in 5 given zidovudine therapy. Progression was related to the initial CD4 count (table). Changes in Karnofsky performance scores did not differ significantly in the actively treated and control patients. Serum levels of HIV antigen decreased significantly in zidovudine-treated patients. Significant anemia and neutropenia occurred in 4% to 5% of the treated group. Fatigue, dyspepsia, and other gastrointestinal effects also were more frequent in the actively treated patients, but there were no adverse effects on cardiopulmonary or renal function. Zidovudine is beneficial to patients having mildly symptomatic HIV infection and is safe. The rate of progression can be slowed in patients who have fewer than 500 CD4 T lymphocytes/mm³.

▶ Zidovudine therapy not only decreased progression to AIDS in this asymptomatically infected cohort, but it also was associated with increased weight gaiin, an increase in CD4 counts, and decreased HIV replication. Because the authors could not demonstrate any benefit for zidovudine therapy in patients with CD4 counts above 500/mm³, the recommendation has been that therapy not be instituted until this level is reached. These results and others using a lower total daily dose of 500–600 mg confirm the appropriateness of this approach.—D.R. Snydman, M.D.

A Pilot Study of Low-Dose Zidovudine in Human Immunodeficiency Virus Infection

Collier AC, Bozzette S, Coombs RW, Causey DM, Schoenfeld DA, Spector SA, Pettinelli CB, Davies G, Richman DD, Leedom JM, Kidd P, Corey L (Univ of Washington; Univ of California, San Diego; Univ of Southern California; Harvard School of Public Health; Natl Inst of Allergy and Infectious Diseases, Bethesda; et al)

N Engl J Med 323:1015–1021, 1990 8–32

Zidovudine delays the progression of HIV infection, but in high dosage it produces hematologic toxicity. Acyclovir reportedly augments the effect of zidovudine on HIV in vitro. The clinical and antiviral effects of varying doses of zidovudine, with and without acyclovir, were compared in an open study of 67 patients with AIDS-related complex.

Twenty-eight patients received zidovudine daily in a dose of 300 mg, and 28 received 600 mg and 15 received 1,500 mg daily. In some cases zidovudine was accompanied by acyclovir in a dose of 4.8 g daily.

Performance scores improved the most with low and medium doses of zidovudine. Those given the lowest dose gained the most weight and had the most improvement in CD4+ lymphocyte counts. There were no dose-related differences in the course of HIV antigenemia or the reduction in plasma viral titers. Acyclovir was well tolerated but did not enhance the antiretroviral effects of zidovudine. High-dose zidovudine produced more toxicity than the medium and low doses, particularly a fall in hemoglobin.

The minimal effective dose of zidovudine remains to be determined, but treatment with 300 mg daily was effective in this study. Use of the lowest feasible dose is both clinically and economically important.

▶ In retrospect, it is easy to wonder how beneficial it might have been if the studies reported in Abstracts 8–25 and 8–26 were combined with this one. Nevertheless, it is hard to escape the conclusion that lower doses of zidovudine than initially employed are indicated.—S.M. Wolff, M.D.

▶ ↓ We do not know whether the lower dose of zidovudine currently employed will be associated with myopathy. However, it is worth noting that 2 patients in this report had exacerbations of their myopathy when retreated at a 400-mg daily dose. D.R. Snydman, M.D.

Mitochondrial Myopathy Caused by Long-Term Zidovudine Therapy

Dalakas MC, Illa I, Pezeshpkour GH, Laukaitis JP, Cohen B, Griffin JL (Natl Inst of Neurological Disorders and Stroke, Bethesda, Md; Armed Forces Inst of Pathology; George Washington Univ; Northwestern Univ)

N Engl J Med 322:1098–1105, 1990 8–33

Myopathic symptoms are developing in an increasing number of patients with HIV infection who receive long-term zidovudine therapy. These symptoms resolve when treatment is withdrawn. Muscle biopsy specimens were obtained from 15 patients with AIDS or AIDS-related complex who had received therapeutic doses of zidovudine for a mean of 13 months and from 5 others not given zidovudine. All of the patients had proximal muscle weakness, myalgia, increased serum creatine kinase levels, and electromyographic evidence of myopathic change.

Abundant ragged-red fibers were present in all biopsy specimens obtained from zidovudine-treated patients but in none of those from untreated patients. Strikingly abnormal mitochondria were confirmed by electron microscopy. The number of ragged-red fibers correlated with the severity of myopathy. All specimens exhibited changes of inflammatory myopathy. Myopathy in zidovudine-treated patients improved when prednisone was given or when zidovudine therapy ceased. Of the 5 patients not treated with zidovudine, 2 responded to prednisone. Counts of CE8+ cells and macrophages were similar in zidovudine-treated patients and those not given the drug.

Long-term zidovudine therapy apparently can produce toxic mitochondrial myopathy. There also may be a T-cell-mediated inflammatory myopathy similar to that associated with primary HIV infection. Initial treatment should be with a nonsteroidal anti-inflammatory drug. If necessary, zidovudine may be discontinued for 3–4 weeks. If the patient improves, a different antiretroviral agent should be tried; otherwise, zidovudine may be resumed with prednisone.

2′,3′-Dideoxyinosine (ddI) in Patients With the Acquired Immunodeficiency Syndrome or AIDS-Related Complex: A Phase I Trial

Lambert JS, Seidlin M, Reichman RC, Plank CS, Laverty M, Morse GD, Knupp C, McLaren C, Pettinelli C, Valentine FT, Dolin R (Univ of Rochester, NY; New York Univ; State Univ of New York, Buffalo; Bristol-Myers Squibb Co, Wallinford, Conn; Natl Inst of Allergy and Infectious Disease, Bethesda, Md)
N Engl J Med 322:1333–1340, 1990 8–34

In a phase I dose-escalation study, 2′,3′-dideoxyinosine (ddI), a potent inhibitor of HIV in vitro, was given to 17 patients with AIDS and to 20 patients with AIDS-related complex (ARC). The drug was administered intravenously every 12 hours for the first 2 weeks, then orally at twice the previous dose every 12 hours. The oral dose ranged from .4 to 66 mg/kg/day. The mean duration of ddI treatment was 17 weeks. Thirty patients had been treated previously with zidovudine for a mean of 8 months.

Intravenous ddI administration was generally well tolerated. The major dose-limiting effects of oral ddI therapy were painful neuropathy in 8 patients and pancreatitis in 5. A statistically significant decrease in the mean p24 antigen serum level and the mean number of CD4+ cells was observed at all dose levels. Twenty-five patients were clinically improved or had a weight gain of 2 kg or more. Thus ddI appears to have promise in the treatment of AIDS and ARC.

Once-Daily Administration of 2',3'-dideoxyinosine (ddI) in Patients With the Acquired Immunodeficiency Syndrome or AIDS-Related Complex: Results of a Phase I Trial

Cooley TP, Kunches LM, Saunders CA, Ritter JK, Perkins CJ, McLaren C, McCaffrey RP, Liebman HA (Boston City Hosp; Boston Univ; Bristol-Myers Squibb Co, Wallingford, Conn)

N Engl J Med 322:1340–1345, 1990 8–35

The clinical and laboratory findings of a phase I open-label, dose-finding trial of ddI in 17 patients with AIDS and 17 patients with severe AIDS-related complex (ARC) were reviewed. Seventeen patients had previously been treated with zidovudine. After 2 weeks of intravenous ddI, a single dose of ddI was given orally at twice the intravenous dose for a median of 12 weeks. Six dose levels, ranging from 1.6 to 30.4 mg/kg/day, were assessed.

After a mean of 15.8 weeks, 24 patients remained in the study. The maximal tolerated dose was 20.4 mg/kg/day. At the 30.4 mg/kg/day dose, pancreatitis developed in 2 patients and painful peripheral neuropathy in 1. Other toxic effects were observed. Treatment with ddI was associated with an increase in the mean number of CD4+ lymphocytes, mean total lymphocyte count, and the mean hemoglobin level. The amount of HIV virus p24 antigen decreased by more than 50% in 14 of 19 patients with detectable antigen, confirming that ddI has antiretroviral activity in patients with AIDS or ARC.

▶ Let's hope that we are beginning to see results of the major efforts during the past 6 or 7 years to find effective agents against HIV-1. Although toxic, ddI, when given in low doses given in combination (not necessarily together) with other agents such as zidovudine, will lead to more effective therapy.—S.M. Wolff, M.D.

Toxicity of Combined Ganciclovir and Zidovudine for Cytomegalovirus Disease Associated With AIDS: An AIDS Clinical Trials Group Study

Hochster H, Dieterich D, Bozzette S, Reichman RC, Connor JD, Liebes L, Sonke RL, Spector SA, Valentine F, Pettinelli C, Richman DD (New York Univ Med Ctr; Univ of California, San Diego; Univ of Rochester, NY; NIAID AIDS Clinical Trials Program, Bethesda, Md)

Ann Intern Med 113:111–117, 1990 8–36

Nearly all adults with AIDS are seropositive for cytomegalovirus and many eventually have active disease. Combined treatment with zidovudine and ganciclovir was evaluated in 40 patients with AIDS-related cytomegalovirus infection. Zidovudine was given in a dose of 100 mg or 200 mg every 4 hours. Ganciclovir was given in a usual induction dose of 5 mg/kg intravenously twice daily for 14 days, then once daily as maintenance 5 days a week.

Hematologic toxicity was frequent (table), even in patients given the

Toxicity by Dose Levels of Zidovudine and Ganciclovir

Characteristics	Zidovudine (1200 mg/d) plus Ganciclovir	Zidovudine (600 mg/d) plus Ganciclovir Induction for 14 d	Zidovudine (600 mg/d) plus Ganciclovir Maintenance
Patients, *n*	10	18	11
Median time to toxicity, *wk (range)*	3 (1 to 11)	4 (2 to 33)	5 (2 to 40)
Median nadir leukocyte count, *$\times 10^9$/L (range)*	1.6 (0.3 to 2.6)	1.8 (0.8 to 3.8)	1.6 (1.3 to 4.4)
Median nadir neutrophil count, *$\times 10^9$/L (range)*	0.82 (0.32 to 2.25)	0.92 (0.29 to 3.03)	0.72 (0.34 to 2.10)
Median nadir hemoglobin, *g/L (range)*	80 (60 to 112)	87 (63 to 117)	103 (72 to 125)
Median fall in hemoglobin, *g/L (range)*	25 (0 to 39)	28 (3 to 70)	17 (0 to 35)
Patients requiring dose reduction, *n(%)*	9/10 (90)	14/18 (82)	9/11 (81)
Grade 3 or 4 leukopenia, *n*	9	9	7
Grade 3 or 4 anemia, *n*	6	7	2
Grade 3 gastrointestinal toxicity, *n*	1	1	1
Grade 4 hepatitis, *n*	1	0	0

(Courtesy of Hochster H, Dieterich D, Bozzette S, et al: *Ann Intern Med* 113:111–117, 1990.)

lower dose of zidovudine. Ten patients had intercurrent infections and 19, progressive cytomegalovirus disease. Pharmacokinetic findings were not altered by combined zidovudine-ganciclovir therapy.

Combined zidovudine and ganciclovir therapy cannot be recommended because of its severe toxic effects. It would, however, be useful to continue anti-HIV treatment while controlling cytomegalovirus disease. It may be feasible to use growth factors to counter severe hematologic toxicity. An alternative is to combine ganciclovir with a nonmyelosuppressive antiretroviral agent.

Failure of Zidovudine Prophylaxis After Accidental Exposure to HIV-1

Lange JMA, Boucher CAB, Hollak CEM, Wiltink EHH, Reiss P, van Royen EA, Roos M, Danner SA, Goudsmit J (Univ of Amsterdam; Netherlands Red Cross Blood Transfusion Service, Amsterdam)

N Engl J Med 322:1375–1377, 1990 8–37

Encouraging results from animal studies prompted a placebo-controlled trial to assess the chemoprophylactic efficacy of zidovudine after occupational or nosocomial exposure to HIV-1. However, this trial will not be completed. Several programs of zidovudine chemoprophylaxis for health care workers exposed to HIV-1 have been implemented. Data on a patient in whom zidovudine prophylaxis administered after accidental HIV-1 exposure did not prevent HIV-1 infection were reviewed.

Man, 58, who was monogamous and heterosexual was accidentally injected with a syringe containing a small amount of blood from a man with HIV-1. Within 45 minutes, zidovudine treatment was initiated. The patient received zidovudine, 500 mg, orally every 6 hours for the first 2 days, 2.5 mg/kg intravenously every 4 hours on days 3–20, then 500 mg orally every 6 hours on days 21–37. Thereafter, the patient took 250 mg of zidovudine orally every 6 hours for another 2 months. On day 30, HIV-1 p24 antigen was detected. Seroconversion for HIV-1 antibodies occurred on day 41; HIV-1 was isolated from peripheral-blood mononuclear cells 58 days after the accident.

Recommendations for prophylaxis with zidovudine have been based on the type of exposure. In patients such as this one, the argument for prophylactic treatment is stronger. Under such circumstances, however, zidovudine may fail to prevent infection.

▶ Did the lawyers in The Netherlands read this case report? Aside from the horror one gets on reading this account, the discouraging aspect is the lack of any prophylactic effect zidovudine had on HIV transmission in this setting. This somber result raises major questions about prophylactic zidovudine for such exposures, although one can argue that the inoculum was likely to be high. Sensitivity testing confirmed that the isolate was sensitive to zidovudine.—D.R. Snydman, M.D.

The Efficacy of Inosine Pranobex in Preventing the Acquired Immunodeficiency Syndrome in Patients With Human Immunodeficiency Virus Infection

Pedersen C, Sandström E, Petersen CS, Norkrans G, Gerstoft J, Karlsson A, Christensen KC, Håkansson C, Pehrson PO, Nielsen JO, Jürgensen HJ, the Scandinavian Isoprinosine Study Group (Hvidovre Hosp, Copenhagen; Södersjukhuset, Stockholm; Bispebjerg Hosp, Copenhagen; Östra Hosp, Göteborg, Sweden; Rigshospitalet, Copenhagen, et al)

N Engl J Med 322:1757–1763, 1990 8–38

TABLE 1.—Base-Line Comparability of the Treatment Groups

Variable	Inosine Pranobex Group (N = 429)	Placebo Group (N = 437)
Medical history — no. (%)		
Temperature >38°C (≥3 wk)	10 (2.3)	9 (2.1)
Weight loss	25 (5.8)	31 (7.1)
Night sweats (≥3 wk)	21 (4.9)	36 (8.2)*
Diarrhea (≥4 wk)	6 (1.4)	11 (2.5)
Herpes simplex infection	37 (8.6)	32 (7.3)
Herpes zoster	3 (0.7)	5 (1.1)
Candida infection	31 (7.2)	37 (8.5)
Hairy leukoplakia	7 (1.6)	12 (2.7)
Physical examination — no. (%)		
Herpes simplex infection	13 (3.0)	4 (0.9)†
Herpes zoster	0 (0.0)	1 (0.2)
Candida infection	29 (6.8)	34 (7.8)
Hairy leukoplakia	5 (1.2)	10 (2.3)
Mean body weight (kg)	71.7	72.3
Mean general well-being score (mm)‡	25.5	24.6
Immunologic measures — mean (range)		
CD4+ cell count ($\times 10^{-6}$/liter)	599 (8–2340)	563 (0–2600)*
CD8+ cell count ($\times 10^{-6}$/liter)	931 (156–2810)	945 (100–3780)
CD4+:CD8+ ratio	0.77 (0.05–3.60)	0.71 (0–4.70)*
CD4+ substratum — no. (%)§		
<200 $\times 10^{6}$/liter	29 (6.8)	31 (7.1)
200–500 $\times 10^{6}$/liter	169 (39.7)	185 (42.6)
>500 $\times 10^{6}$/liter	228 (53.5)	218 (50.2)
Clinical staging — no. (%)		
CDC Group II or III	384 (89.5)	381 (87.2)
CDC Group IV without AIDS	44 (10.5)	54 (12.4)
AIDS (1987 definition)‖	1 (0.2)	2 (0.5)

*.05 < P < .10.
†P = .03.
‡As measured with use of a visual-analogue scale. Lower values indicate a better level of general well-being.
§For 3 patients in the inosine pranobex group and 3 in the placebo group, CD4+ cell counts at baseline were not available.
‖Two of these patients had AIDS according to the 1985 definition.
(Courtesy of Pedersen C, Sandström E, Petersen CS, et al: *N Engl J Med* 322:1757–1763, 1990.)

Inosine pranobex, or isoprinosine, enhances immune function in vitro and in vivo, and as such may have clinical application in immunocompromised patients infected with the HIV. A randomized, double-blind, placebo-controlled trial was performed to assess the efficacy and safety of isoprinosine therapy in HIV-infected patients.

Of 866 patients with HIV infection but without manifestations of AIDS, 429 received isoprinosine 1 g 3 times a day, and 437 were given matching placebo for 24 weeks. The treatment groups were compared (Table 1). Efficacy could be assessed in 412 isoprinosine-treated patients and 421 placebo-treated patients.

Acquired immunodeficiency syndrome developed in 17 placebo-treated

TABLE 2.—Disease Progression According to Baseline CD4+ Cell Count

CD4+ Cell Count at Base Line*	Inosine Pranobex Group			Placebo Group†			P Value
	Group II or III	Group IV without AIDS	AIDS	Group II or III	Group IV without AIDS	AIDS	
	number of patients (percent)						
<200	16 (57.1)	11 (39.3)	1 (3.6)	11 (35.5)	14 (45.2)	6 (19.4)	0.11
200 to 500	121 (73.8)	42 (25.6)	1 (0.6)	115 (65.3)	54 (30.7)	7 (4.0)	0.07
>500	169 (77.9)	48 (22.1)	0 (0.0)	160 (76.2)	46 (21.9)	4 (1.9)	0.06
Total	306 (74.8)	101 (24.7)	2 (0.5)	286 (68.6)	114 (27.3)	17 (4.1)	

*Values shown are $\times 10^{-6}$/L. At baseline, there were 28 patients in the inosine pranobex group with CD4+ cell counts < 200, 164 with counts from 200 to 500, and 217 with counts > 500. In the placebo group, the numbers were 31, 176, and 210, respectively. For 3 patients in the inosine pranobex group and 3 in the placebo group, CD4+ cell counts at baseline were not available.

†One patient with AIDS according to the 1987 Centers for Disease Control definition at entry is not included.

(Courtesy of Pedersen C, Sandström E, Petersen CS, et al: *N Engl J Med* 322:1757–1763, 1990.)

patients and 2 isoprinosine-treated patients. There were no significant differences between the groups with respect to changes in CD4+ cell count, (Table 2) as a beneficial effect of isoprinosine was seen irrespective of baseline CD4+ cell counts. There were no significant differences between groups for the development of other HIV-related conditions, except that fewer isoprinosine-treated patients had thrush. No serious side effects occurred. Thus, isoprinosine therapy in HIV-infected patients appears to delay progression to AIDS.

▶ Several promising agents are undergoing clinical trials to confirm data suggesting that they favorably alter the course of HIV infection. One such agent is isoprinosine. The carefully controlled trial reported by Pedersen and colleagues in Scandinavia suggests that, indeed, the drug delays progression to AIDS. These results have not been confirmed. No changes in CD4 cells or virus markers have been shown, however, and the mechanism by which the drug favorably affects the course of HIV infection, if real, remains unknown. Another recent study (1) involved 15 men with early asymptomatic HIV infection given ribavirin as well as isoprinosine. No beneficial effect was found over a short observation period of up to 3 months. However, the combination did result in a significant generalized lymphopenia. Further study of this agent appears to be warranted, but only under carefully controlled clinical trial protocols.—G.T. Keusch, M.D.

Reference

1. Schulof RS: *J AIDS* 3:485, 1990.

9 Sexually Transmitted Diseases

The Limited Value of Symptoms and Signs in the Diagnosis of Vaginal Infections

Schaaf VM, Perez-Stable EJ, Borchardt K (Univ of California, Berkeley and San Francisco; San Francisco State Univ)

Arch Intern Med 150:1929–1933, 1990 9–1

Despite relatively discrete constellations of symptoms and signs for various vaginal infections, many women remain without a diagnosis. Lack of agreement on the cause and diagnostic criteria for bacterial vaginosis and the infection vs. colonization controversy compound the diagnostic difficulty, as does the inability of traditional symptoms and signs to predict specific causes. To explore the correlation between clinical findings and microbiological conclusions, data were reviewed on 123 women with vaginal complaints.

To elicit clinical symptoms, a standardized questionnaire was administered that reflected all relevant symptoms reported in the literature and included a free-form question on symptoms. Urinary tract infection was evaluated by the leukocyte-esterase-nitrite dipstick test on a clean-catch urine specimen. Patients with negative urine test results underwent pelvic examination. Swabs of vaginal discharge were obtained for microbiological analysis. Vaginal odor, discharge pH, color, consistency, and odor when mixed with 10% potassium hydroxide were noted.

Trichomonas vaginalis, Candida albicans, or bacterial vaginosis was diagnosed in 49% of the women; the cause was not determined in 51%. Of the 60 patients with definite diagnoses, 53 (88%) had 1 infection and 7 (12%) had 2 infections. *Candida albicans* was cultured in 32 patients and *T. vaginalis* was cultured in 8. No patients had these 2 infections simultaneously. Using as a criterion the presence of 3 of 4 clinical signs, bacterial vaginosis was found in 27 women; 13% had 5–7 symptoms; 72% had 2–4 symptoms; and 15% had only 1 symptom. Symptoms did not differ among the 3 infections, and lack of vaginal odor in yeast infection was the only physical sign that differed significantly. Itching was the only symptom found more frequently among those with a definite diagnosis. Trichomonads were seen on microscopy in 75% of culture-positive specimens; yeast was seen in 63% of these specimens. There were no significant clinical criteria for vaginosis. Presenting signs and symptoms have limited value in evaluating vaginitis. For half of the women with vaginitis, a microbiologic diagnosis may be lacking.

▶ This report has 2 major messages: that a microbiological diagnosis can be made in only half of the women with vaginitis, and that presenting signs and symptoms have little predictive value for the specific cause. This report is consistent with the frustration experienced by many physicians and patients in dealing with this illness.—M.J. Barza, M.D.

Erythromycin for Persistent or Recurrent Nongonococcal Urethritis: A Randomized, Placebo-Controlled Trial

Hooton TM, Wong ES, Barnes RC, Roberts PL, Stamm WE (Harborview Med Ctr, Seattle; Univ of Washington)

Ann Intern Med 113:21–26, 1990 9–2

The treatment of persistent or recurrent nongonococcal urethritis is frustrating. Because up to 40% of these cases are believed to be caused by tetracycline-resistant *Ureaplasma urealyticum,* treatment with erythromycin has been recommended.

In a prospective, randomized double-blind trial the efficacy of a 3-week regimen of erythromycin in treating persistent or recurrent nongonococcal urethritis in men was evaluated. Seventy-seven sexually active men (mean age, 28 years) who had objective evidence of nongonococcal urethritis, a median duration of urethritis of 3 months, and previous treatment with at least 1 course of tetracycline or erythromycin received either erythromycin, 500 mg, or placebo 4 times daily for 3 weeks.

At enrollment 79% of the men had an urethral discharge and 87% had a leukocyte count of at least $10/mm^3$ in first-voided urine. Urine cultures grew *U. urealyticum* in 12% of patients, *Mycoplasma hominis* in 4%, α-streptococci in 9%, and *Gardnerella vaginalis* in 7%.

Erythromycin was more effective than placebo in resolving urethral symptoms and urethritis (e.g., urethral discharge and leukocytosis) as determined after 2 weeks of treatment and at 2, 4, and 8 weeks of follow-up, but most of these differences were not statistically significant (table). However, erythromycin caused a significantly greater reduction in pyuria than placebo; the median leukocyte count in first-voided urine decreased by 89% in the erythromycin group, compared with 23% in the placebo group. This effect was especially prominent in men with prostatic inflammation, in whom urinary leukocyte counts decreased by a median of 94% in those treated with erythromycin, compared with a 46% increase in patients treated with placebo. Side effects with erythromycin were mild and included gastrointestinal symptoms. The findings indicate a beneficial effect of a 3-week regimen of erythromycin in men with persistent or recurrent nongonococcal urethritis, particularly among those with prostatic inflammation.

Resolution of Urethral Discharge and Leukocytosis During and After Treatment With Erythromycin or Placebo

Treatment Group	**Visit**		
	2 Weeks	**4 Weeks**	**8 Weeks***
Erythromycin			
Number†, *n/n* (%)	**15/25 (60)**	**15/34 (44)**	**10/26 (38)**
95% CI, %	**40 to 79**	**27 to 61**	**20 to 57**
Placebo			
Number†, *n/n* (%)	**15/34 (44)**	**14/38 (37)**	**8/36 (22)**
95% CI, %	**27 to 61**	**22 to 52**	**9 to 36**
Difference (95% CI), %	**16 (−10 to 41)**	**7 (−15 to 30)**	**16 (−6 to 39)**

*Evaluable patients at 8 weeks include those who were retreated at earlier visit and those who returned for 8-week visit.

†Number of patients with resolution compared with number evaluable. Resolution was defined as resolution of both urethral discharge and leukocytosis and no previous retreatment.

(Courtesy of Hooton TM, Wong ES, Barnes RC, et al: *Ann Intern Med* 113:21–26, 1990.)

▶ The interpretation of this study is a bit confusing, although the issue being addressed, the treatment of persistent or recurrent nongonococcal urethritis, is clinically important. The authors presumed that erythromycin might work because many of the cases could be caused by tetracycline-resistant strains of *U. urealyticum.* However, only 12% of cultures grew that species at enrollment. Aside from certain significant imbalances in the groups (erythromycin-treated patients were younger, less likely to be white, and more likely to have had a previous episode of urethritis) and of reinfection, which the authors note, it is not clear how compliant the patients were in taking their medication. Many patients cannot take 2 g of erythromycin per day for more than a few days. To me, the paper suggested no impressive benefit of erythromycin; 1 week after the end of treatment symptoms had resolved in 41% of patients taking erythromycin and in 31% of those taking placebo (which may be good news for placebo manufacturers).—M.J. Barza, M.D.

National Surveillance of Antimicrobial Resistance in *Neisseria gonorrhoeae*

Schwarcz SK, Zenilman JM, Schnell D, Knapp JS, Hook EW III, Thompson S, Judson FN, Holmes KK, and The Gonococcal Isolate Surveillance Project (Ctrs for Disease Control, Atlanta; Baltimore City Health Dept; Emory Univ; Denver Public Health Dist; Univ of Washington)

JAMA 264:1413–1417, 1990 9–3

Although the incidence of gonorrhea has decreased since 1975, infections caused by antimicrobial-resistant gonococci are increasing. The Gonococcal Isolate Surveillance Project is a national sentinel surveillance system developed to estimate levels and monitor trends of antimicrobial resistance in prospectively collected isolates of *Neiserria gonorrhoeae.* Data on the 6,204 isolates from 21 clinic sites evaluated from September

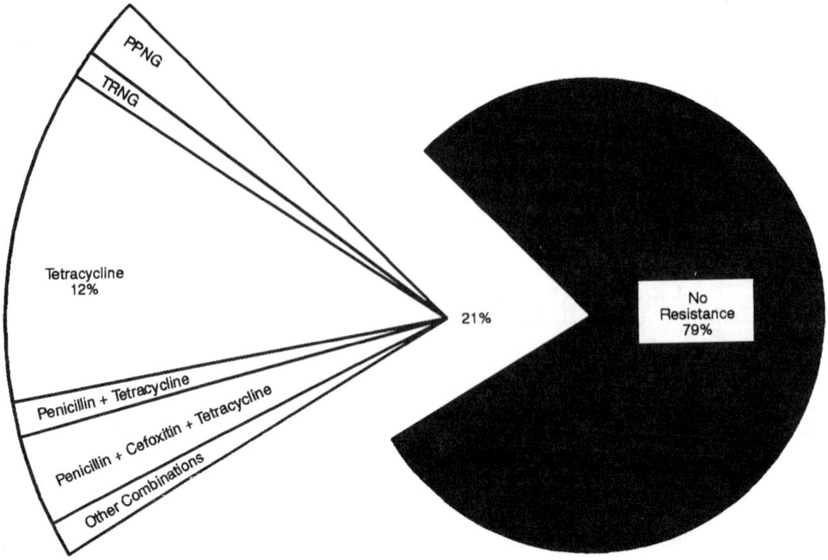

Fig 9–1.—Types of resistance in the Gonococcal Isolate Surveillance Project, 1987–1988. *PPNG* indicates plasmid-mediated penicillin-resistant *Neisseria gonorrhoeae; TRNG,* plasmid-mediated tetracycline-resistant *N. gonorrhoeae;* and others, chromosomally mediated resistant *N. gonorrhoeae.* (Courtesy of Schwarcz SK, Zenilman JM, Schnell D, et al: *JAMA* 264:1413–1417, 1990.)

1987 to December 1988 were reviewed. The sample was limited to males with urethritis.

Overall, 21% of the isolates met at least 1 of the surveillance criteria for resistance to penicillin, tetracycline, cefoxitin, or spectinomycin (Fig 9–1). Antimicrobial resistance was caused by plasmid-mediated penicillinase production (PPNG) in 2.2% of the isolates, high-level plasmid-mediated tetracycline resistance (TRNG) in 1%, and chromosomally mediated resistance (defined as a minimum inhibitory concentration 2 μg/mL or greater) to penicillin, tetracycline, or cefoxitin. Three isolates were resistant to spectinomycin. All isolates were susceptible to ceftriaxone. All forms of antimicrobial resistance were widespread, but PPNG appeared to be more common in coastal areas and tetracycline-resistant isolates were more prevalent in cities east of the Mississippi River. There was no correlation between the prevalence of PPNG isolates and the prevalence of chromosomally mediated resistance (Fig 9–2). Patient demographics and behavioral characteristics were not predictive of resistant infection.

These data document the high prevalence of antimicrobial-resistant *N. gonorrhoeae* in the United States. Guided by these surveillance data, the Centers for Disease Control in 1989 revised the national treatment protocol for gonococcal infections. For uncomplicated gonorrhea, the current first-line therapy is a single dose of ceftriaxone, 250 mg given intramuscularly, combined with doxycycline, 100 mg given orally twice daily

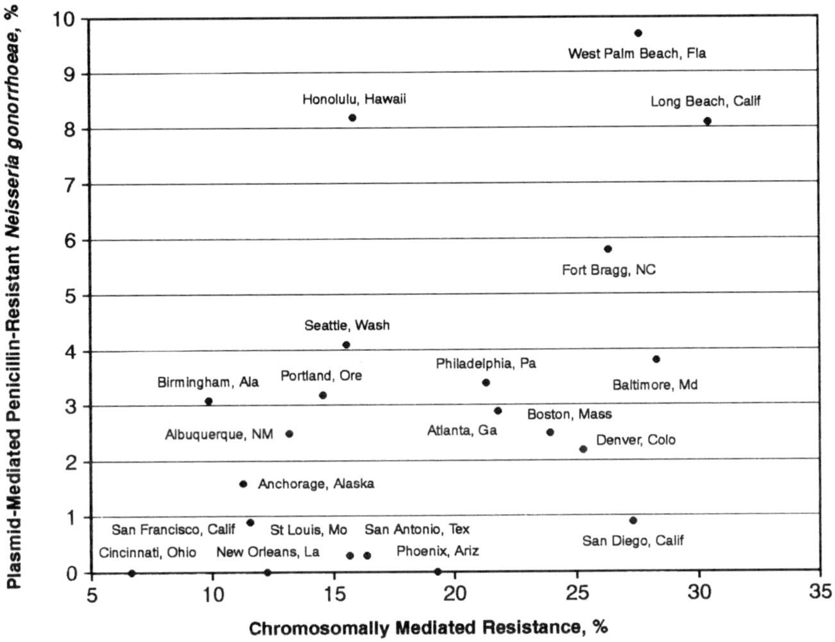

Fig 9–2.—Gonococcol Isolate Surveillance Project, 1987–1988; scattergram comparing the percentage of isolates that had plasmid-mediated penicillin resistance to the percentage of isolates that had chromosomally mediated resistance in each participating city. (Courtesy of Schwarcz SK, Zenilman JM, Schnell D, et al: *JAMA* 264:1413–1417, 1990.)

for 7 days. Penicillin and tetracycline are no longer recommended as first-line therapies for gonococcal infection.

▶ As the authors note, since preparation of their manuscript, data from 1989 have been published, demonstrating a further increase in the incidence of PPNG in reporting clinics (e.g., 32% in Long Beach, 18% in Atlanta, and 15% in Boston). These figures are worrisome, if not unexpected, and show the utility of the national gonococcal surveillance project for monitoring trends in resistance.—M.J. Barza, M.D.

Escherichia coli Bacteriuria and Contraceptive Method

Hooton TM, Hillier S, Johnson C, Roberts PL, Stamm WE (Univ of Washington; Harborview Med Ctr, Seattle)

JAMA 265:64–69, 1991 9–4

Both sexual intercourse and diaphragm use predispose young women to urinary tract infection. However, it is not known whether these 2 factors are truly independent or by what mechanism these associations occur. To test the hypothesis that diaphragm-spermicide use or spermicide

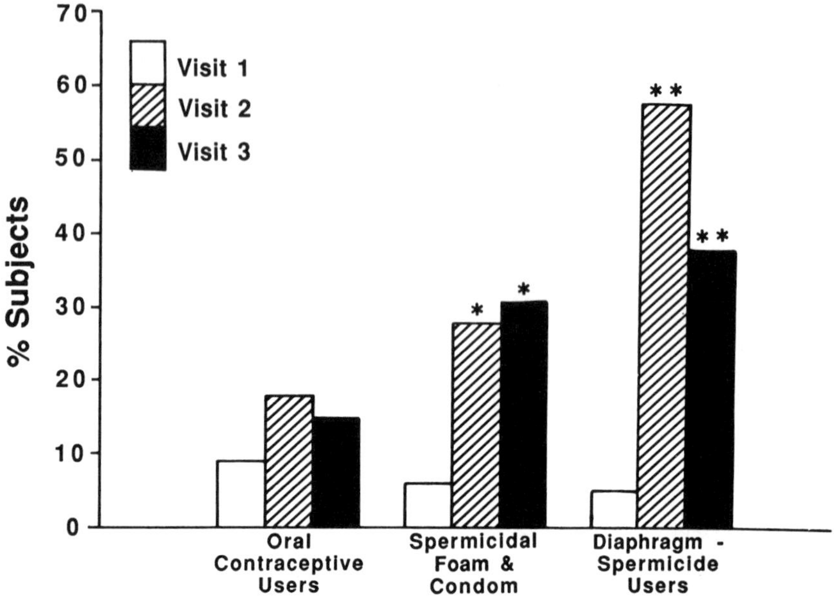

Fig 9–3.—Prevalence of bacteriuria with *E. coli* before and after intercourse in oral contraceptive users, spermidical foam and condom users, and diaphragm-spermicide users. Bars show percentage of subjects who had at least 10^2 colony-forming units of *E. coli* per milliliter of midstream urine at each visit. Visit 1 was before intercourse, visit 2 was morning after intercourse, and visit 3 was 24 hours later. $^*P < .01$ for comparison with prevalence at visit 1; $^{**}P < .001$. (Courtesy of Hooton TM, Hillier S, Johnson C, et al: *JAMA* 265:64–69, 1991.)

use alone increased the risk of vaginal colonization and bacteriuria with *Escherichia coli,* 104 sexually active women older than age 18 years were assessed before having sexual intercourse, the morning after intercourse, and 24 hours later.

The prevalence of *E. coli* bacteriuria increased slightly in oral contraceptive users after sexual intercourse and dramatically in foam, condom, and diaphragm-spermicide users (Fig 9–3). The prevalence of bacteriuria remained significantly increased 24 hours later in the latter 3 groups, and vaginal colonization with *E. coli* was also more dramatic and persistent (Fig 9–4). Vaginal colonization with *Candida* organisms, enterococci, and staphylococci was also elevated significantly in diaphragm-spermicide users after intercourse.

The use of a diaphragm with spermicidal jelly or the use of a spermicidal foam with a condom greatly affects normal vaginal flora. Users of such contraceptives are strongly predisposed to vaginal colonization and bacteriuria with *E. coli.*

▶ This is a provocative study. The explanations of the findings are not obvious. The authors suggest that among the effects of the spermicide could be an alteration of the vaginal flora or because of a detergent effect, a stripping away

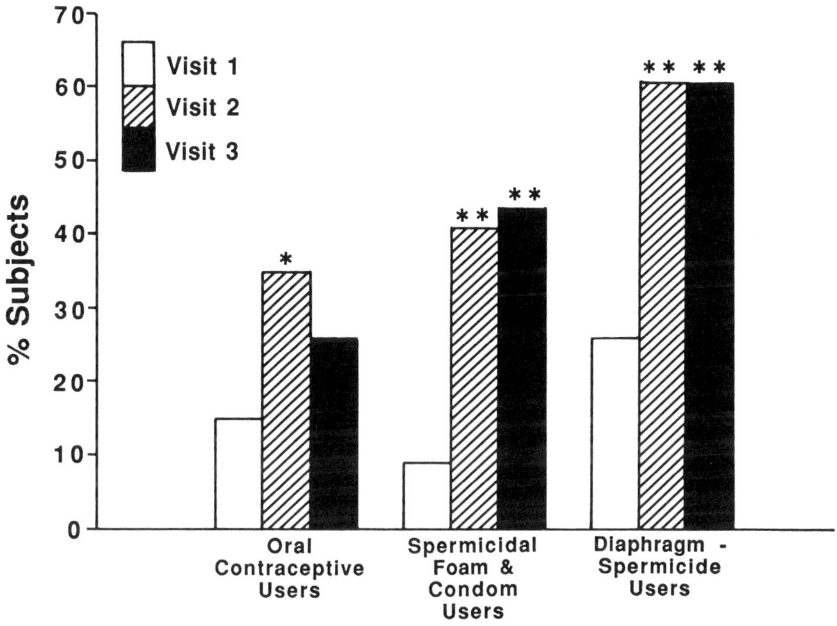

Fig 9–4.—Prevalence of vaginal colonization with *E. coli* before and after intercourse in oral contraceptive users, spermicidal and condom users, and diaphragm-spermicide users. Bars show percentage of subjects who had vaginal colonization with *E. coli* at each visit. Visit 1 was before intercourse, visit 2 was morning after intercourse, and visit 3 was 24 hours later. *$P < .05$ for comparison with prevalence at visit 1; **$P < .001$. (Courtesy of Hooton TM, Hillier S, Johnson C, et al: *JAMA* 265:64–69, 1991.)

of protective mucosal coatings, either of which could predispose to colonization of the vagina by *E. coli*. The effect of the diaphragm is probably related to low-grade urethral outlet obstruction. Oral contraceptives seem not to predispose to introital colonization with *E. coli* or bacteriuria.—M.J. Barza, M.D.

Ciprofloxacin Compared With Doxycycline for Nongonococcal Urethritis: Ineffectiveness Against *Chlamydia trachomatis* Due to Relapsing Infection

Hooton TM, Rogers ME, Medina TG, Kuwamura LF, Ewers C, Roberts PL, Stamm WE (Univ of Washington; Tacoma-Pierce County Sexually Transmitted Disease Clinic, Tacoma Wash)
JAMA 264:1418–1421, 1990 9–5

Men with nongonococcal urethritis are commonly treated with tetracycline congeners or erythromycin. However, alternative treatments are desirable because at least 30% of men have persistent or recurrent disease after treatment with these regimens. *Chlamydia trachomatis* causes up to 50% of these infections; therefore, alternative treatments must be effective against chlamydial infections.

TABLE 1.—Eradication of *Chlamydia trachomatis* at Each Posttreatment Visit Among Men Who Initially Had Cultures Positive for *Chlamydia*

	No. (%) of Chlamydia-Negative/Assessable Patients*		
Posttreatment Visit	**Ciprofloxacin, 750 mg (n = 26)**	**Ciprofloxacin, 1000 mg (n = 21)**	**Doxycycline (n = 13)**
2-3 d	26/26 (100)	18/20 (90)	12/12 (100)
2 wk	11/20 (55)	13/18 (72)	9/9 (100)*
4 wk	10/21 (48)	10/16 (62)	10/10 (100)†

Note: Assessable patients include those who initially had cultures positive for *Chlamydia* who returned for given visit or who had *Chlamydia* reisolated at previous visit.
**P* = .03 compared with ciprofloxacin, 750 mg; *P* = .14 compared with ciprofloxacin, 1,000 mg.
†*P* = .005 compared with ciprofloxacin, 750 mg; *P* = .05 compared with ciprofloxacin, 1,000 mg.
(Courtesy of Hooton TM, Rogers ME, Medina TG, et al: *JAMA* 264:1418–1421, 1990.)

A series of 178 men with objective evidence of urethral discharge or urethral inflammation or urethral culture positive for *C. trachomatis* were randomized to receive 750 mg of ciprofloxacin, 1,000 mg of ciprofloxacin, or 100 mg of doxycycline. All treatments were given twice daily for 7 days.

At 2 weeks and 4 weeks after treatment, resolution of nongonococcal urethritis was comparable in all 3 treatment groups. Doxycycline was significantly more effective in eradicating *C. trachomatis* than either ciprofloxacin regimen at 4 weeks after treatment (Table 1). Treatment outcome at 4 weeks in those who were initially culture negative for *Chlamydia* was not significantly different in the 3 treatment groups (Table 2). In patients with initial cultures positive for *Chlamydia, C. trachomatis* was reisolated in cultures within 4 weeks after treatment in 52% of patients treated with 750 mg of ciprofloxacin and in 38% of those treated with the 1,000-mg dose. Recurrent strains were identical in serotype to the initial infecting strain. Relapsing infection with *C. trachomatis* was not found in any patient treated with doxycycline.

Ciprofloxacin is ineffective in treating chlamydial urethritis, even in doses as high as 2 g daily, therefore, this drug is not suitable for treating

TABLE 2.—Resolution of Nongonococcal Urethritis 4 Weeks After Treatment

	No. (%) of Resolved/Assessable Patients *		
Microbiologic Findings at Enrollment	**Ciprofloxacin, 750 mg**	**Ciprofloxacin, 1000 mg**	**Doxycycline**
Positive for chlamydia	6/17 (35)†	8/16 (50)	8/11 (73)
Negative for chlamydia, positive for *Ureaplasma*	2/6 (33)	6/12 (50)	5/12 (42)
Negative for chlamydia, negative for *Ureaplasma*	12/15 (80)	7/13 (54)	7/13 (54)

Note: Analysis includes only those who had objective evidence of nongonococcal urethritis at enrollment.
*Assessable patients include those who returned for 4-week visit or who were retreated for nongonococcol urethritis at previous visit.
†*P* = .05 compared with the doxycyeline group; *P* = .05 compared with patients who had cultures negative for *Chlamydia* treated with this regimen.
(Courtesy of Hooton TM, Rogers ME, Medina TG, et al: *JAMA* 264:1418–1421, 1990.)

men with nongonococcal urethritis. However, because the overall clinical cure rate for doxycycline was only 56% in this study, further studies of other quinolones or other newer oral agents are warranted.

▶ Because previous studies of ciprofloxacin, 500 mg or 750 mg twice daily, had not been highly effective in eradicating chlamydial infection in patients with nongonococcal urethritis, the authors tried the higher dosage of 1,000 mg twice daily as well as 750 mg twice daily. The eradication rates were still unacceptably low. The reasons for the poor results with ciprofloxacin in this infection are not clear but do not seem to relate to the development of drug resistance or to reinfection. Persistence or relapse was most notable in patients whose secretions contained high numbers of chlamydial inclusion bodies at enrollment, suggesting an "inoculum effect"; such an effect, combined with the relatively modest antichlamydial activity of ciprofloxacin in relation to serum levels of the drug, constitutes the best explanation.—M.J. Barza, M.D.

10 Nosocomial Infections

Risk of Exposure of Surgical Personnel to Patients' Blood During Surgery at San Francisco General Hospital

Gerberding JL, Littell C, Tarkington A, Brown A, Schechter WP (Univ of California, San Francisco; San Francisco Gen Hosp)

N Engl J Med 322:1788–1793, 1990 10–1

Assessments of the Centers for Disease Control guidelines for prevention of hepatitis B virus (HBV) and HIV infection in surgical personnel have been lacking. The intraoperative exposures to blood and other body fluids were evaluated in a hospital in which a high proportion of patients had HBV or HIV infection.

A total of 1,307 consecutive operating room procedures performed during a 2-month period were reviewed. Circulating nurses were asked to record parenteral and cutaneous exposures to blood and to note information about all procedures. These data were analyzed to determine factors that might predict such exposures and thereby identify interventions that could reduce their frequency. An additional follow-up validation study was also done to verify the accuracy of the data collected by the nurses. In that study, 50 randomly selected surgical procedures were observed and 960 gloves examined to determine the rate of glove perforation.

During 84 of the 1,307 procedures (6.4%) there were 117 accidental

Parenteral and Cutaneous Exposures Observed During 1,307 Surgical Procedures

Parenteral Exposures (22 Events in 22 Cases)		Cutaneous Exposures (95 Events in 62 Cases)	
Needle sticks	11	Hands	32
Suture needle	10	Glove tear	26
Hollow needle	1	Other	6
Lacerations	6	Face	25
Mucous-membrane splashes	4	Foot	5
Open-wound contamination	1	Other sites	33

Case exposure rate, parenteral exposures:
22 procedures with parenteral exposure divided by 1307 procedures = 1.7 percent

Case exposure rate, cutaneous exposures:
62 procedures with cutaneous exposure divided by 1307 procedures = 4.7 percent

(Courtesy of Gerberding JL, Littell C, Tarkington A, et al: *N Engl J Med* 322:1788–1793, 1990.)

exposures to parenteral or cutaneous blood (table). The total rate of exposure to parenteral blood was 1.7%. The risk of exposure was increased in procedures that lasted longer than 3 hours, in patients who lost more than 300 mL of blood, and in cases of major intravascular and intra-abdominal gynecologic surgery. Exposure could not be prevented by knowledge of diagnosed HIV infection or of the patient's risk for infection. Double-gloving technique was successful in preventing perforations of the inner glove and cutaneous exposures of the hand.

Intraoperative exposure to blood is a risk for surgical personnel. Double gloving and the increased use of waterproof garments and face shields can prevent mucocutaneous exposures to blood. Preoperative testing for HIV infection would probably not reduce the frequency of accidental exposures to blood.

▶ There are still many who argue that it would be helpful to identify those patients infected with HBV or HIV. This study and Abstract 10–3 argue that this is not the case, i.e., that the rate of exposures is the same whether or not the patient is known or perceived to be infected by these agents. However, in this study, which was done at the San Francisco General Hospital, the prevalence of HIV infection in the population is sufficiently high that it may be that surgeons routinely operate at the highest level of awareness. Double gloving, as used at this hospital, appeared to reduce the rate of perforations of the inner glove by more than 60% and reduced the rate of cutaneous exposure to blood. Elsewhere, preliminary reports suggest that gloves reduce the amount of blood that might be introduced on a penetrating suture needle by 50%.—M.J. Barza, M.D.

The Direct Costs of Universal Precautions in a Teaching Hospital

Doebbeling BN, Wenzel RP (Univ of Iowa)

JAMA 264:2083–2087, 1990 10–2

In 1987 the Centers for Disease Control emphasized the importance of routinely using a barrier method to minimize exposure to blood and

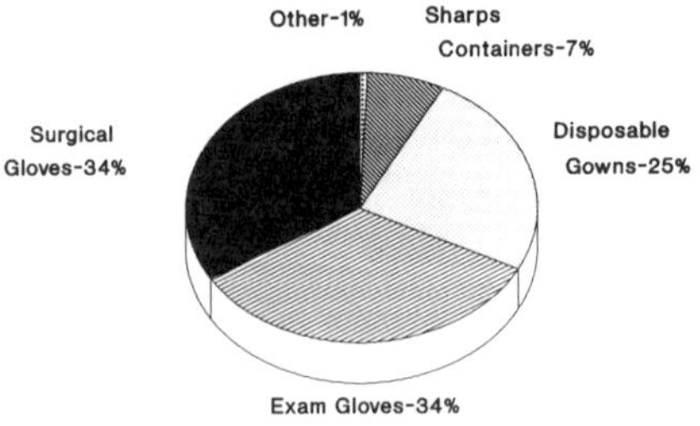

Fig 10–1.—Increased costs for isolation materials. Percentages are the increment in hospital expenditures for isolation materials in fiscal year 1989 compared with fiscal year 1987, ajusted for inflation. Percentages do not add to 100% because of rounding. (Courtesy of Doebbeling BN, Wenzel RP: *JAMA* 264:2083–2087, 1990.)

body fluids. Since then there have been frequent shortages of isolation materials, as well as price increases. The cost of implementing the new guidelines of the Centers for Disease Control was estimated by comparing expenditures for barrier isolation materials before and after instituting universal precautions at a 900-bed university hospital.

The use of rubber gloves increased from 1.6 to 2.8 million pairs annually after universal precautions began. The total annual costs for isolation materials increased by $351,000 (Fig 10–1). The increase per admission, after adjusting for inflation, was 60%. Costs for outpatient visits increased by more than 90%, mostly because of the use of rubber gloves.

The estimated cost of universal precautions in the United States in fiscal year 1989, adjusting for inflation, was at least $336 million. The higher costs cannot be explained by an increase in nosocomial infections. It will be important to evaluate various ways of controlling costs of isolation materials.

▶ If the rate of compliance with universal precautions is as low as suggested by other articles such as Abstract 10–3, the authors may have severely underestimated the true cost of barrier precautions. Even so, their estimate is greatly in excess of the Occupational Safety and Health Administration (OSHA) estimates. Most infection control workers I have spoken to also thought the OSHA estimates too low.—M.J. Barza, M.D.

HIV, Trauma, and Infection Control: Universal Precautions Are Universally Ignored

Hammond JS, Eckes JM, Gomez GA, Cunningham DN (Univ of Miami-Jackson Mem Med Ctr, Miami)

J Trauma 30:555–561, 1990 10–3

The medical, legal, and ethical problems associated with routine HIV screening have prompted the recommendation that all patients be presumed seropositive, thus protective measures should be adopted by all health care workers. However, this philosophy of "universal precautions" has been hard to adhere to and enforce. In some trauma population subsets, the prevalence of HIV seropositivity runs as high as 19%. To judge compliance with a strict universal precautions protocol, trauma nurse coordinators observed surgical residents engaged in trauma room resuscitations.

Eighty-one trauma rooms were observed for a 2-month period. Eighteen house officers were involved. The overall compliance with strict universal precautions was only 16%. The most common variations involved sharps technique. Although glove use was nearly universal, protective eye wear, ankle and foot protection, and body protection such as gowns or aprons were commonly ignored. Compliance was less than 40% even in the presence of invasive procedures such as endotracheal intubation or insertion of chest tubes. The reasons most often given for the lapse in protocol were not knowing the protocol, forgetting it, or not having time to implement it. Even with the 9 patients whom residents suspected of being in a high-risk group, the protocol was strictly adhered to only once.

Even under the best of circumstances compliance with universal precautions is difficult to attain. Passive informational measures cannot be assumed to achieve this goal. Active infection control surveillance and ongoing housestaff inservice training are needed to minimize the risk of inadvertent injury or contamination.

▶ The title of this article is ironic, but its import is all too familiar to those of us interested in the spread of infection within the hospital. The thrust of the article is that there is a low rate of compliance with universal precautions, an observation that has been made in several other studies. However, I think it is important that glove use was nearly universal and sharps techniques were violated in only 3% of instances; these measures strike me as among the most important in the reduction of significant exposures. Most of the violations were in the area of masks, ankle protection, and using gloves and gowns, which may be less important (although the authors do not make this suggestion). They raise the argument that universal precautions may be an impractical goal, and that routine testing for HIV infection of patients to whom exposure will be prolonged may be more effective. However, their own study showed that there was virtually no adherence to universal precautions even for patients known to be HIV positive. Finally, as the authors remind us, only 40% of the exposures of health care workers are preventable. Although education and surveillance appear to increase compliance with universal precautions, the increase is likely to be modest and transitory. It appears to me that our efforts may be better put into technical advances such as automatic sheathing devices to prevent needlesticks.—M.J. Barza, M.D.

A Surgeon With AIDS: Lack of Evidence of Transmission to Patients

Mishu B, Schaffner W, Horan JM, Wood LH, Hutcheson RH, McNabb PC (Ctrs for Disease Control, Atlanta; Vanderbilt Univ; Tennessee Dept of Health and Environment, Nashville; Univ of Tennessee, Memphis)

JAMA 264:467–470, 1990 10–4

The identity of a surgeon in whom AIDS was diagnosed was reported in 1988. Because concern about transmission of HIV from this surgeon to his patients persisted, a collaborative effort was undertaken by the 3 hospitals where the surgeon had practiced to offer free HIV antibody testing and counseling to that surgeon's former patients.

A total of 2,160 patients who had been operated on by the surgeon since 1982 were identified. None of these patients had been reported to Tennessee's AIDS registry. Of the 264 patients who had died, none died of AIDS or other HIV-related diseases; 1,652 of the remaining 1,896 patients were contacted, and 616 (37%) were tested. Only 1 patient who was positive for HIV antibody was an intravenous drug user and may have already had AIDS at the time of his surgery.

Precisely quantifying the risks of HIV transmission from infected surgeons to patients may not be possible because of the inability to do prospective studies. However, this retrospective study is the largest of its type to date and may provide the best information for some time to come. The risks to patients operated on by HIV-infected surgeons are most likely quite low.

▶ Although this study reassures us that HIV infection may not be easily transmitted by an HIV-infected surgeon during surgery, the recent report of an HIV-infected oral surgeon transmitting infection to 4 patients makes this selection somewhat "passe" (1). The guidelines for the management of the HIV-infected health care worker are undergoing revision and scrutiny. Unfortunately, all of the decisions that institutions may be forced to make may not be totally rational. This paper at least provides a counterpoint to dentist-associated cases.—D.R. Snydman, M.D.

Reference

1. From the CDC: *JAMA* 265:563, 1991.

Prospective, Controlled Study of Vinyl Glove Use to Interrupt *Clostridium difficile* Nosocomial Transmission

Johnson S, Gerding DN, Olson MM, Weiler MD, Hughes RA, Clabots CR, Peterson LR (VA Med Ctr, Minneapolis; Univ of Minnesota)

Am J Med 88:137–140, 1990 10–5

Clostridium difficile diarrhea-colitis is a nosocomial infection, yet its mode of transmission remains unclear. Because *C. difficile* has been recovered from the hands of hospital personnel, it is possible that they could represent an important mode of transmission that could be interrupted by their use of gloves when handling body substances.

To test this hypothesis, the incidence of *C. difficile*-associated diarrhea was monitored for 6 months before and after institution of an intensive program of disposable vinyl glove use on 2 hospital wards in a controlled trial. The intensive education program included initial and periodic in-services, posters, and placement of boxes of gloves at each patient's bedside. Two comparable wards where no special interventions were undertaken served as controls.

The incidence of *C. difficile* diarrhea was significantly reduced from 7.7/1,000 patient discharges during the 6 months before the intervention to 1.5/1,000 during the 6 months of intensive gloving (table). In contrast, no significant change in incidence was observed in the control wards during the same time period or in the hospital as a whole. Although there was a trend toward lower point prevalence of asymptomatic *C. difficile* carriage on all 4 wards, the reduction in *C. difficile* colonization was significant on the glove wards only. A total of 61,500 gloves were used in

Incidence of *Clostridium difficile* Diarrhea and Carriage Prevalence Before and After Institution of Intensive Use of Vinyl Gloves on Glove Wards

	Six Months Before		Six Months After		
Wards	CD Diarrhea Incidence*	CD Carriage Prevalence†	CD Diarrhea Incidence‡	CD Carriage Prevalence§	p Value
Glove wards					
5B	5/488	5/14	1/473	1/16	
5AW	4/683	5/23	1/892	3/27	
Total		10/37		4/43	0.029
Total	9/1,171		2/1,365		0.015
Control Wards					
3A	3/438	1/11	2/339	1/18	
6B	4/792	4/19	3/853	4/31	
Total		5/30		5/49	NS
Total	7/1,230		5/1,192		NS

Abbreviations: CD, C. difficile; NS, not significant.
*Cases of CD per patient discharge from July 1, 1986, to December 31, 1986.
†Point prevalence of CD carriage by patients on December 29, 1986.
‡Cases per patient discharge from January 22, 1987, to July 31, 1987.
§Point prevalence or CD carriage by patients on August 5, 1987.
(Courtesy of Johnson S, Gerding DN, Olson MM, et al: *Am J Med* 88:137–140, 1990.)

the glove wards for a cost of $2,768, compared with a cost of $1,895 for 42,100 gloves used in the control wards.

In this study the use of disposable vinyl gloves was associated with a reduced incidence of *C. difficile* diarrhea. This finding provides indirect evidence that personnel hand carriage is an important mode of nosocomial transmission of *C. difficile.*

▶ The incidence of *C. difficile* diarrhea and carriage was significantly lower on the glove ward during the period of glove use than on the same ward before the intervention. However, the incidence did not differ significantly between the glove ward and the control ward during the intervention period because the incidence figures had fallen somewhat on the control ward during that period. This finding must be somewhat disquieting to those of us who have tried measures to control the spread of *C. difficile* and found our hopes raised falsely by the unexplained fluctuations in the incidence of this infection. Interestingly, with the advent of universal precautions, the use of gloves has increased in general, and some authors have suggested that failure to change gloves between patients may be a substantial hazard for the transmission of *C. difficile.*—M.J. Barza, M.D.

Risk Factors for *Clostridium difficile* Carriage and *C. difficile*-Associated Diarrhea in a Cohort of Hospitalized Patients

McFarland LV, Surawicz CM, Stamm WE (Univ of Washington)

J Infect Dis 162:678–684, 1990 10–6

Age-Adjusted Relative Risks (aRR) for *Clostridium difficile* Carriage or Diarrhea

	aRR (95% CI)	
	Carriage	Diarrhea
Host factors		
History of laxative abuse	4.24 (1.93, 9.31)	3.92 (1.10, 13.9)
Other nosocomial infections	1.75 (1.01, 3.03)	3.44 (1.79, 6.63)
Hypochlorhydria	2.40 (1.43, 4.04)	1.33 (0.71, 2.49)
Immunocompromised	1.52 (0.88, 2.65)	1.85 (0.82, 4.19)
Medications		
Stool softeners	2.30 (1.39, 3.80)	1.69 (0.88, 3.26)
Antacids	2.10 (1.32, 3.32)	1.48 (0.77, 2.83)
Gastrointestinal stimulants	IN	5.18 (2.76, 9.72)
Laxatives	1.77 (1.07, 2.91)	1.46 (0.76, 2.67)
Procedures		
Nasogastric tube (>1 week)	2.36 (1.32, 4.23)	3.76 (1.88, 7.51)
Enemas	2.27 (1.21, 4.26)	2.36 (1.05, 5.32)
Nongastrointestinal surgery	2.11 (1.18, 3.80)	2.34 (1.20, 4.56)
Endoscopy	1.84 (0.87, 3.92)	2.71 (1.22, 6.02)
Antibiotics		
Vancomycin	2.06 (0.88, 4.84)	3.08 (1.17, 8.13)
Ampicillins	1.92 (1.19, 3.10)	1.38 (0.70, 2.73)
Other penicillins	1.32 (0.85, 2.03)	2.63 (1.31, 5.29)
Cephalosporins	1.58 (0.88, 2.86)	2.43 (1.29, 4.58)
TMP/SMX	1.20 (0.59, 2.46)	2.67 (1.37, 5.21)

Abbreviations: IN, insufficient numbers; *CI,* confidence interval; *TMP-SMX,* trimethoprim-sulfamethoxazole.

Note: Antibiotics were multiple agents (i.e., not mutually exclusive categories).

(Courtesy of McFarland LV, Surawicz CM, Stamm WE: *J Infect Dis* 162:678–684, 1990.)

Clostridium difficile occurs frequently in hospitalized patients. Its presentation can range from asymptomatic carriage to colitis. An attempt was made to identify risk factors associated either with asymptomatic carriage of *C. difficile* or with the occurrence of associated diarrhea in a prospective study of 399 patients admitted consecutively to a single ward.

All had negative cultures for *C. difficile.* Rectal specimens were obtained within 48 hours of admission and every 3–4 days thereafter. Patients were considered to be carriers if they had at least 1 positive culture but no diarrheal symptoms. Patients with a positive culture, diarrhea, and no other possible causes for diarrhea were classified as having *C. difficile*-associated diarrhea.

Eighty-three patients acquired *C. difficile* after hospitalization; 52 were asymptomatic carriers, 26 had antibiotic-associated diarrhea, and 5 had diarrhea with no associated antibiotic use. Increased age, severity of underlying disease, and length of stay were significantly related to *C. difficile* infection, according to univariate analysis. After age adjustment, a number of other factors were found to be associated with *C. difficile* carriage and C. *difficile*-associated diarrhea (table). Multivariate analysis of risk factors revealed that exposure to stool softeners and antacids was significantly associated with C. *difficile* carriage. Risk factors for the associated diarrhea, in addition to older age and more severe underlying illness, were the use of cephalosporin, penicillin, enemas, gastrointestinal stimulants, and stool softeners.

The latter 5 factors can alter the normal gastrointestinal flora. Intrinsic host factors also play a part in the risk of acquisition of C. *difficile* in the hospital. More stringent infection control measures are recommended as a means of reducing the nosocomial transmission of C. *difficile.*

▶ Most hospital epidemiologists reading this article will readily accept the likely importance of the risk factors identified. Unfortunately, none of the studies of this frustrating nosocomial infection has come up with effective and economically reasonable measures to interrupt transmission beyond the standard recommendations of handwashing, use of gloves, and environmental decontamination. These measures are clearly important, but some institutions using good practices continue to have high rates of nosocomial infection.—M.J. Barza, M.D.

Nosocomial Maxillary Sinusitis During Mechanical Ventilation: A Prospective Comparison of Orotracheal Versus the Nasotracheal Route for Intubation

Salord F, Gaussorgues P, Marti-Flich J, Sirodot M, Allimant C, Lyonnet D, Robert D (Hôp de la Croix-Rousse, Lyon, France)
Intensive Care Med 16:390–393, 1990 10–7

The incidence of nosocomial maxillary sinusitis was compared in patients in an intensive care unit who were undergoing mechanical ventilation through the orotracheal (OTI) or nasotracheal (NTI) route. During a 6-month period, 111 consecutive adult patients requiring endotracheal intubation were randomly allocated to OTI or NTI groups. All had a nasogastric feeding tube. The diagnosis of nosocomial maxillary sinusitis was radiologic. The 2 patient groups were similar in age, duration of mechanical ventilation, and severity index.

Maxillary sinusitis developed in 26 patients, 25 of whom were in the NTI group. Most episodes occurred during the first 2 weeks after admission. Most episodes of nosocomial maxillary sinusitis had a favorable outcome, but 4 patients died of septic complications. Sinus drainage, performed in 14 patients, yielded a fluid purulent with altered polynuclear cells. Tube removal, initially performed in 17 patients, was successful in 12 patients. Although the OTI group had significantly more incidents related to the route for long-term intubation, none proved fatal. Long-term OTI clearly reduces the incidence of maxillary sinusitis compared with NTI.

▶ As more and more of our consults are for patients in the intensive care unit, well-done prospective studies that provide clean answers to important problems are especially welcome. In this series, sinusitis developed in 43% of those patients who were intubated via the nasal-tracheal route, but in only 1.8% of those who had oral-tracheal intubation. Not only is the difference striking, but the absolute incidence in those patients who had nasal-tracheal intubation is extraordinary. Of perhaps greater concern was the incidence of nosocomial pneumonia, which occurred in 14 of the 26 patients who had maxillary sinusitis and only in 4 of the 85 patients who did not have sinusitis. Although the advantages of oral-tracheal intubation are clear from an infectious disease standpoint, more complications of intubation occur via this route. These include greater rates of self-extubation and selective intubation of the right mainstem bronchus, greater difficulty in tube fastening, pressure necrosis on the inferior portion of the lip, and tube biting, especially in patients with neurologic disorders. However, it seems that all of these complications are avoidable and, given the choice, oral-tracheal intubation seems to be a far safer way to go.—M.S. Klempner, M.D.

Sternal Wound Complications After Isolated Coronary Artery Bypass Grafting: Early and Late Mortality, Morbidity, and Cost of Care

Loop FD, Lytle BW, Cosgrove DM, Mahfood S, McHenry MC, Goormastic M, Stewart RW, Golding LAR, Taylor PC (Cleveland Clinic Found)

Ann Thorac Surg 49:179–187, 1990 10–8

Data were reviewed on sternal wound complications (mediastinitis or dehiscence, or both) and their outcome in 6,504 consecutive patients who underwent isolated coronary artery bypass grafting from 1985 through 1987.

Among the 5,369 patients who had a first-time coronary artery bypass 15 women and 40 men (1%) (median age, 62 years) had sternal wound complications. Among the 1,135 patients who underwent reoperation 3 women and 14 men (1.5%) (median age, 59 years) experienced wound complications. All 72 patients with sternal wound complications were followed up.

When grouped by type of conduit used in primary grafting, wound complication rates were .9% for vein grafts only, .9% for 1 internal thoracic artery, and 1.6% for bilateral internal thoracic artery grafts. There were no significant differences in wound complication rates between patients who had primary and reoperation procedures. The mean interval between operation and diagnosis of a wound complication was 11 days.

Wound cultures were negative in 11 patients and positive in 61. Forty-one cultures grew *Staphylococcus* species and 17 grew *Enterobacteriaceae*. Ten patients with wound infections (14%) died in the hospital of multisystem failure. Two additional patients died of renal failure in the first postoperative year.

Univariate analysis identified 12 variables that achieved significance in the calculation of risk factors for sternal wound complications. Subsequent multivariate analysis identified 4 clinical factors that were predictive of an increased risk of wound complication after isolated coronary bypass grafting: operating time, bilateral internal thoracic artery grafting in the presence of diabetes, obesity, and the number of blood units or blood products received before the diagnosis of a wound complication.

The median charge for all 72 patients with wound complications was $58,092 (range, $16,966 to $408,632), which was 2.8 times that of patients with uncomplicated cases. These charges do not include physician's fees. Hospital charges incurred were not significantly different among conduit groups or between primary and reoperation cases with wound complications.

▶ This study is a useful reference for hospital epidemiologists and others interested in wound infections related to cardiothoracic surgery. However, the study appears to have been retrospective, and it seems that infection rates in retrospective studies are usually lower than in prospective ones. Although the type of graft did not generally influence the rate of infection, bilateral internal thoracic artery grafting in diabetic patients had a relative risk of fivefold. The literature on this issue has been controversial. The authors contend that continued vigilance and regular feedback to surgeons of infection rates for their own patients are beneficial in keeping the rates low.—M.J. Barza, M.D.

Catheter-Related Sepsis: Prospective, Randomized Study of Three Methods of Long-Term Catheter Maintenance

Eyer S, Brummitt C, Crossley K, Siegel R, Cerra F (St. Paul-Ramsey Med Ctr, Minn)

Crit Care Med 18:1073–1079, 1990 10–9

Indwelling vascular catheters may be used for drug infusions, blood products, hemodynamic monitoring, nutrition, or dialysis. Catheter longevity, construction, and techniques of placement and care influence the rate of infectious complications, which has ranged as high as 19% in some studies. The management of long-term indwelling catheters was evaluated in terms of mechanical complications and episodes of catheter-related sepsis (CRS).

The catheters in 112 patients were changed to a new site every 7 days with percutaneous puncture, exchanged through guidewire exchange every 7 days at the same site, or managed with no change at all unless clin-

Catheter-Related Sepsis Episodes

	GWX	PERC	NWC
Percent patients with CRS	15%	16%	13%
CRS episode/patient	0.17	0.22	0.16
CRS episode/catheter cultured	0.024	0.038	0.041
CRS episode/patient-catheter day	0.004	0.005	0.003

(Courtesy of Eyer S, Brummitt C, Crossley K, et al: *Crit Care Med* 18:1073–1079, 1990.)

ically indicated. In all groups, a catheter change was mandatory for a positive blood culture, skin site infection, or sepsis without a likely source.

The lowest number of CRS episodes was in the no-change group, with .16 CRS episodes per patient; the highest number (.22 episodes per patient) was in the group having percutaneous puncture. In the guidewire exchange group the number of episodes per patient was .17 (table). Regardless of management, the chance of CRS developing was .3% to .5% per catheter per day. The similar rates of infectious risk suggest that the method associated with least complications and expense should be used. General guidelines are to avoid routine changing of catheters, exchanging guidewires when catheters are changed, and catheterizing at a new site if skin infection is present.

▶ It seems to be a relatively unusual circumstance in contemporary medicine when the least expensive and most convenient approach (in this case, not changing long-term intravenous catheters until there was a clinical indication to do so) is as effective and safe as the other options. In fact, the incidence of episodes of CRS was slightly, but not significantly, lower when catheters were changed only as clinically indicated rather than every 7 days (whether over a guidewire or to a new site).—M.J. Barza, M.D.

Antibiotic Therapy of Catheter Infections in Patients Receiving Home Parenteral Nutrition

Miller SJ, Dickerson RN, Graziani AA, Muscari EA, Mullen JL (Univ of Pennsylvania)

J Parenter Enteral Nutr 14:143–147, 1990 10–10

Previous studies have documented that staphylococcal species are most commonly responsible for catheter-related infections in patients who are receiving long-term parenteral nutrition. Because the number of available catheter sites is obviously limited, extraordinary care is taken to preserve the central venous catheter. However, the efficacy of antibiotic therapy of catheter infections while the catheter remains in place has not been well studied.

A review of the medical records of all patients who received home parenteral nutrition between 1983 and 1987 yielded 58 episodes of documented catheter-related sepsis in 21 patients. Parenteral nutrition was administered either via a silicone catheter or a permanently implanted device. Among the 81 organisms isolated from blood culture, 47 were gram-positive cocci, 20 were gram-negative bacilli, and 13 were yeasts. Infectious episodes were initially treated empirically at home with 1 g of cefazolin, administered intravenously every 12 hours.

Of the 12 episodes of gram-negative infection treated initially with cefazolin, 11 (92%) resulted in hospitalization and 6 (50%) resulted in catheter removal (table). Gram-positive infections in 30 episodes resulted in 17 hospitalizations (57%) and 7 catheter removals (23%). All 11 epi-

Episodes Resulting in Hospitalization and Catheter Removal

	No. episodes (%) requiring hospitalization	No. episodes (%) requiring catheter removal
Gram-positive cocci		
Coagulase-negative staph (N = 23)	11 (48)	5 (22)
Group D streptococcus (N = 2)	2 (100)	1 (50)
Staphylococcus aureus (N = 4)	3 (75)	1 (25)
Others (N = 1)	1 (100)	0 (0)
Total Gram-positive (N = 30)	17 (57)	7 (23)
Gram-negative bacilli		
Total Gram-negative (N = 12)	11 (92)	6 (50)
Yeast*		
Total yeast (N = 11)	11 (100)	11 (100)
Nonfungal polymicrobial (N = 5)	5 (100)	2 (40)
Totals		
All Episodes (N = 58)	44 (76)	26 (45)

*All episodes in which fungi were isolated are included in this category.

(Courtesy of Miller SJ, Dickerson RN, Graziani AA, et al: *J Parenter Enteral Nutr* 14:143–147, 1990.)

sodes of yeast infection required immediate hospitalization and catheter removal. The average duration of therapy was 12 days for cefazolin failures and 25 days for successful cefazolin therapy. Eleven cefazolin failures were subsequently treated with vancomycin, which was unsuccessful in 5 cases. Overall, patients required hospitalization in 44 of the 58 episodes of catheter-related sepsis (76%), with catheter removal in 26 episodes (45%). Treatment algorithms for coagulase-negative staphylococcal infections and gram-negative infections are shown in Figures 10–2 and 10–3.

Because attempts at treating catheter-associated infections in patients who receive home parenteral nutrition have been largely unsuccessful, patients are now routinely admitted for clinical evaluation and aggressive antibiotic therapy. Vancomycin is presently the preferred drug for treatment of these infections.

▶ Like most studies of infections related to intravenous catheters, this one suffers from being retrospective and not highly informative. Although the authors describe treatment algorithms relating to the choice of antibiotic and the decisions to hospitalize the patient and remove the catheter, these decisions were made arbitrarily by the physicians and without a protocol. The main messages are that outpatient treatment (cefazolin, 1 g every 12 hours) was usually unsucessful, even in patients with infections caused by susceptible organisms, and that the need for catheter removal was very high (100%) with fungal infection, moderate (50%) with gram-negative bacillary infection, and lowest (23%)

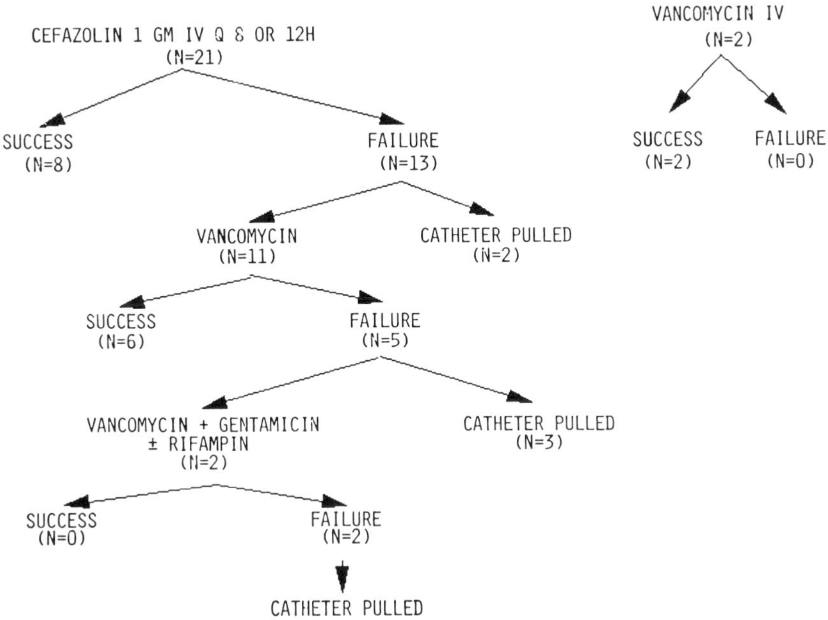

Fig 10–2.—Treatment algorithm for coagulase-negative staphylococcal infections. (Courtesy of Miller SJ, Dickerson RN, Graziani AA, et al: *J Parenter Enter Nutr* 14:143–147, 1990.)

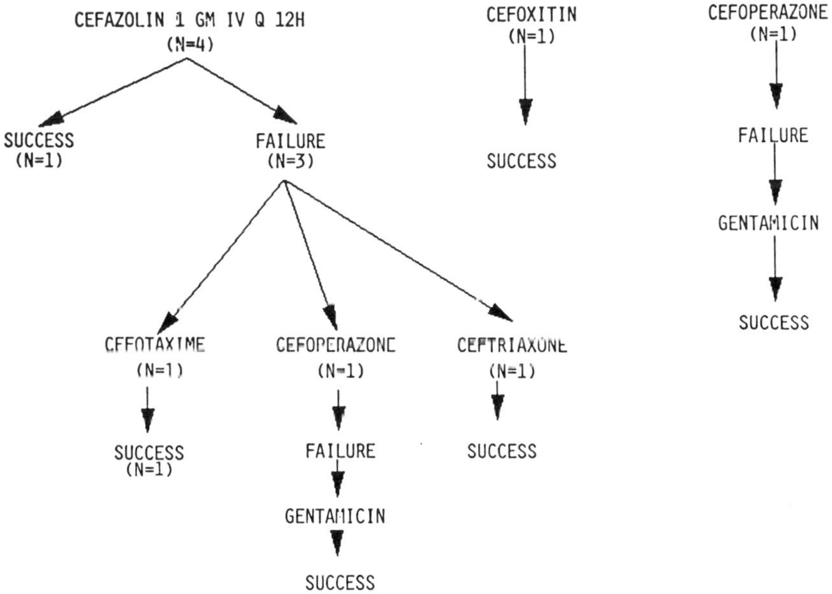

Fig 10–3.—Treatment algorithm for gram-negative infections. (Courtesy of Miller SJ, Dickerson RN, Graziani AA, et al: *J Parenter Enter Nutr* 14:143–147, 1990.)

with infection by gram-positive cocci. However, even these data are difficult to interpret because the criteria for each decision were established retrospectively and some of the outcomes were predetermined, e.g., the finding of fungal infection automatically dictated removal of the catheter, I, for one, remain unsure as to which catheters need to be removed and which infections can be cured without removal of the catheter.—M.J. Barza, M.D.

Outpatient Percutaneous Central Venous Access in Cancer Patients

Broadwater JR, Henderson MA, Bell JL, Edwards MJ, Smith GJ, McCready DR, Swanson RS, Hardy MER, Shenk RR, Lawson M, Ota DM, Balch CM (Univ of Texas, Houston)

Am J Surg 160:676–680, 1990 10–11

Cancer patients usually require central venous access for safe delivery of chemotherapy. Because of the manpower requirements for intraoperative insertion in traditional methods of central venous catheterizations, such as tunneled catheters, percutaneous catheterization was instituted for outpatient care of cancer patients. During a 1-year period 664 consecutive outpatients with cancer underwent 763 attempts at percutaneous subclavian catheter insertions, mostly for delivery of chemotherapy. An infusion therapy team at the clinic provided intensive education for catheter care to all patients and their families.

Catheter insertion was successful in 722 attempts (95%). Insertion complications included pneumothorax in 13 patients (2%); 30 catheters (4%) required repositioning. The average duration of catheterization was 193 days (range, 0 to 892 days). Fifty-six catheters (8%) were removed for suspected infection, but only 21 patients (3%) had documented infection (Table 1). Eight patients (1%) had catheter site infection. Thus only

TABLE 1.—Indications for Catheter Removal

Indication for Removal	No.	%
Treatment completed	310	43
Death	140	19
Sepsis suspected	56	8
Sepsis proven	21	3
Catheter thrombosis	21	3
Catheter removed accidentally	11	2
Site infection	8	1
Malposition	7	1
Malfunction	7	1
Insertion complication	4	1
Reason unknown	34	5
Total	619	87*

*At time of chart review 103 catheters (14%) remained in place.

(Courtesy of Broadwater JR, Henderson MA, Bell JL, et al: *Am J Surg* 160:676–680, 1990.)

TABLE 2.—Estimated Cost by Central Venous Catheterization Technique

Charge (in dollars)	Percutaneous Silicone Catheter	Tunneled Catheter	Reservoir
Insertion charges			
Physician	265	450	500
Anesthesia	NA	350	350
Operating room	NA	336	336
Radiology	77	181	181
Nursing	37	NA	NA
Clinic visit *	112	NA	NA
Catheter	23	54	339
Supplies	48	32	32
Total	562	1,403	1,738

Abbreviation: NA, not applicable.
Note: Costs estimated from routine hospital charges.
*Insertion requires 4 clinic visits.
(Courtesy of Broadwater JR, Henderson MA, Bell JL, et al: *Am J Surg* 160:676–680, 1990.)

.22 infection per catheter year occurred during the 382 catheter-years' experience. The estimated cost of the percutaneous technique was about one third of the insertion cost for a tunneled catheter or for a reservoir device (Table 2).

These data show that percutaneous subclavian catheterization is a reliable and cost-effective method for central venous access, with a frequency of catheter-related infections similar to that for tunneled or reservoir devices. A detailed educational program that involves the patients and their families is an important element in the success of this program. Percutaneous catheterization should be the method of choice in centers where a large number of patients require central venous access.

▶ The cost of insertion of the percutaneous catheters in this series was about one third that of tunneled catheters or subcutaneous reservoir catheters. The authors argue that the rate of infection with percutaneous catheters was probably no higher than what one would expect with tunneled catheters, and that tunneled catheters have no distinct advantage over percutaneous catheters. It should be noted that all percutaneous catheters in the study were implanted by surgical housestaff; infusions were given only by the infusion therapy team, and patients underwent a program of education regarding the maintenance of the catheters. In contrast to tunneled or percutaneous catheters, reservoir (subcutaneous) catheters require no external catheter or dressing changes and heparin injection is needed only once each month. These may be the preferred catheters in children and patients with more active life-styles. For others, at least in centers with large numbers of patients requiring central venous catheters, the percutaneous catheter may be preferred on the grounds of cost.—M.J. Barza, M.D.

Association of Intravenous Lipid Emulsion and Coagulase-Negative Staphylococcal Bacteremia in Neonatal Intensive Care Units

Freeman J, Goldmann DA, Smith NE, Sidebottom DG, Epstein MF, Platt R (Brigham and Women's Hosp, Boston; Brockton/West Roxbury VA Med Ctr, W Roxbury, Mass; Children's Hosp, Boston; Harvard School of Public Health, Boston)

N Engl J Med 323:301–308, 1990 10–12

Coagulase-negative staphylococci are the leading cause of bacteremia in neonatal intensive care units (NICUs). A case-control study of 882 infants treated in 2 NICUs during 1982 was conducted to determine potential risk factors for this nosocomial infection. Of the infants, 45 had nosocomial bacteremia with coagulase-negative staphylococci; 38 were included in the study after excluding neonates with birth weights of less than 700 g. The 76 control infants without bacteremia were matched according to hospital, birth weight, and date of discharge.

The 38 patients and the 76 matched controls were similar with respect to 27 indicators of the severity of the underlying illness. Of the 20 therapeutic measures that were possible risk factors for nosocomial bacteremia, only the intravenous administration of lipid emulsion and the use of nonumbilical central venous catheters were strongly associated with nosocomial bacteremia caused by coagulase-negative staphylococci. Infants with coagulase-negative staphylococcus were 5.8 times as likely as controls to have been given lipid emulsion before the onset of bacteremia. Infants with bacteremia were also 3.5 times as likely as controls to have had a percutaneously inserted central venous catheter. Because intravenous lipid emulsion was used frequently (68.4%), 56.6% of all cases of nosocomial bacteremia could be attributed to lipid administration, whereas the attributable risk to exposure to nonumbilical central venous catheters was 14.9%.

The induction time for bacteremia after lipid administration, usually through peripheral catheters, was less than 1 day, compared with 5.5 days with the use of central venous catheters not associated with lipid administration. A strong and independent association of coagulase-negative staphylococcal bacteremia with intravenously administered lipid emulsion was also confirmed on a similar analyses of data on another 31 neonates treated in 1988. The relative odds of bacteremia developing was 5.3.

These data indicate that the risk of coagulase-negative staphylococcal bacteremia in infants in NICUs can be attributed primarily to intravenous lipid administration. Because lipids are critical for the nutritional support of premature neonates, further studies are warranted to determine the pathogenesis and prevention of lipid-association bacteremia.

▶ Documentation of this association has another parallel, as pointed out by the authors, in *Malassezia furfur* infection in neonates receiving lipids.

The mechanism wherein lipid emulsions may be associated with coagulase-negative staphylococcal bacteremia include the impedance of neutrophil and macrophage function, provision of a nutrient growth medium, a mechanical effect of lipids, or an increased risk of contamination and manipulation in the system. The authors discount this latter possibility, citing the measures they used to prevent contamination. This complication needs further mechanistic elucidation in order to enable implementation of appropriate control measures.—D.R. Snydman, M.D.

Rapid Dissemination of β-Lactamase-Producing, Aminoglycoside-Resistant *Enterococcus faecalis* Among Patients and Staff on an Infant-Toddler Surgical Ward

Rhinehart E, Smith NE, Wennersten C, Gorss E, Freeman J, Eliopoulos GM, Moellering RC Jr, Goldmann DA (Children's Hosp, Boston; Brockton-West Roxbury VA Hosp, W Roxbury, Mass; New England Deaconess Hosp, Boston)
N Engl J Med 323:1814–1818, 1990 10–13

There is an increasing incidence of infections caused by enterococci with high-level aminoglycoside resistance. Also, a few aminoglycoside-resistant strains of *Enterococcus faecalis* that produce β-lactamases have also been reported. In an infant-toddler surgical ward, rapid spread of a multiply resistant *E. faecalis* was observed that prompted a prospective microbiologic and epidemiologic investigation.

In July 1987, a β-lactamase-producing gentamicin-resistant *E. faecalis* isolate was identified in the index child who had been hospitalized in the infant-toddler surgical ward since birth. In addition, 10 of his roommates or other children who had been on the ward for at least 3 days and 4 of 11 nurses had positive stool cultures. No definite infections occurred. Another 63 of 1,028 patients admitted to the ward in 1988 and 8 of 33 employees with at least 1 positive stool culture were identified in the prospective study.

In a case-control study, independent risk factors associated with colonization included care by nurse 3, hospitalization in the nursery, and bowel preparation for surgery (table). Despite intensive efforts to control the outbreak and relocation to another hospital facility, further improvement was not observed until nurse 3 was removed from clinical duty. Furthermore, restriction-endonuclease digestion of plasmid DNA demonstrated identical patterns from isolates of *E. faecalis* from the index patient and other colonized patients during the outbreak, and isolates of materials cultured from nurse 3's hands and damaged thumbnail.

Gentamicin-resistant strains of *E. faecalis* that produce β-lactamase have the potential for rapid dissemination among susceptible hospitalized children. Although the strain of *E. faecalis* isolate in this outbreak produced remarkably little disease, other strains of β-lactamase-positive strains of *E. faecalis* have been shown to be virulent.

▶ One of the remarkable features of this study is the role that a nurse who was a chronic carrier to β-lactamase-producing enterococci played in the colonization of these infants. There were a number of independent risk factors, but

Independent Factors Associated With Colonization of Patients With β-Lactamase-Positive, Gentamicin-Resistant *E. faecalis*

Study Variable	No. of Patients Exposed	Odds Ratio†	95% Confidence Interval‡
Assignment to nursery	28	10.8	1.9–60.2
Care by Nurse 3	26	11.6	2.2–62.9
Bowel preparation	10	12.9	2.4–68.5
Oral feedings	37	0.1	0.03–0.4
Dilute-formula feedings	25	0.4	0.1–1.4

*Variables were adjusted for the effect of the other variables as well as for weight, duration, and study period. According to the multiple regression model, weights were divided into 5 strata: 1–4 kg, 5–8 kg, 9–12 kg, 13–16 kg, and 17–20 kg; duration of exposure was divided into 4 strata: 1–2 days, 3–22 days, 23–40 days, and 41–53 days.

†Mantel-Haenszel summary-adjusted estimates of odds ratios.

‡Chi and test-based 95% confidence intervals.

(Courtesy of Rhinehart E, Smith NE, Wennersten C, et al: *N Engl J Med* 323:1814–1818, 1990.)

until she was removed the epidemic of colonization could not be controlled. One can only wonder how commonly carriers of other organisms, not so readily recognized, contribute to transmission of antibiotic resistance in the hospital. Fortunately for the nurse, these investigators were able to eliminate fecal carriage with oral vancomycin, 500 mg 4 times daily, and rifampin, 300 mg twice daily, for 14 days along with 2% total body chlorhexidine bathing.—D.R. Snydman, M.D.

▶ ↓ This is the second report in this year's Year Book in which a chronically colonized nurse was associated with transmission of an unusual organism. Several factors led to recognition of this outbreak, including the holding of plates for 5 days.—D.R. Snydman, M.D.

A Cluster of *Rhodococcus (Gordona) bronchialis* Sternal-Wound Infections After Coronary-Artery Bypass Surgery

Richet HM, Craven PC, Brown JM, Lasker BA, Cox CD, McNeil MM, Tice AD, Jarvis WR, Tablan OC (Ctrs for Disease Control, Atlanta; Infections Limited, Tacoma, Wash)

N Engl J Med 324:104–108, 1991 10–14

Rhodococcus species are gram-positive aerobic actinomycetes that colonize and infect animals but rarely cause infections in humans. A hospital outbreak of surgical wound infections occurred, caused by a single genetically distinct strain of *Rhodococcus (Gordona) bronchialis.*

Sternal wound infections caused by *R. bronchialis* occurred in 7 patients who had undergone open-heart surgery between May 1 and December 31, 1988. Infection occurred at a mean 53 days (range, 30–102) after surgery. All patients were treated initially with antimicrobial agents, but 4 subsequently required surgical débridement. Only 3 patients improved with antimicrobial therapy alone, with treatment lasting for 74–122 days. No relapses occurred.

When compared with randomly selected controls, the only factor that was significantly associated with sternal wound infection caused by *R. bronchialis* was the presence of the operating room nurse A. Procedural and microbiologic investigations indicated that the presence of nurse A was associated with an increased risk of *R. bronchialis* surgical wound infection after open-heart surgery alone, and not with other procedures in which nurse A was present as well. The mode of transmission was apparently through the use of the water bath for the activated clotting-time test in the operating room.

Rhodococcus (Gordona) bronchialis grew in cultures of materials obtained from nurse A's hands, scalp, and vagina, and from the neck-scruff skin of 2 of nurse A's 3 dogs. All isolates cultured from the patients, nurse A, and her dogs were morphologically and biochemically similar and matched the mycolic-acid profile of the ATCC type strain *R. bronchialis* W4157. Plasmid studies, restriction-endonuclease analysis, and ribosome typing indicated that the strains of *R. bronchialis* isolated from nurse A were genetically related to those isolated from the patients. There were no further cases in the 12 months after the outbreak when nurse A was reassigned to noncardiac surgical procedures. The nurse's dogs were most likely the source of the outbreak strain.

A Cluster of *Legionella* Sternal-Wound Infections Due to Postoperative Topical Exposure to Contaminated Tap Water

Lowry PW, Blankenship RJ, Gridley W, Troup NJ, Tompkins LS (Stanford Univ)

N Engl J Med 324:109–113, 1991 10–15

Extrapulmonary *Legionella* infections are uncommon, and nosocomial clusters of these infections are even more rare. A cluster of 3 patients with sternal wound infections caused by *Legionella* was identified.

In May 1989, 2 patients in the intensive care unit contracted *Legionella* infections after cardiac surgery. One had sternal wound infection (patient 1, table) and the other had pleural effusion (patient 4). Two additional patients with *Legionella* sternal wound infections were identified retrospectively (patients 2 and, table). All 3 patients with sternal wound infections had evidence of unusual sternal disruption. *Legionella dumoffi* was isolated in patient 1, *Legionella pneumophila* in patient 2, and both *L. dumoffi* and *L. pneumophila* in patient 3.

A case-control study indicated that cases were more likely to have had 2 or more sternotomies and more sternal wound dressing changes during the first week of surgery. Investigation showed that most nurses routinely used tap water to bathe patients after cardiovascular surgery. The sternal wounds may have been exposed to tap water during patient bathing, as evidenced by a fluorescein study. The 2 *Legionella* strains were detected only in the taps of patient sinks in the intensive care unit. Restriction endonuclease digestion analysis showed that *L. dumoffi* isolated from pa-

Clinical Features of 3 Patients With *Legionella* Sternal Wound Infections

Patient No.	Sex/Age	Type of Surgery (Date)	Perioperative Events	Positive Cultures	Treatment	Outcome
1	F/85 yr	Aortic-valve replacement (4/24/89)	Required chest compressions for bradyarrhythmia and repair of sternal bleeding during first 24 hr after operation	Two colonies of *L. dumoffii* isolated from blood (5/3/89) and sternum (5/4/89)	Mediastinal exploration (5/4/89); erythromycin, 4 g per day intravenously	Died after 7 days of erythromycin
2	F/3 wk	Norwood procedure for hypoplastic left ventricle (3/3/88)	Required repair of suture-line bleeding 2 days after operation; underwent intrathoracic cardiac massage 2 and 8 days after operation	*L. pneumophila* isolated from mediastinal tissue (3/22/88) and lung (3/25/88)	Mediastinal exploration (3/2/88)	Died; diagnosis made post mortem
3	M/27 yr	Third aortic-valve replacement (11/7/86)	Two previous aortic-valve replacements; mediastinal fibrosis and sternal bleeding noted at surgery (11/7/86)	*L. dumoffii* and *L. pneumophila* isolated from sternal "cyst" (1/14/87); *L. dumoffii* isolated from aortic valve (1/29/87)	Aspiration of sternal "cyst" (1/14/87); 4th aortic-valve replacement (1/29/87); erythromycin, 2 g per day intravenously, plus rifampin, 1200 mg per day orally, for 9 mo	Cured after 9 mo of antibiotic therapy

Note: A fourth patient (patient 4) had *L. dumoffii* isolated from pleural fluid but did not have a sternal wound infection.
(Courtesy of Lowry PW, Blankenship RJ, Gridley W, et al: *N Engl J Med* 324:109–113, 1991.)

tients 1, 3, and 4 had the same digestion pattern as the *L. dumoffi* isolates from tap water. Similarly, isolates of *L. pneumophila* serogroup 1 recovered from patients 2 and 3 were identical to isolates of *L. pneumophila* cultured from tap water. *Legionella* sternal wound infections in these patients after cardiac surgery are attributed to direct contact of the wounds with contaminated tap water during bathing or changing of dressings.

▶ Several years ago we reviewed the report of *Legionella* endocarditis from this institution (1). The source may well have been the tap water described in this outbreak! One moral from this outbreak is avoid using tap water on fresh surgical wounds. Another aspect for consultants to remember is to consider *Legionella* in culture-negative wound infections.—D.R. Snydman, M.D.

Reference

1. 1990 Year Book of Infectious Diseases, pp 8–9.

11 Pediatric Infections

Mycoplasmal Infections of Cerebrospinal Fluid in Newborn Infants From a Community Hospital Population

Waites KB, Duffy LB, Crouse DT, Dworsky ME, Strange MJ, Nelson KG, Cassell GH (Univ of Alabama, Birmingham; Alabama Neonatology Assoc, Birmingham; Neonatal Unit AMI Brookwood Med Ctr, Birmingham)

Pediatr Infect Dis J 9:241–245, 1990 11–1

In a previous study, *Mycoplasma hominis* or *Ureaplasma urealyticum* was isolated from the CSF of 13 preterm newborn infants among 100 tested in a university hospital. These infants were derived from a high-risk obstetric population consisting predominantly of women of lower income and socioeconomic status who had little or no prenatal care. To determine whether such infections occur with the same frequency in the general population, CSF cultures were performed in 318 infants born to women cared for mainly through private obstetric practices and who delivered in 4 suburban community hospitals.

During an 8-month period, *M. hominis* was isolated from 9 (2.8%) and *U. urealyticum* was isolated from 5 (1.6%) CSF cultures. Most of these infants were born at or near term, and only 1 had a birth weight of less than 1,000 g (Table 1). Spontaneous eradication of the infecting organism was documented in 5 infants. In most infants, CSF pleocytosis was minimal or absent (Table 2). Except for 1 infant, none received spe-

TABLE 1.—Demographic Features of Infants With Positive CSF Cultures

Case	Sex	Race	Birth Weight (g)	Gestation (Weeks)	Delivery	Membrane Rupture (Hours)	Maternal Complications
Mycoplasma hominis							
1	M	W	4080	39	Cesarean	0	None
2	F	W	1500	32	Cesarean	0	Hypertension
3	M	W	2700	33	Vaginal	9	Preterm labor
4	F	B	3500	42	Cesarean	8	Fetal distress
5	M	B	1120	28	Cesarean	Unknown	Placenta previa
6	M	W	2750	35	Vaginal	Unknown	None
7	M	W	2440	32	Cesarean	21	Preterm labor
8	M	B	2950	37	Cesarean	Unknown	None
9	M	W	1800	33	Vaginal	Unknown	Preterm labor
Ureaplasma urealyticum							
10	M	W	2865	40	Vaginal	Unknown	None
11	F	W	630	24	Vaginal	Unknown	Amnionitis
12	F	W	3800	42	Vaginal	<4	None
13	F	W	2990	37	Vaginal	Unknown	None
14	M	W	4330	42	Cesarean	10	Amnionitis

Abbreviations: *W*, white; *B*, black.

(Courtesy of Waites KB, Duffy LB, Crouse DT, et al: *Pediatr Infect Dis J* 9:241–245, 1990.)

TABLE 2.—Clinical and CSF Findings in Infected Infants

Case and Organism	Age (Days)	*Mycoplasma* Culture *	Protein (mg/dl)	WBC (Cells/mm³)	RBC (Cells/m³)	Treatment
Mycoplasma hominis (Cases 1–9)						
1†	1	+ (10^1)	140	3	0	None
2	1	+ (10^4)	90	0	0	None
	5	–	110	10	395	
3	1	+ (10^1)	120	0	514	None
4	1	+ (10^5)	63	0	889	None
5 †	1	–	n.a.	n.a.	n.a.	
	16	–	96	1	9	
	21	+ (10^4)	87	3	1	None
6'†	32	+ (10^2)	170	500'‡	30,000	None
	36	–	n.a.	n.a.	n.a.	
7	1	+ (10^4)	140	6	717	None
8 †	3	+ (10^3)	100	2	3	Clindamycin
	6	–	150	0	59	
	12	–	180	10	330	
9 §	1	+ (10^2)	170	8	4050	None
	23	–	78	4	1	
Ureaplasma urealyticum (Cases 10–14)						
10	1	+ (10^4)	110	5	900	None
	23	–	n.a.	n.a.	n.a.	
11	1	+ (10^5)	150	240 ‖	2000	None
12	1	+ (10^1)	90	5	0	None
13	1	+ (10^2)	130	10	0	None
14	1	+ (10^1)	79	36 ‡	21	None
	10	–	n.a.	n.a.	n.a.	

Abbreviations: WBC, white blood cells; *RBC,* red blood cells.

*Numbers in (parentheses) color change units per mililiter of organisms present in CSF. A color change unit refers to the minimum inoculum required to produce a color change in the medium indicative of growth.

†Endotracheal aspirate culture for mycoplasms performed but negative.

‡White blood cells predominantly mononuclear cells.

§Endotracheal aspirate culture positive for *M. hominis* at age 1 day.

‖White blood cells predominantly polymorphonuclear cells.

(Courtesy of Waites KB, Duffy LB, Crouse DT, et al: *Pediatr Infect Dis J* 9:241–245, 1990.)

cific treatment for mycoplasma. There was a good perinatal outcome in 12 infants. There were 2 deaths, the cause of which was systemic infection with *Hemophilus influenzae* in 1 infant and extreme prematurity, intraventricular hemorrhage, and possible ureaplasmal meningitis in the other.

These data suggest that mycoplasmas are common causes of neonatal infections, not only in high-risk populations, but also in the general population. Although the infections appear to be innocuous in some infants, further studies are warranted to define the significance and natural history of mycoplasma infections.

▶ I wonder how many pediatricians or infectious disease specialists would list mycoplasma as the number 1 organism isolated in CSF specimens obtained from newborns. That was the conclusion of a previous study of these authors in high-risk premature infants. They now find a similar result in neonates delivered by private obstetricians in 4 suburban community hospitals. They make a convincing case that we must be missing a number of these infections because most of the neonates have otherwise normal CSF findings. A critical question is what to do with a positive culture. Only 1 of the 14 patients with a positive culture for *M. hominis* or *U. urealyticum* received specific treatment for mycoplasmas. And the 2 deaths that occurred were in infants in whom there were other explanations. Whether or not there will be long-term sequelae to neonatal CSF infections with mycoplasma will be an important follow-up study from these authors.—M.S. Klempner, M.D.

Maternal Colonization by Group B Streptococci and Puerperal Infection: Analysis of Intrapartum Chemoprophylaxis

Matorras R, García-Perea A, Madero R, Usandizaga JA (Hosp La Paz, Madrid; Autonomous Univ of Madrid, Spain)

Eur J Obstet Gynecol Reprod Biol 38:203–207, 1990 11–2

The importance of group B streptococci in neonatal sepsis has been well documented. The significance of group B streptococcal maternal colonization during pregnancy in the genesis of puerperal infection was studied using data obtained from 1,011 puerperal women.

Of these, 121 were streptococcal carriers during pregnancy. They were randomly assigned to receive either ampicillin, 500 mg intravenously every 6 hours during delivery, or no chemoprophylaxis. When compared with noncarriers, the carriers who received no prophylaxis had a significant increase in mild puerperal infective morbidity, defined as the proportion of women with an index fever of 10 or greater. The increased incidence of premature rupture of the membranes among carriers and of other possible morbidity factors made it impossible to identify the role of group B streptococci.

In this series, mild puerperal infective morbidity in carriers who were given prophylaxis was lower than in those without prophylaxis, being very similar to that in noncarriers. The use of chemoprophylaxis to prevent neonatal sepsis would probably be associated with reduced infectious puerperal morbidity.

▶ The usual focus of discussions involving group B streptococci is what happens to the neonate when the mother has vaginal colonization. This study examines what happens to the mother and the effect of antibiotic prophylaxis administered to carriers. In general, women who were carriers had the same morbidity from puerperal infections as did noncarriers. Indeed, there were no statistically significant differences in puerperal infection rates, the occurrence of fever, or the requirement for antibiotic therapy in the perinatal period of carriers and noncarriers. Although those carriers who received ampicillin prophylaxis experienced fewer infections and required less perinatal antibiotics, these differences were not statistically significant. A previous report by Boyer et al. (1) did not find a significant reduction of puerperal morbidity in carriers who received intrapartum antibiotic prophylaxis.—M.S. Klempner, M.D.

Reference

1. Boyer KM, et al: *J Infect Dis* 148:810, 1983.

Efficacy of Adenoidectomy for Recurrent Otitis Media in Children Previously Treated With Tympanostomy-Tube Placement: Results of Parallel Randomized and Nonrandomized Trials

Paradise JL, Bluestone CD, Rogers KD, Taylor FH, Colborn DK, Bachman RZ, Bernard BS, Schwarzbach RH (Children's Hosp of Pittsburgh; Univ of Pittsburgh)

JAMA 263:2066–2073, 1990 11–3

Adenoidectomy long has been done to lower the risk of otitis media in children, but its efficacy is unproved. Parallel trials of adenoidectomy, 1 randomized and the other not, were evaluated in children who previously had received a tympanostomy tube for persistent and/or recurrent otitis media and had otitis after extrusion of the tube (Fig 11–1). Ninety-nine

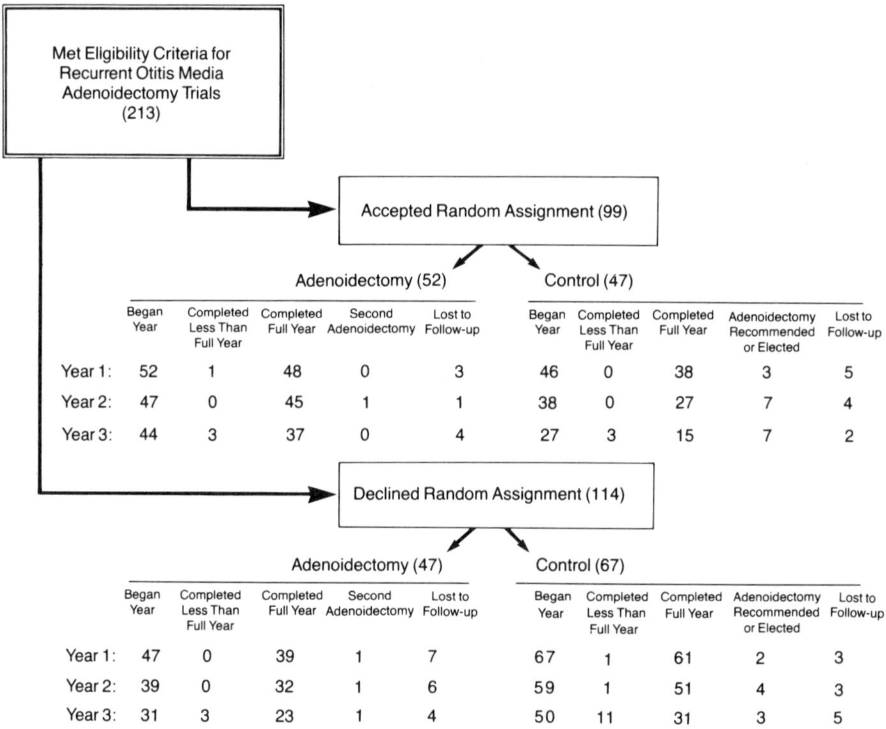

Accepted Random Assignment (99)

	Adenoidectomy (52)					Control (47)				
	Began Year	Completed Less Than Full Year	Completed Full Year	Second Adenoidectomy	Lost to Follow-up	Began Year	Completed Less Than Full Year	Completed Full Year	Adenoidectomy Recommended or Elected	Lost to Follow-up
Year 1:	52	1	48	0	3	46	0	38	3	5
Year 2:	47	0	45	1	1	38	0	27	7	4
Year 3:	44	3	37	0	4	27	3	15	7	2

Declined Random Assignment (114)

	Adenoidectomy (47)					Control (67)				
	Began Year	Completed Less Than Full Year	Completed Full Year	Second Adenoidectomy	Lost to Follow-up	Began Year	Completed Less Than Full Year	Completed Full Year	Adenoidectomy Recommended or Elected	Lost to Follow-up
Year 1:	47	0	39	1	7	67	1	61	2	3
Year 2:	39	0	32	1	6	59	1	51	4	3
Year 3:	31	3	23	1	4	50	11	31	3	5

Fig 11–1.—Assignment of subjects to treatment groups and subsequent changes in status. Second adenoidectomies were performed because of recurrent nasal obstruction in 3 subjects (1 randomized) and persistent nasal obstruction in 1 subject (nonrandomized). Seventeen subjects (11 randomized) were withdrawn from control status to receive adenoidectomy at the study team's recommendation, and 9 (6 randomized) at parental request. Adenoidectomy was recommended because of unremitting otitis media in 9 subjects (6 randomized) and persistent nasal obstruction in 7 subjects (4 randomized) and in conjunction with tonsillectomy that was considered advisable in 1 subject (randomized). (Courtesy of Paradise JL, Bluestone CD, Rogers KD, et al: *JAMA* 263:2066–2073, 1990.)

Typanostomy-Tube Procedures, Episodes of Secondary Otorrhea, Days With Ear Pain, and Days With Antimicrobial Treatment in Randomly Assigned Subjects, According to Whole Follow-up Year and Treatment Group

	Follow-up Year					
	1		2		3	
Outcome Measure	Adenoidectomy Group (n = 48)	Control Group (n = 38)	Adenoidectomy Group (n = 45)	Control Group (n = 27)	Adenoidectomy Group (n = 37)	Control Group (n = 15)
Tympanostomy-tube procedures*						
Mean No. per subject (range)	0.13 (0-1)	0.29 (0-1)	0.13 (0-2)	0.26 (0-2)	0.08 (0-1)	0.13 (0-1)
Episodes of secondary otorrhea						
Mean No. per subject (range)	0.13 (0-1)	0.13 (0-2)	0.09 (0-1)	0.04 (0-1)	0.05 (0-1)	0.07 (0-1)
Days with ear pain:†						
Mean No. per subject (range)	3.99 (0-21)	4.54 (0-22)	4.21 (0-27)	4.28 (0-15)	3.94 (0-20)	5.08 (0-20)
Proportion of subjects with ≥4 %	32‡	55‡	40	41	34	42
Days with antimicrobial treatment:†						
Mean No. per subject (range)	30.7 (0-130)	43.2 (0-124)	28.6 (0-104)	45.3 (0-128)	30.8 (0-138)	25.8 (0-105)
Proportion of subjects with ≥15, %	60‡	89‡	63	85	66	58

*Limited to procedures performed after the trial starting point. The proportion of procedures each year that involved bilateral tube placement ranged from 33% to 100% in the adenoidectomy group and from 50% to 64% in the control group.

†For subjects with fewer than 365 days of reportage in a follow-up year, the number of days was standardized on the basis of 365 days. During the first, second, and third follow-up years, respectively, the mean numbers of days of reportage were 334, 334, and 342 in adenoidectomy subjects and 343, 346, and 344 in control subjects.

‡Adenoidectomy vs. control; $P \leq .05$ by a χ^2 analysis of distribution of subjects.

(Courtesy of Paradise JL, Bluestone CD, Rogers KD, et al: *JAMA* 263:2066–2073, 1990.)

children were randomly assigned to adenoidectomy or a control group, and 114 others whose parents refused randomization were assigned according to parental preference.

Although both trials were biased by the removal of some severely affected patients from the control group, adenoidectomy was associated with a better outcome in the first 2 years of follow-up (table). In the first year of the randomized trial, adenoidectomy patients had 47% less time with otitis than controls and 28% fewer suppurative episodes. The comparable figures in the second year were 37% and 35%.

Adenoidectomy is warranted on an individual basis for children who have recurrent otitis media after tympanostomy tubes extrude. Countering the decision to operate are the small risk of adverse effects and the tendency for otitis to decline with advancing age.

▶ In their introduction the authors cite 17 previous reports published in the past 25 years in which the role of adenoidectomy in children with recurrent otitis media was studied. Is there any wonder that there is no clear answer? In this 18th study, the authors find that in a specific subset of patients who continue to have recurrent otitis even after tube placement, adenoidectomy offers benefit for at least 2 years. However, they also conclude that decisions regarding the performance of adenoidectomy will be influenced by individual factors, including the degree of morbidity to the patient, the child's tolerance of antimicrobial agents, the nature of available anesthesia, the impact of the child's recurrent otitis on the family, and the presence or absence of adenoid related disorders. It sounds to me like a consensus panel would be useful.—M.S. Klempner, M.D.

Otitis Media in Infancy and Intellectual Ability, School Achievement, Speech, and Language at Age 7 Years

Teele DW, Klein JO, Chase C, Menyuk P, Rosner BA, and the Greater Boston Otitis Media Study Group (Boston City Hosp; Boston Univ; Harvard Med School)

J Infect Dis 162:685–694, 1990 11–4

Children with frequent episodes of acute otitis media and effusions of the middle ear (MEE) experience some degree of conductive hearing loss during their illness. In young children such hearing loss occurs during the time when language and other skills are acquired. Because previous studies that related MEE to later delay or impairment of speech, language, or cognitive abilities have been inconclusive, 194 children with a history of MEE were evaluated at age 7 years.

The children were stratified by estimated time spent with MEE during the first 3 years of life: fewer than 30 days, 30–129 days, or 130 days or more. The third group had a disproportionate number of boys, children with siblings, and those who had ventilation tubes.

After controlling for confounding variables, a significant association was observed between estimated time spent with MEE during the first 3

TABLE 1.—Cognitive Ability at Age 7 Years by Estimated Days With Middle Ear Effusion (MEE) During First 3 Years of Life

IQ test	Estimated days with MEE <30	30–129	≥130
Full scale	113.1*†	107.5*	105.4†
Verbal	111.5‡§	106.5‡	105.8§
Performance	112.2†‖	108.3‖	104.1†

Note: Cognitive ability is expressed as mean IQ by Wisc-R after adjusting for socioeconomic status and gender (general linear model procedure SAS-GLM). Time spent with middle ear effusion is natural log of time with effusion (days, +1). Intervals with MEE were selected to produce 3 groups of about equal size.
*P = .007.
†P = .001.
‡P = 0.26.
§P = .008.
‖Not significant.
(Courtesy of Teele DW, Klein JO, Chase C, et al: *J Infect Dis* 162:685–694, 1990.)

years of life and lower scores on tests of cognitive ability (Table 1), speech and language, and school performance at age 7 years (Table 2). Children with MEE during the first 3 years of life had significantly lower scores in mathematics and reading on the Metropolitan Achievement Test. Articulation and the use of morphological markers were similarly affected. Scores on the full-scale WISC-R were lowest for children who spent the most time with MEE (105.4) and highest for those who spent the least time (113.1).

The hearing loss experienced by children with MEE appears to have an effect on later intellectual ability, success in school, and in using speech and language. Time with MEE after age 3 years did not significantly affect these measures. Thus effective intervention to prevent MEE in infancy may help children reach their intellectual and linguistic potential.

▶ This study was well done and the interpretations are appropriately cautious. Whatever the mechanism, there appears to be an inverse relationship between

TABLE 2.—School Achievement at Age 7 Years and Estimated Days With Middle Ear Effusion (MEE) During First 3 Years of Life

Test part	Estimated days with MEE <30	30–129	≥130
Mathematics	472.6*†	452.9*	440.7†
Reading	541.2*‡	519.2*	502.6‡

Note: Scores are means on Metropolitan Achievement Test after adjusting for socioeconomic status and gender (general linear model procedure SAS-GLM). Time spent with middle ear effusion is natural log of time with effusion (days, +1). Intervals were selected to produce 3 groups of about equal size.
*P not significant.
‡P = .009.
‡P = .045.
(Courtesy of Teele DW, Klein JO, Chase C, et al: *J Infect Dis* 162:685–694, 1990.)

the time spent with MEE in the first 3 years of life and later intellectual performance. Interestingly, there were significantly *fewer* firstborn children among those with the highest number of days with effusions. I thought there was some evidence that firstborns score higher on IQ tests than subsequent children, but the authors do not address this possibility.—M.J. Barza, M.D.

Management of Infants at Risk for Occult Bacteremia: A Decision Analysis

Downs SM, McNutt RA, Margolis PA (Univ of North Carolina, Chapel Hill)

J Pediatr 118:11–20, 1991 11–5

As many as 12% of febrile infants with no apparent source of infection have bacteremia, and in some of them serious complications develop. Occult bacteremia may be difficult to detect clinically. The method of decision analysis was used to assess various alternative means of management for a child aged 2–24 months who had a rectal temperature of 39° C or higher without an identifiable source of bacterial infection.

The alternatives considered were blood culture with empirical antibiotic treatment; laboratory testing and treatment of those whose leukocyte count was at least 15,000/μL; and watchful waiting (follow-up in 24 hours). Probabilities were estimated from both published studies and expert opinion.

Empirical antibiotic treatment of all febrile infants had the highest expected utility. The difference in days of life between treating all patients and testing them was only 4. The difference between treatment and discharge was 11 days. Empirical treatment involved treating nearly fourfold more patients than the test strategy, but it prevented many hospitalizations. Death or permanent disability was least frequent with empirical treatment. This decision analysis study strongly supports empirical antibiotic therapy for all infants at risk of occult bacteremia.

Strategies for Diagnosis and Treatment of Children at Risk for Occult Bacteremia: Clinical Effectiveness and Cost-Effectiveness

Lieu TA, Schwartz JS, Jaffe DM, Fleisher GR (Univ of Pennsylvania; Univ of Toronto; Harvard Med School)

J Pediatr 118:21–29, 1991 11–6

The optimal management of a febrile child without an obvious focus of bacterial infection remains controversial. Decision analysis was used to evaluate the probable health benefits, complications, and costs of 6 management strategies for febrile children at risk for occult bacteremia. These strategies included no intervention, treatment alone with a 2-day course of oral amoxicillin, blood culture alone, blood culture plus a 2-day oral course of amoxicillin, obtaining a leukocyte count and providing patients with a count of at least 10,000/mm^3 with a 2-day oral course of amoxicillin, and clinical judgment. The decision model used data from the lit-

TABLE 1.—Health Outcomes for a Hypothetical Cohort of 100,000 Febrile Children Without Focus of Infection

	Blood culture +treatment	Leukocyte count	Blood culture alone	Clinical judgment	Treatment alone	No intervention
Complications of occult bacteremia						
Patients with major infections	312	320	390	400	480	600
Major infections prevented						
No.	288	280	210	200	120	0
%	48	47	35	33	20	0
Complications of antibiotic allergy						
Patients with rash	4049	2389	86	1840	4029	36
Avoidable rashes*	(4013)	(2353)	(50)	(1804)	(3993)	(0)
Patients with anaphylaxis	4.3	2.7	0.6	2.1	4.2	0.2
Avoidable anaphylactic reactions*	(4.1)	(2.4)	(0.3)	(1.9)	(4.0)	(0)
Hospitalizations						
Patients with major infection	312	320	390	400	480	600
Patients with *H. influenzae* bacteremia	353	351	336	280	0	0
Patients with *S. pneumoniae* bacteremia	151	206	714	105	0	0
TOTAL HOSPITALIZATIONS	816	877	1440	785	480	600

*Antibiotic complications were potentially avoidable when patients without major focal infection were treated presumptively.
(Courtesy of Lieu TA, Schwartz JS, Jaffe DM, et al: *J Pediatr* 118:21–29, 1991.)

erature and from a 1987 prospective study of occult bacteremia in 955 children.

The strategy in which all patients had blood culture plus antibiotic treatment prevented the highest number of major infections (Table 1) and

TABLE 2.—Cost Effectiveness for Each Strategy Under Baseline Assumptions

	Strategy					
Cost-effectiveness ratio	**Blood culture + treatment**	**Leukocyte count**	**Blood culture alone**	**Clinical judgment**	**Treatment alone**	**No intervention**
Average cost per patient* ($)	145.45	146.60	149.34	133.20	80.11	79.94
Cost per major infection prevented ($)	50,503	52,357	71,114	66,600	66,758	NA
Rashes per major infection prevented	14.0	8.5	0.4	9.2	33.6	NA
Anaphylactic reactions per major infection prevented	0.0150	0.0096	0.0027	0.0106	0.350	NA
Hospitalizations per major infection prevented	2.8	3.1	6.9	3.9	4.0	NA

Abbreviation: NA, not applicable.

*Average overall financial cost per person, including cost of follow-up visits and hospitalizations. For example, average cost per patient with treatment alone was only 17 cents more per patient than no intervention strategy because it saved costs of 120 hospitalizations for major infections, compared with no intervention strategy.

(Courtesy of Lieu TA, Schwartz JS, Jaffe DM, et al: *J Pediatr* 118:21–29, 1991.)

resulted in the lowest cost per major infection prevented (Table 2). The leukocyte count strategy had clinical effectiveness and cost effectiveness roughly equal to that of blood culture plus treatment and also had the advantage of averting many antibiotic complications. Blood culture alone was the third most clinically effective strategy but was the least cost effective. Treatment alone with a 2-day oral course of amoxicillin resulted in the lowest average cost per febrile patient, but it was the least effective clinically. However, the low degree of effectiveness of empiric treatment alone was based on the assumption that oral amoxicillin therapy was only 20% effective in preventing major infections after bacteremia. At higher estimates of effectiveness, treatment alone became a more viable strategy. Approaches that combine blood culture and empiric antibiotic treatment provide the most clinically effective and most cost-effective option for treating febrile children at risk for occult bacteremia.

Bacteremia in an Ambulatory Setting: Improved Outcome in Children Treated With Antibiotics

Woods ER, Merola JL, Bithoney WG, Spivak H, Wise PH (Children's Hosp; Massachusetts Dept of Public Health, Boston)

Am J Dis Child 144:1195–1199, 1990 11–7

To evaluate the initial presentation, treatment, and outcomes of children with ambulatory bacteremias, data were reviewed on 167 children (mean age, 20.8 months) with *Hemophilus influenzae* and 247 with *Streptococcus pneumoniae* bacteremia treated in a 4-year period. More than half (58.2%) of the patients were treated in the ambulatory setting; the rest hospitalized at the initial visit. Antibiotics were used to treat 60.6% of the ambulatory patients.

Children with *H. influenzae* appeared more ill to clinicians and were more likely to have a clear bacterial source evident at presentation than those with *S. pneumoniae*. The necessity for initial hospital admission, a higher clinical scale, and a lower number of polymorphonuclear leukocytes were all significant predictors of finding *H. influenzae* on blood culture. Although patients initially treated had more potential bacterial diagnoses, they were less likely than untreated children to have otitis media and had fewer new foci of infection, positive blood cultures at follow-up, and hospital admissions.

Meningitis developed significantly more often in patients with *H. influenzae* than in those with *S. pneumoniae*. In agreement with a previous study, a significant association was noted between the performance of an lumbar puncture at initial presentation and the subsequent development of meningitis. The effect of treatment was greater in patients with *S. pneumoniae*.

▶ The first 2 studies (Abstracts 11–5 and 11–6) address the problem of how to manage a young child (2–24 months in the first study and 3–36 months in the second study) who is febrile without an identifiable source. As Downs et al. point out, to answer this question with a prospective randomized trial would require a study of more than 35,000 infants. As such a study will almost surely never be done, we are left with the somewhat unsatisfying answers that are provided by the decision analysis model. The good news is that both papers agree that in the absence of a test that can predict bacteremia better than the ones we currently have (e.g., white count), it is cost effective and fully justified to treat empirically with antibiotics. The third study (Abstract 11–7) looks at this problem from a different viewpoint. When children with bacteremia caused by *H. influenzae* or *S. pneumoniae* are evaluated retrospectively, are there differences in outcome between those who did and did not receive empirical antibiotic treatment? The answer is that treated patients had fewer new serious foci of infections, fewer subsequent positive blood cultures, and were more likely to be well at follow-up.

So, despite all of these papers beginning with a statement about how controversial empirical antibiotics are for children with fever caused by an unidentifiable source, they all conclude that it's the correct thing to do. Let's end the controversy!—M.S. Klempner, M.D.

Invasive Disease Due to Multiply Resistant *Streptococcus pneumoniae* in a Houston, Tex, Day-care Center

Rauch AM, O'Ryan M, Van R, Pickering LK (Univ of Texas Med School at Houston)

Am J Dis Child 144:923–927, 1990 11–8

Data were reviewed on 2 children with invasive disease caused by a multiply resistant *Streptococcus pneumoniae* during an outbreak in a day-care center (DCC). In July 1988, 2 toddlers aged 12 and 14 months attending the same DCC were hospitalized within 24 hours of each other. One had sepsis and the other had sepsis and meningitis caused by a multiply-resistant *S. pneumoniae*. Nasopharyngeal cultures were performed in 82 of 85 DCC children, in 26 of 29 DCC staff, and in 28 of 31 family members. *Streptococcus pneumoniae* grew from 29 (35%) cultures from DCC children, and 10 (34%) of these were resistant to sulfamethoxazole-trimethoprim, oxacillin, and tetracycline, and were relatively resistant to penicillin. Only 1 household contact and none of the staff members had positive cultures (table). The multiply resistant isolates were all serotype 14 and had the same pattern of antimicrobial susceptibility.

Rifampin, 10 mg/kg, was administered twice daily for 2 days to 97%

Nasopharyngeal Carriage of Multiply Resistant *Streptococcus pneumoniae* in Houston Day-Care Center Children and Staff

Day-care Population	Individuals With *S pneumoniae* (%)	Individuals With Susceptible *S pneumoniae* (%)	Individuals With Multiply Resistant *S pneumoniae* (%)
Infants	7/35 (20)	6/35 (17)	1/35 (3)
Toddlers	22/47 (47)	13/47 (28)	9/47 (19)
Staff	0/26 (0)	0/26 (0)	0/26 (0)
Total	**29/108** (27)	**19/108** (18)	**10/108** (9)

(Courtesy of Rauch AM, O'Ryan M, Van R, et al: *Am J Dis Child* 144:923–927, 1990.)

of the DCC children and staff members and household contacts with positive cultures. Treatment resulted in a 70% reduction in positive nasopharyngeal cultures for *S. pneumoniae*. Despite treatment, 3 additional children and 1 family contact were identified at follow-up nasopharyngeal cultures. No new patients with invasive disease caused by multiply resistant *S. pneumoniae* were identified during a 9-month observation period.

This is the first report in the United States of an outbreak of invasive disease caused by multiply resistant *S. pneumoniae*. Nasopharyngeal colonization is common among exposed children in the DCC, but not in the staff and household contacts. Treatment with rifampin for 2 days only partially eradicates the organism from colonized individuals.

▶ This is 1 of 2 papers by Dr. Rauch in this volume of YEAR BOOK OF INFECTIOUS DISEASES. No, he is not my brother-in-law, but he is working in the modern-day version of the pediatric infectious diseases gold mine, the DCCs. If you are there, and have your eyes open, events, outbreaks, and organisms will come and go, and you can collect data, affect outcome, and publish papers. In this instance, a multiply-drug-resistant *Pneumococcus* outbreak resulted in invasive disease in 2 children and a large number of asymptomatic pharyngeal infections in others, but not in staff members at the center, including one third carrying the resistant type 14 strains. Rifampin prophylaxis resulted in eradication of carriage in 7 of 10 infected with the resistant isolate and did not induce subsequent rifampin resistance. No additional invasive illnesses occurred. It is not clear what the difference was between the 2 children who became sick and the large number of others who did not. What is clear is that antibiotic resistance among type 14 pneumococci, the most prevalent serotype in invasive pediatric infections, may spell trouble down the line, and that line may be rather short. It is timely that pneumococcal polysaccharide-protein conjugate vaccines are in late stages of development and may become available in the new few years for immunization in the first few months of life.—G.T. Keusch, M.D.

Pneumococcal Revaccination of Splenectomized Children

Konradsen HB, Pedersen FK, Henrichsen J (Statens Seruminstitut; Rigshospitalet, Copenhagen)
Pediatr Infect Dis J 9:258–263, 1990 11–9

Children who have undergone splenectomy have similar response to pneumococcal vaccination as normal children and adults. However, because of individual variation in response to vaccination, a decrease in antibody concentration over the years, and the continuing risk of infections throughout life, revaccination may be necessary to provide sufficient protection. The need and proper time for revaccination in these children were ascertained.

Forty-three children received a single subcutaneous dose of a 14-valent pneumococcal vaccine either before or up to several years after splenectomy. Blood samples were taken before and at 4 weeks and 5 years after vaccination. Depending on the pneumococcal antibody status 5 years af-

TABLE 1.—Comparison of Concentrations of Antibody Against 14 Pneumococcal Polysaccharide Antigens 4 Weeks and 5 Years After Pneumococcal Vaccination in 27 Splenectomized Children*

Pneumococcal Type	Geometric Mean Type-Specific Antibody Concentrations 5 Years After Vaccination (% of Antibody Concentrations) 4 Weeks After Vaccination	
	Group A†	Group B
1	18	53‡
2	34	63§
3	2	12‡
4	48	73‖
6A	34	52
7F	64	66
8	24	56
9N	33	40
12F	59	85
14	88	69
18C	100	130
19F	49	73
23F	43	66
25	31	76
Mean	45	66

*Antibody concentrations were measured by enzyme-linked immunosorbent assay.

†In group A, the log sum of the enzyme-linked immunosorbent assay values of all 14 types is <.29.1; those with a log sum <30.9 are also included if >3 single values are <100. In group B, the log sum of the enzyme-linked immunosorbent assay values for all 14 types is either between 29.1 and 30.9 and <3 single values are <100 or the log sum is >30.9.

‡Significantly higher than group A (P = .01).

§Significantly higher than group A (P = .003).

‖Significantly higher than group A (P = .04).

(Courtesy of Konradsen HB, Pedersen FK, Henrichsen J: *Pediatr Infect Dis J* 9:258–263, 1990.)

ter primary vaccination, the children were either revaccinated with a new 23-valent pneumococcal vaccine or scheduled for reexamination later. An enzyme-linked immunosorbent assay was used to measure total pneumococcal antibody concentrations and antibodies against each of the pneumococcal capsular polysaccharide antigens.

Based on arbitrarily chosen enzyme-linked immunosorbent assay values, 15 splenectomized children were revaccinated (group A) and 12 were reexamined later (group B). The remaining 16 patients who had no antibody concentration measurements in relation to their primary vaccination but with low antibody concentrations before revaccination (same as group A) were also revaccinated (group C). There were no significant differences in mean age among the 3 groups. Compared with group B, splenectomized children in group A had significantly lower antibody concentrations before and at 4 weeks and 5 years after primary vaccination (Table 1) and significantly higher combined mean antibody fold increase af-

TABLE 2.—Adverse Reactions to Pneumococcal Revaccination in 20 Splenectomized Children

Type of Reaction	Duration of Reaction (Days)			
	1 or less	2	3	>3
Local redness >5 cm at injection site		2 (10)*	2 (10)	
Induration >5 cm at injection site			1 (5)	
Pain at injection site		2 (10)	2 (10)	1 (5)
Fever >38°C	1 (5)			
Fever <38°C	3 (15)			
Feeling tired and dizzy	2 (10)			

*Numbers in parentheses, percent.
(Courtesy of Konradsen HB, Pedersen FK, Henrichsen J: *Pediatr Infect Dis J* 9:258–263, 1990.)

ter vaccination. The combined antibody concentration before vaccination strongly correlated with the combined geometric mean fold increase after vaccination in group A, but not in group B. Adverse reactions to revaccination were mild, and no serious reactions were observed (Table 2). In splenectomized children with low antibody concentrations 5 years after primary pneumococcal vaccination, revaccination is safe and results in satisfactory antibody response.

▶ This study suggests that certain splenectomized children respond less well to pneumococcal polysaccharide vaccines and demonstrate a more rapid decline in postimmunization antibody levels as well. Nevertheless, such children respond to reimmunization, albeit less well than to primary immunization. The study was carried out in Denmark, and no sickle cell patients were involved, the majority having idiopathic thrombocytopenic purpura or hereditary spherocytosis as the cause of splenectomy. The authors cite unpublished data of their own that demonstrate the impact of immunization in splenectomized children on subsequent invasive pneumococcal infections (15 invasive infections in 10 years among 456 splenectomized children before the vaccine program vs. none in 292 immunized since 1978). Thus preventive immunization appears worthwhile. The imminent introduction of polysaccharide conjugate vaccines that induce memory response capacity may change the need for follow-up of antibody titors and reimmunization in the future. In the meantime, current pneumococcal vaccines can be recommended as the details of follow-up and the need for subsequent immunization are sorted out.—G.T. Keusch, M.D.

Safety and Immunologic Response to *Haemophilus influenzae* Type b Oligosaccharide-CRM$_{197}$ Conjugate Vaccine in 1- to 6-Month-Old Infants

Madore DV, Johnson CL, Phipps DC, Pennridge Pediatric Assocs, Popejoy LA, Eby R, Smith DH (Praxis Biologics Inc, Rochester, NY; Pennridge Pediatrics, Sellersville, Pa; Temple Univ; St Christopher's Hosp for Children, Philadelphia; William Beaumont Army Med Ctr, El Paso, Texas)

Pediatrics 85:331–337, 1990 11–10

The predominant cause of bacterial meningitis in infants and young children is *Hemophilus influenzae* type b. Although several vaccines have been licensed in the United States for use in children aged 18 months and older, the peak incidence of disease caused by *H. influenzae* type b occurs between the ages of 6 and 12 months. The safety and immunogenicity of *H. influenzae* type b oligosaccharide-CRM_{197} conjugate (HbOC) were evaluated in 432 infants aged 1–6 months.

The multicenter study involved 10 sites in 6 states. The healthy infants were vaccinated with 3 doses of 10 μg of HbOC, which were given at 2-month intervals and administered in the anterolateral thigh. The diphtheria, tetanus, pertussis vaccine was given at the same time, but in the opposite thigh, to 122 of the infants. Serum specimens were collected immediately before each of the 3 vaccinations, at 1 and 6 months after the third vaccination, and at age 2 years.

The vaccine was well tolerated. Mild side effects were reported in approximately 2% of the infants and included temperature elevation or localized reactions which were much less frequent and less severe than those associated with the diphtheria, tetanus, pertussis vaccination. More than 90% of infants of all ages responded after 2 doses. After the third dose more than 98% had anti-*H. influenzae* type b capsular polysaccharide (HbPs) levels of antibody of at least 1 μg/mL. This level of anti-HbPs antibody was retained in more than 94% of the infants 6 months after the third dose and in more than 80% of the infants at age 2 years.

The data indicate that HbOC safely primed and boosted the immune system of young infants, offering long-lasting protective levels of anti-HbPs antibodies. Predominantly IgG, rather than IgM, anti-HbPs antibodies were generated. Older infants had the greatest response to the first dose. The largest increase in anti-HbPs levels occurred after the second dose.

▶ The formulation of polysaccharide-protein conjugate vaccines with enhanced antigenicity, especially for young children who did not normally respond well to polysaccharides, has reached a state of technological development suggesting that these will (very) soon replace the polysaccharides themselves. This study reports on the antigenicity of one of several versions of *H. influenzae* type b (Hib)-conjugate vaccine (others use tetanus toxoid as the protein component, for example) and, compared to PRP alone, demonstrates its superiority in young children, as well as its ability to generate IgG antibody and a memory response resulting in a booster effect with subsequent injections. The formulation and schedule are compatible with diphtheria/tetanus/pertussis vaccination. There is little question that this represents an advance that deserves widespread use to close the current window of susceptibility in the months between the waning of maternal-derived immunity and the earliest use of Hib polysaccharide vaccine. The question now will be refinement of the data to help in the selection of which vaccine to use. For example, are there any significant differences in immune response to the different preparations (how many respond, how soon, how high the titer, how long)? Are there any surprises in reactogenicity or side effects? Will there be big differences in cost? Even to ask these questions is a big advance.—G.T. Keusch, M.D.

Adenovirus Types 40 and 41 and Rotaviruses Associated With Diarrhea in Children From Guatemala

Cruz JR, Cáceres P, Cano F, Flores J, Bartlett A, Torún B (Inst of Nutrition of Central America and Panama, Guatemala City, Guatemala; Natl Insts of Health, Bethesda, Md; Johns Hopkins Univ)
J Clin Microbiol 28:1780–1784, 1990 11–11

Adenovirus type 40 (Ad40) and type 41 (Ad41) are important causes of gastroenteritis in young children, especially in temperate climates. The prevalence of adenoviruses and rotaviruses was determined in 194 healthy and sick children, aged 0–35 months, living in a rural Guatemalan community with a high diarrhea mortality rate, and 57 children, aged 6–31 months, who were hospitalized with diarrhea.

Field workers visited the children's homes twice a week to watch for diarrheal illnesses. Whenever a child had diarrhea, the date of onset was recorded and a stool specimen was collected. Sick children were visited every other day until they recovered. Treatment included oral rehydration and antibiotics in children with *Shigella* infection. Of the 57 hospitalized children, 10 came from rural areas and 47 came from poor families living in urban areas. Stool specimens were collected on 2 consecutive days after hospital admission. All collected stool specimens were cultured and examined for serotype by enzyme-linked immunosorbent assay.

The study material consisted of 458 fecal specimens obtained from 143 rural children during 385 episodes of diarrhea and 191 stool specimens taken from 128 of those same children when they were healthy and from another 51 children who did not have diarrhea. Forty-three (22.2%) children excreted adenoviruses and 20 (10.3%) shed rotaviruses. Adenovirus type 40 and Ad41 were associated with 54 (14%) illnesses and rotavi-

TABLE 1.—Distribution of Infections Caused by Ad40 and Ad41 and Rotaviruses, by Age

Age (mo)	No. with the following infections: Ad40 and Ad41		Rotavirus		No. of specimens examined
	Diarrhea present	Asymptomatic	Diarrhea present	Asymptomatic	
0–5	4	6	1	2	111
6–11	14	1	3	0	125
12–17	15	1	6	0	136
18–23	14	1	6	0	120
≥24	7	0	2	0	149
Total	54	9	18	2	649*

*In 8 instances the exact age of the child was not recorded.
(Courtesy of Cruz JR, Cáceres P, Cano F, et al: *J Clin Microbiol* 28:1780–1784, 1990.)

TABLE 2.—Characteristics of Infections Caused by Ad40 and Ad41 and Rotaviruses

Type of infection	Infections caused by Ad40 and Ad41					Infections caused by rotaviruses				
	No.	Median duration (days)	Age (mo)		No. with coinfection	No.	Median duration (days)	Age (mo)		No. with coinfection
			Median	Range				Median	Range	
Symptomatic										
Total	54	10	17	0–34	27	17	8	17	4–26	6
Duration <14 days	33	6	14	0–33	11	12	4	17	4–26	2
Duration >14 days	21	20	18	6–34	16	5	26	15	8–21	4
Asymptomatic	9		3	1–22	1[a]	2			0, 3	1*

*Ad40 and Ad41 and rotavirus.
(Courtesy of Cruz JR, Cáceres P, Cano F, et al: *J Clin Microbiol* 28:1780–1784, 1990.)

ruses were associated with 18 (4.7%) illnesses. Nine children with asymptomatic Ad40 and Ad41 infections, and 2 had asymptomatic rotavirus infections (Table 1). Of the 385 episodes of diarrhea, 301 lasted 1–13 days and 84 lasted 2 weeks or longer (Table 2).

Thirty-six (63.2%) of the 57 hospitalized children had viral infections of which 29 (50.9%) were rotavirus infections and 15 (31.2%) were Ad40 and Ad41 infections. Eight children had dual infections. Of 22 typeable rotavirus strains, 9 were serotype 1, 12 were serotype 2, and 1 was serotype 3. All children with serotype 2 rotavirus infections were coinfected with other enteric pathogens, whereas only 3 of those children with rotavirus serotype 1 infection excreted another enteric pathogen. Adenoviruses and rotaviruses are important causes of diarrheal illness in ambulatory and hospitalized Guatemalan children.

▶ Dr. Cruz and colleagues have carried out the "Son of the Santa Maria Cauque" study (to the uninitiated, the Santa Maria Cauque study carried out by Leonardo Mata and colleagues is the prototype of the prospective cohort study of infection and illness in populations living in natural conditions in the community). This is without doubt just one of many papers likely to appear from this study defining the risk and significance of individual pathogens. In this rural highland Indian community, adenoviruses 40 and 41 were more commonly associated with diarrhea than rotavirus, whereas the reverse was true in a hospitalized population studied as well. Either the epidemiology of viral diarrhea is different among the primarily urban children in the hospital population, or rotavirus is more likely to cause severe diarrhea requiring hospitalization. It is not clear which is correct, although the urban poor are usually more malnourished and poorly cared for than are the rural poor living in cultural communities such as the Mayan Indians in Guatemala. At any rate, adenovirus appears to be a very significant diarrheal pathogen in children in Guatemala.—G.T. Keusch, M.D.

Hypoglycemia During Diarrhea in Childhood: Prevalence, Pathophysiology, and Outcome

Bennish ML, Azad AK, Rahman O, Phillips RE (Internatl Centre for Diarrhoeal Disease Research, Bangladesh, Dhaka; Tufts-New England Med Ctr, Boston; Harvard Univ; Univ of Oxford, England)

N Engl J Med 322:1357–1363, 1990 11–12

Diarrhea is the major cause of death among children in some of the developing countries, even in areas where oral rehydration therapy is widely used. The lethal complications of diarrhea other than dehydration remain poorly understood. Hypoglycemia is a known potentially fatal complication of infectious diarrhea in both well nourished and poorly nourished children. A prospective study was performed to determine the frequency and outcome of hypoglycemia during diarrhea in children.

During an 8-month study period, 2,003 children younger than age 15 years were hospitalized with severe diarrhea at a special diarrhea treat-

TABLE 1.—Clinical Characteristics at Admission of 46 Hypoglycemic Patients and 25 Normoglycemic Patients With Diarrhea

Characteristic	Hypoglycemic Patients	Normoglycemic Patients
Age (mo)	48 (24–168)	48 (24–120)
Male — no. (%)	23 (50)	17 (68)
Duration of diarrhea (hr)	12 (3–360)	72 (3–360)†
Time since last feeding (hr)	18 (1–48)	9 (2–96)†
Weight for age (% of NCHS median)	61 (34–99)	59 (38–81)
Weight for height (% of NCHS median)‡	81 (56–103)	78 (57–102)
Fever (rectal temperature >38.0°C) — no. (%)	19 (41)	12 (48)
Moderate or severe dehydration — no. (%)	17 (37)	6 (24)
Convulsions — no. (%)	16 (35)	2 (8)†
Stool pathogen — no. (%)		
Shigella species	16 (35)	8 (32)
V. cholerae 01	6 (13)	6 (24)
Other pathogen	9 (20)	4 (16)
No pathogen identified	15 (33)	7 (28)
White cells in stool (per high-powered field)	20 (0–>200)	20 (0–80)
Red cells in stool (per high-powered field)	0 (0–>200)	1 (0–80)
Hematocrit	0.36 (0.22–0.46)	0.35 (0.25–0.44)
Leukocyte count ($\times 10^{-9}$/liter)	16 (5–40)	18 (5–49)

*All values are medians, with the range shown in parentheses, unless otherwise noted. The normoglycemic patients were matched with the first 25 hypoglycemic patients on the basis of age and weight for age. *Abbreviation: NCHS,* National Center for Health Statistics.

†$P \le .05$ for the comparison with the hypoglycemic patients.

‡Data on weight for height were available for 22 of the hypoglycemic patients (48%) and 14 of the normoglycemic patients (56%).

(Courtesy of Bennish ML, Azad AK, Rahman O, et al: *N Engl J Med* 322:1357–1363, 1990.)

ment center in Dhaka, Bangladesh. Hypoglycemia was defined as a capillary blood glucose concentration of less than 2.2 mmol/L.

Of the 2,003 hospitalized children, 91 (4.5%) had hypoglycemia and 1,912 did not. Thirty-nine (42.9%) hypoglycemic children and 122 (6.4%) normoglycemic children died while in the hospital. Thus, 39 (24.2%) of the 161 children who died had hypoglycemia. Plasma levels of glucoregulatory hormones and gluconeogenetic substrates were measured in 46 hypoglycemic children with a mean age of 48 months and 25 age- and weight-matched normoglycemic children (Table 1). Both groups had similar nutritional status at admission and similar pathogens identified in the stool.

Hypoglycemic children had been ill with diarrhea for a significantly shorter period than normoglycemic children, but the time since the last feeding was significantly longer in the former. All hypoglycemic children had appropriately low plasma C-peptide levels and elevated plasma glucagon and epinephrine levels, excluding failure of glucose counterregulation as a cause of hypoglycemia. Both groups had similar alanine and β-hydroxybutyrate concentrations. These data suggest failure of gluconeogenesis as a causative mechanism (Table 2). Infusion of 5.6 mmol of dextrose per kg resulted in a prompt and sustained increase in the plasma glucose concentration.

Patients with convulsions had a significantly lower median plasma glucose concentrations and a higher median plasma lactate concentration. Patients who died had a significantly lower median weight for age.

A comparison of 18 severely malnourished hypoglycemic children and 26 better-nourished hypoglycemic children revealed that malnourished children had been ill longer and had reduced alanine but normal lactate plasma levels, whereas the better-nourished children with hypoglycemia had normal alanine but a significantly elevated lactate concentration, suggesting impairment of hepatic enzymes involved in gluconeogenesis.

In addition to dehydration, hypoglycemia is a major cause of death in

TABLE 2.—Clinical Characteristics and Biochemical and Hormonal Findings at Admission in Patients With Hypoglycemia and Diarrhea, According to Nutritional Status

Variable	Severely Malnourished (<60% of Median Weight for Age; N = 18)		Better Nourished (≥60% of Median Weight for Age; N = 26)	
	No. tested		No. tested	
Age (mo)	—	48 (24–96)	—	48 (24–168)
Duration of diarrhea (hr)	—	18 (4–360)	—	10 (3–24)†
Time since last feeding (hr)	—	20 (1–48)	—	18 (10–29)
Fever (rectal temperature >38.0°C) — no. (%)	—	2 (11)	—	16 (62)†
Glucose (mmol/liter)	18	0.62 (0.15–1.95)	26	0.74 (0.05–2.17)
C peptide (nmol/liter)	18	0.02 (0–0.29)	24	0.04 (0–0.20)
Cortisol (nmol/liter)	16	1381 (738–>1380)	24	858 (180–>1380)†
Growth hormone (mU/liter)	18	26.5 (4.0–60.0)	26	26.5 (3.0–>60.0)
Glucagon (pmol/liter)	18	27 (8–123)	25	64 (1–193)†
Epinephrine (pmol/liter)	18	3100 (900–34,000)	26	3400 (300–44,000)
Norepinephrine (pmol/liter)	18	5300 (200–31,700)	26	8500 (200–26,000)
β-Hydroxybutyrate (μmol/liter)	17	1303 (148–11,130)	26	1075 (159–5810)
Lactate (mmol/liter)	18	1.9 (1.2–7.0)	26	3.9 (1.2–15.0)†
Alanine (μmol/liter)	18	173 (67–568)	26	293 (88–966)†
Albumin (g/liter)	16	28 (16–43)	23	32 (20–43)†
Bilirubin (μmol/liter)	12	6 (1–66)	23	6 (1–38)
Aspartate aminotransferase (U/liter)	12	80 (33–351)	23	101 (64–489)

*Values are medians, with the range shown in parentheses, unless otherwise indicated. Information on 2 patients for whom weight was not recorded was not included in this analysis.

†$P \leq .05$ for the comparison with the severely malnourished patients.

(Courtesy of Bennish ML, Azad AK, Rahman O, et al: *N Engl J Med* 322:1357–1363, 1990.)

children with diarrhea. Hypoglycemia in these patients appears most often caused by the failure of gluconeogenesis rather than by the failure of glucose counterregulation, as had been suggested in earlier studies.

▶ The World Health Organization has made the use of an oral rehydration solution in dehydrated patients the single most important strategy to reduce diarrhea mortality in developing countries. This study shows that nearly 5% of children admitted to a research hospital in Bangladesh have significant hypoglycemia, apparently primarily because of failure of the gluconeogenic response to keep up with needs. Whatever the mechanism, the mortality rate in hypoglycemic children was 7 times that in normoglycemic children. Overall, mortality was associated with hypoglycemia in almost 25% of the patients who died. Altered consciousness or convulsions in children with diarrhea may be caused by electrolyte abnormalities (e.g., hyponatremia) or hypoglycemia, but both are associated with increased fatality rates. Case management strategies need to take these biochemical findings into consideration, even when laboratory support is not available to define the abnormality present. Hypoglycemia may also be an important factor in death attributable to other infectious diseases in the developing world, conditioned in part by the level of malnutrition. A more general strategy to deal with this problem is needed.—G.T. Keusch, M.D.

Acute Hematogenous Pelvic Osteomyelitis in Infants and Children

Mustafa MM, Sáez-Llorens X, McCracken GH Jr, Nelson JD (Univ of Texas, Dallas)

Pediatr Infect Dis J 9:416–421, 1990 11–13

Hematogenous osteomyelitis in children most commonly involves the metaphyses of long bones and rarely involves the pelvic bones. The early diagnosis of pelvic osteomyelitis is difficult, and appropriate treatment may be delayed. A review was made of the case reports of 82 children with a diagnosis of acute hematogenous pelvic osteomyelitis or sacroiliitis. Thirty-nine of these were treated at Children's Medical Center and Parkland Memorial Hospital in Dallas, and 43 were described in the literature.

The most common clinical findings were pain in the affected hip or groin, fever, and gait disturbances. Only 20 children had abnormal admission radiographs, but most had radiographic evidence of osteomyelitis later in the course of disease (Table 1). Only 10 of 64 patients (16%) had an admission diagnosis of pelvic osteomyelitis. The most common initial diagnosis was septic hip (Table 2). The correct diagnosis was established within 1 week in 55 (72%) patients and within 2 weeks in 66 (86%). However, 11 patients (14%) had a delay in diagnosis of 2–3 weeks. Bacteriologic confirmation was obtained for 29 patients. *Staphylococcus aureus* was the most commonly isolated pathogen (Table 3).

Initial treatment was empiric and consisted of intravenous antibiotic

TABLE 1.—Laboratory and Radiologic Findings at the Time of Admission

Clinical Characteristic	No. of Patients with the Finding/ No. Tested*		
	Present series (39 patients)	Other series (43 patients)	Combined (82 patients)
Total WBC count			
<10 000	11/39	19/43	30/82 (37)†
≥10 000	28/39	24/43	52/82 (63)
ANC			
≤6000	9/39	1/6	10/45 (22)
>6000	30/39	5/6	35/45 (78)
WBC count >10 000 or ANC > 6000 or both	32/39	5/6	37/45 (82)
Erythrocyte sedimentation rate (mm/hour)			
<20	4/34	0/42	4/76 (5)
≥20	30/34	42/42	72/76 (95)
20–50	5/30	7/25	12/55 (22)
≥50	25/30	18/25	43/55 (78)
Hemoglobin concentration (g/dl)			
Below normal for age	5/39	3/21	8/60 (13)
Appropriate for age	34/39	18/21	52/60 (87)
Abnormal roentgenograms	7/38	13/43	20/81 (25)

*There were no significant differences between the 2 groups of patients.
†Numbers in parentheses are percentages.
(Courtesy of Mustafa MM, Sáez–Llorens X, McCracken GH Jr, et al: *Pediatr Infect Dis J* 9:416–421, 1990.)

therapy. Twenty children (24%) required surgical drainage and débridement of necrotic tissue. Seventy-nine children (96%) recovered without significant long-term sequelae. The other 3 patients had serious morbidity after delays in diagnoses ranging from 120 to 190 days.

TABLE 2.—Admitting Diagnoses*

Diagnosis	No. of Patients with Diagnosis		
	Present series (39 patients)	Other series (25 patients)	Both combined (64 patients)
Septic hip	25	8	33 (52) †
Pelvic osteomyelitis	3	7	10 (16)
Osteomyelitis, unspecified site	11	—	11 (17)
Sacroiliitis	2	—	2 (3)
Toxic synovitis of the hip	2	2	4 (6)
Myositis/collagen-vascular	3	—	3 (5)
Cellulitis (buttock or thigh)	1	3	4 (6)
Others	4‡	5§	9 (14)

*Patients may have more than 1 admitting diagnosis.
†Numbers in parentheses are percentages.
‡Four patients in the present series had the admitting diagnoses of Legg-Calvé-Perthes disease; sickle cell pain crisis, rheumatic fever, and rhabdomyosarcoma.
§Five patients had the admitting diagnosis of nephrolithiasis, acute abdomen, Bartholin abscess, inguinal lymphadenitis, or Kawasaki disease.
(Courtesy of Mustafa MM, Sáez–Llorens X, McCracken GH Jr. et al: *Pediatr Infect Dis J* 9:416–421, 1990.)

TABLE 3.—Bacteriologic Results in Infants and Children With Pelvic Osteomyelitis

Specimen	No. of Positive Results/No. Tested			Pathogen Recovered (No. of Cultures)	
	Present series	Other series	Both		
Blood	17/39	19/38	36/77 (47)*	*Staphylococcus aureus*	33 (91)
				Haemophilus influenzae type b	1 (3)
				Streptococcus pneumoniae	1 (3)
				Streptococcus pyogenes	1 (3)
Bone/joint/soft tissue aspirate†	22/25	20/38	42/63 (67)	*Staphylococcus aureus*	31 (74)
				Salmonella enteritidis	4 (10)
				Haemophilus influenzae type b	1 (2)
				Streptococcus pyogenes	1 (2)
				Streptococcus pneumoniae	1 (2)
				Streptococci (nonhemolytic)	1 (2)
				Mycobacterium tuberculosis	1 (2)
				Gram-negative bacilli	1 (2)
				Micrococcus	1 (2)
Any site	29/39	29/43	58/82 (71)		

*Numbers in parentheses are percentages.
†Significantly more patients in the present series had organisms recovered from bone/joint/soft tissue aspirate compared to the other series (88% vs. 53%, $P = .006$).
(Courtesy of Mustafa MM, Sáez–Llorens X, McCracken GH Jr, et al: *Pediatr Infect Dis J* 9:416–421, 1990.)

The prognosis of acute hematogenous pelvic osteomyelitis in infants and children is good provided the definitive diagnosis is not delayed. Modern imaging techniques are useful in establishing the correct diagnosis.

▶ This review serves as a good reminder that the long bones are not the only site of hematogenous osteomyelitis in kids. In fact, the pelvis is not an uncommon site, with 6% of the patients seen at UT-Southwestern Medical Center, Dallas, over time having evidence of pelvic disease. Children who appear to have supportive hip infections, but who have minimal abnormalities in passive range of motion, and especially with tenderness of the pelvic bones or a lack of referred pain in the knee, are more likely to have pelvic bone infection. The diagnosis should be considered in all patients admitted with possible suppurative hip infection, and they should be evaluated by appropriate imaging techniques if hip infection is not substantiated. The pathogenesis in most cases seems to be via the hematogenous route, and *S. aureus* remains the most common pathogen. Given the availability of good drugs and the ability of otherwise healthy children to respond quickly and fully to treatment, the prognosis is excellent.—G.T. Keusch, M.D.

12 Clinical Diagnosis

Prevalence and Diagnosis of *Legionella* Pneumonia: A 3-Year Prospective Study With Emphasis on Application of Urinary Antigen Detection

Ruf B, Schürmann D, Horbach I, Fehrenbach FJ, Pohle HD (Rudolf Virchow Univ Hosp; Freie Univ; Robert Koch Inst, Berlin)

J Infect Dis 162:1341–1348, 1990 12–1

Urinary antigen detection was compared with serologic tests and the examination of respiratory secretions in the diagnosis of *Legionella* pneumonia. Legionellosis was diagnosed in 56 of 1,243 patients with pneumonia. Legionellosis accounted for 5.9% of nosocomial pneumonias and 3.4% of community-acquired pneumonias. No yearly, seasonal, or monthly pattern was seen. *Legionella pneumophila* was identified in 55 patients and *Legionella dumoffi* in 1 patient. The mortality rate associated with legionellosis was 39%.

Each clinical test was assessed for its rate of positive results (table). Detection of *L. pneumophila* serogroup 1 antigen in urine had the highest sensitivity, with 86% of patients with culture-proven disease being positive. The rates of positive results were 36% for serology and 26% for examination of respiratory secretions.

For the optimal diagnosis of legionellosis, a broad spectrum of tests

Diagnostic Results in 53 Patients With *Legionella* Pneumonia Evaluated by Single Tests and Test Combinations

Tests	Total no. of cases	No. of positive cases (% of total tested): Total	Serum antibody detection	Urinary antigen detection	Respiratory secretions: Total	Culture	DFA
S	47	–	17 (36)	–	–	–	–
U	40	–	–	32 (80)	–	–	–
U^SG1	33	–	–	29 (88)	–	–	–
C/D	27	–	–	–	7 (26)	3 (11)	6 (22)
S + U + C/D	17	16 (94)	7 (41)	12 (71)	4 (24)	2 (12)	3 (18)
S + U + C/D^SG1	15	14 (93)	5 (33)	12 (80)	4 (27)	2 (13)	3 (20)
S + U	36	33 (92)	13 (36)	28 (78)	–	–	–
S + U^SG1	30	27 (90)	7 (23)	26 (87)	–	–	–
U + C/D	18	14 (78)	–	13 (72)	5 (28)	2 (11)	4 (22)
U + C/D^SG1	15	14 (93)	–	13 (87)	5 (33)	2 (13)	4 (27)
S + C/D	23	10 (43)	8 (35)	–	5 (22)	2 (9)	4 (17)

Abbreviations: DFA, direct fluorescent antibody test; *S,* serum antibody detection; *U,* urinary antigen detection; *C/D,* culture and DFA of respiratory secretions.

Note: Patients with *L. pneumophila* serogroup 1 pneumonia who had urine samples tested for *Legionella* antigen were evaluated separately regarding the fact that an assay for detection of *L. pneumophila* SG1 antigen was applied (indicated by index^{SG1} assigned to the tests).

(Courtesy of Ruf B, Schürmann D, Horbach I, et al: *J Infect Dis* 162:1341–1348, 1990.)

must be performed. Urine antigen detection has a high sensitivity and allows early diagnosis. Postmortem examination of lung tissue is important for estimating the prevalence of the disease and assessing the diagnostic significance of clinical tests.

▶ This study suffers from the fact that not all patients underwent investigation by all 3 techniques (urinary antigen detection, serologic testing, and culture and immunofluorescence of respiratory secretions). However, it has the advantage that it involved a relatively large number of patients in a "real world" situation. The urinary antigen test appears to me to be the most sensitive and specific test now available for the diagnosis of legionnaires' disease. It is my understanding that several commercial laboratories offer the test at an affordable price and with a rapid turnaround time. One defect of the test is that it detects only serogroup I of *L. pneumophila,* but this is the most prevalent cause of infection in humans.—M.J. Barza, M.D.

Evaluation of Urinary Antigen ELISA for Diagnosing *Legionella pneumophila* Serogroup 1 Infection

Birtles RJ, Harrison TG, Samuel D, Taylor AG (Central Public Health Lab, London)

J Clin Pathol 43:685–690, 1990 12–2

Several enzyme-linked immunosorbent assays (ELISAs) have been described for the detection of *Legionella* antigen in the urine of patients with legionnaires' disease, but none has been thoroughly evaluated. An ELISA that used a monoclonal antibody (LKC2b) was applied to detect a soluble antigen in the urine of patients with legionnaires' disease caused by *Legionella pneumophila* subgroup 1 (L.pn 1). A fluorescein–isothiocyanate (FITC)–anti-FITC system was used to amplify the signal. Urine samples from 120 patients with confirmed legionnaires' disease and 80 patients with infections caused by agents other than *Legionella* were evaluated by urinary antigen ELISA.

The reproducibility of the ELISA was very good for specimens examined within the same batch. The L.pn 1 antigen was not detected in an samples from patients with infections other than L.pn 1 pneumonia. Thus the calculated specificity was 100%. The L.pn 1 antigen was detected in 93 (77%) of 120 patients with confirmed legionnaires' disease. No antigen was detected in the 3 patients with legionnaires' disease caused by *L. pneumophila* of a serogroup other than serogroup 1. The diagnostic sensitivity of the assay decreased as the time between onset of symptoms and urine collection increased (table). The sensitivity decreased significantly over time, from 86% for urine collected within 7 days of the onset of symptoms to 64% for urine collected after this time. When the antigen was detected, it was present in all but 1 of the first urine samples. For the exception, antigen was detected in a sample collected 5 days after onset of symptoms. Antigen was detected as early as 2 days after the onset of symptoms in 2 patients and persisted for at least 60 days in another patient, but more than half of the patients had stopped producing detectable antigen within 14 days of the onset of symptoms.

The urinary antigen ELISA is a relatively simple procedure that can prove beneficial in the diagnosis of very acute stages of L.pn 1 infection. Its overall sensitivity of 77% compares favorably with that reported for previously described ELISAs and serologic tests. When legionnaires' disease is suspected, urine should be collected as early as possible after the onset of symptoms.

▶ When a commercially available ELISA becomes available, *Legionella* urinary antigen detection will become the diagnostic method of choice.—D.R. Snydman, M.D.

Rapid Diagnosis of Herpes Simplex Encephalitis by Nested Polymerase Chain Reaction Assay of Cerebrospinal Fluid

Aurelius E, Johansson B, Sköldenberg B, Staland Å, Forsgren M (Central Microbiological Lab, Stockholm; Karolinska Inst, Danderyd Hosp, Danderyd, Sweden)
Lancet 337:189–192, 1991 12–3

Early and specific detection of herpes simplex virus encephalitis or demonstration of viral antigen previously necessitated invasive and potentially risky brain biopsy. The polymerase chain reaction (PCR) technique with nested primers has made amplification of virus-specific target DNA sequences possible with increased specificity and sensitivity.

This assay was applied to 151 samples of CSF from 43 consecutive patients with herpes simplex encephalitis and compared to the assay of 87 samples of CSF from 60 patients with acute febrile focal encephalopathy. The PCR procedure detected herpes simplex virus (HSV) DNA in 42 of 43 patients with proved herpes simplex encephalitis (Fig 12–1).

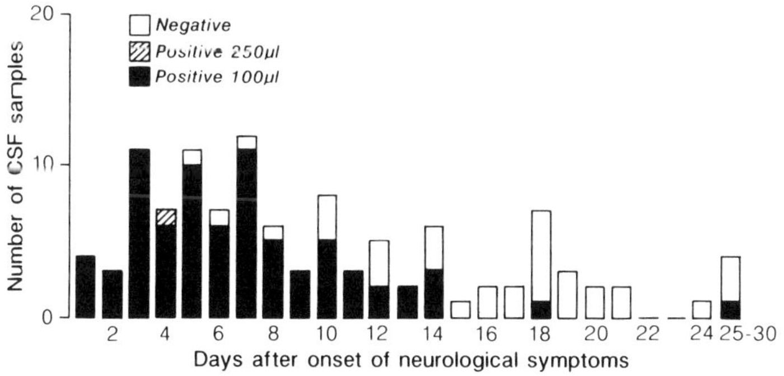

Fig 12–1.—Results of PCR in relation to time from onset of neurologic symptoms in samples of CSF from 42 PCR-positive patients with herpes simplex encephalitis. None of 36 samples taken at 30 days or more was positive. (Courtesy of Aurelius E, Johansson B, Sköldenberg G, et al: *Lancet* 337:189–192, 1991.)

The PCR was negative in 1 patient treated with acyclovir within 20 hours of onset of symptoms. The 87 control samples and all contamination controls were PCR negative. The results of PCR remained positive in samples drawn up to 27 days after the onset of neurologic symptoms.

The PCR technique may be difficult to master but the reproducibility is very high. It may be useful to include a weak positive sample in each run and to analyze duplicate samples. Specificity and sensitivity of the PCR assay are enhanced through the nested approach. This reaction provides a rapid and noninvasive diagnostic method for herpes simplex encephalitis.

▶ If confirmed in additional studies, and when non–radioisotopic techniques can be applied, the use of PCR for encephalitis caused by herpes simplex virus may become the diagnostic method of choice. However, as pointed out by Pershing, there are many pitfalls to overcome (1).—D.R. Snydman, M.D.

Reference

1. Pershing DH: *J Clin Microbiol* 29:1281, 1991.

Inappropriate Testing for Diarrheal Diseases in the Hospital

Siegel DL, Edelstein PH, Nachamkin I (Hosp of the Univ of Pennsylvania; Univ of Pennsylvania)

JAMA 263:979–982, 1990 12–4

At many centers, stool cultures and ova-parasite studies are ordered on all symptomatic patients apart from the pretest likelihood of diarrhea being caused by various organisms. A retrospective study was done to estimate the yield of these tests on specimens from outpatients and hospital patients as a function of time after admission.

Only 1 of 191 positive stool cultures obtained in a 3-year period was from a patient whose stool specimen was submitted after 3 days in hospital. None of 90 positive ova-parasite studies was from such patients. Nevertheless, specimens from this group constituted nearly half of all specimens received each year (Fig 12–2). About one fourth of the samples were positive for *Clostridium difficile* toxin, regardless of admission status, and about one fifth of the diarrheas were ascribed to *C. difficile* infection.

If routine stool cultures and ova-parasite studies on hospital patients were eliminated, costs would decline significantly without adversely affecting patient care. Exceptions may reasonably include patients with cryptosporidiosis and epidemiologic evidence of an increased diarrhea attack rate.

▶ This study confirms what all of us have intuitively felt regarding the rote, global work-up of stools from patients who develop diarrhea in hospital. Far too

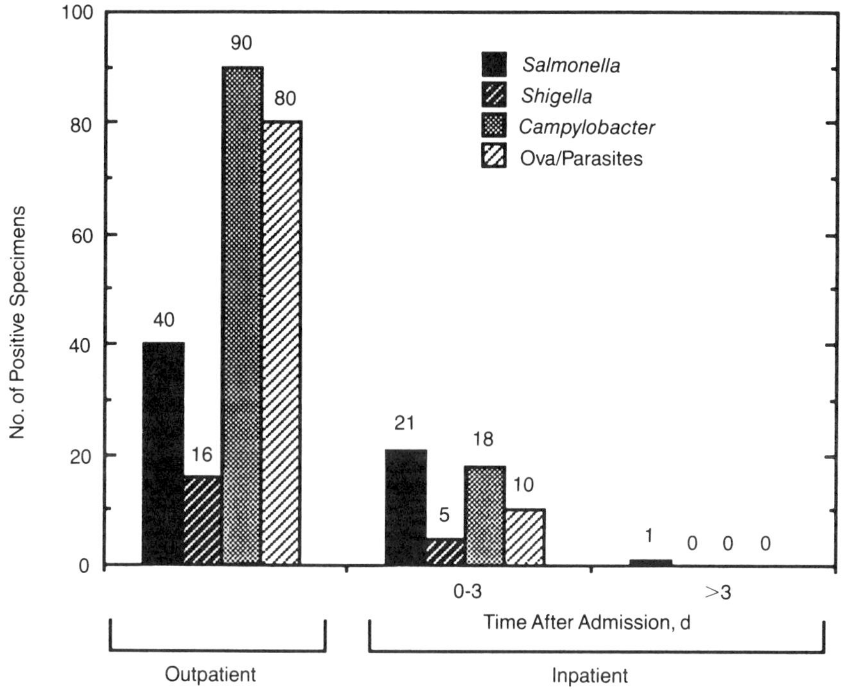

Fig 12–2.—Summary of positive stool cultures and ova and parasite examinations with positive results across outpatient and inpatient groups during 3-year period. (Courtesy of Siegel DL, Edelstein PH, Nachamkin I: *JAMA* 263:979–982, 1990.)

many physicians or house officers check the slip to rule out all potential pathogens. These investigators have shown that these specimens are rarely, if ever, positive for anything except *C. difficile* toxin. The positive predictive value of any test rests on the *a priori* probability of the patient having the disease. Given these studies, all hospital laboratories should follow the recommendations of these authors. I applaud their study. We have instituted this restrictive policy in our laboratory.—D.R. Snydman, M.D.

Value of Antigen Detection in Predicting Invasive Pulmonary Aspergillosis
Rogers TR, Haynes KA, Barnes RA (Charing Cross and Westminster Med School, London)
Lancet 336:1210–1213, 1990 12–5

In severely neutropenic patients, *Aspergillus* species is a significant pathogen. It is difficult to establish a clinical or microbiologic diagnosis of invasive pulmonary aspergillosis (IPA), and delay in starting antifungal therapy may be fatal. An alternative approach to diagnosis is through demonstration of *Aspergillus* antigen in serum, urine, or bronchoalveolar lavage fluid. Polyclonal and monoclonal inhibition enzyme-linked immunosorbent assays were used to establish the value of antigen detection in diagnosis of aspergillosis.

The presence of the antigen correctly predicted development of IPA in 19 of 20 patients. In 2 patients, antigen appeared after the clinical diagnosis was made. In 11 of 13 episodes of clinically suspected fungal infection, antigen was detected before clinical diagnosis. Antigen was detected in 1 of 90 patients who had no evidence of IPA. Both assays had positive and negative predictive values for IPA of more than 95%. Neutropenic patients may be screened for *Aspergillus* antigen and given antifungal therapy if antigen is detected, thereby increasing their chances of survival.

▶ There has been considerable interest in recent years in the diagnosis of invasive fungal infections by detection of antigen or antibody in serum and urine. *Candida, Aspergillus,* and *Blastomyces* infections have been studied in this way. Clearly, antigen detection has advantages over antibody detection, especially in immunocompromised patients. However, there has been much disappointment because the tradeoff between the sensitivity and specificity of the assays has proven poor. Admittedly, the assay described in this paper appears promising, although it would probably not be suitable for routine hospital laboratories. However, given the experience with other antigen assays for fungal infection, I would wait for further reports before concluding that this assay will be clinically useful.—M.J. Barza, M.D.

Infection Due to *Leuconostoc* Species: Six Cases and Review

Handwerger S, Horowitz H, Coburn K, Kolokathis A, Wormser GP (Mount Sinai School of Medicine, New York; New York Med College, Valhalla; Albert Einstein College of Medicine, New York)

Rev Infect Dis 12:602–610, 1990 12–6

Leuconostoc species, members of the family *Streptococcaceae,* are recognized as potential pathogens. *Leuconostoc* bacteremia was diagnosed in 6 patients, and data on 11 previously reported patients with *Leuconostoc* infection were reviewed.

The patients' ages ranged from 1 day to 78 years; the group included 6 children aged 6 months or less. Fifteen patients had bacteremia associated with fever, leukocytosis, or gastrointestinal complaints (table). The most striking feature among patients with *Leuconostoc* bacteremia was the degree of host-defense impairment. Almost all had significant underlying disease, including gastrointestinal disease in 7 patients. Many were critically ill before the onset of *Leuconostoc* infection. Ten of the bacteremic patients had received previous antibiotic therapy, and many had undergone invasive procedures that interrupted the normal integumentary host defense. In contrast, several children were not immunocompromised, 2 were asymptomatic, and 3 had received no antibiotic therapy previously.

Leuconostoc species were isolated in the blood of 15 patients, in the

Clinical Features of *Leuconostoc* Infection

Case no.	Organism isolated	Site	Temperature (°C)	Associated symptoms	No. of WBC/μL	Treatment	Outcome
1	L. para	Blood	38.1	. . .	14,000	Penicillin, catheter removal	Improved
2	L. mes sub. mes	Blood	38.6	Abdominal pain	18,000	Nafcillin	Improved
3	L. para	Blood	38.0	. . .	17,000	Catheter removal	Improved
4	L. para	Blood	40.0	. . .	8,000	Gentamicin, catheter removal	Died
5	L. mes sub. mes	Blood	40.0	Diarrhea, vomiting	14,200	Penicillin	Improved
6	L. para	Blood	39.0	. . .	11,600	Catheter removal	Improved
7	L. mes sub. dex	Blood	39.0	NA	NA	Gentamicin	Died
8	L. spp.	Blood	NA	NA	NA	Penicillin	Improved
9	L. spp.	Blood	37.9	Vomiting	22,000	Penicillin, gentamicin	Improved
10	L. mes	Blood	fever	NA	NA	Penicillin, catheter care	Improved
11	L. spp.	Blood	NA	Lethargy	9,700	Clindamycin	Improved
12	L. spp.	Blood	NA	Ileus	NA	None	Improved
13	L. spp.	Blood	NA	. . .	NA	None	Improved
14	L. spp.	Blood	37.8	Pneumonia	NA	Penicillin	Improved
15	L. spp.	Blood	NA	Diarrhea, ileus	NA	Trimethoprim-sulfamethoxazole	Died
16	L. spp.	CSF	37.8	Headache, meningismus	18,200	Penicillin	Improved
17	L. mes sub. dex	PD	NA	NA	NA	NA	NA

Abbreviations: L. para—L. paramesenteroides; L. mes sub. mes—L. mesenteroides subspecies *mesenteroides; L. mes sub. dex—L. mesenteroides* subspecies *dextranicum; NA,* not available; *L. spp.—Leuconostoc,* not futher speciated; *L. mes—Leuconostoc mesenteroides; PD,* peritoneal dialysate fluid.

(Courtesy of Handwerger S, Horowitz H, Coburn K, et al: *Rev Infect Dis* 12:602–610, 1990.)

CSF of 1, and in the peritoneal fluid of 1. Of the 15 patients with bacteremia, 8 had polymicrobial bacteremia. *Staphylococcus* was identified as the second organism in 7 of these patients. Clinical isolates of *Leuconostoc* were frequently misidentified, usually as viridans streptococci. All clinical isolates tested demonstrated high resistance to vancomycin. Successful therapy for *Leuconostoc* infection included high-dose penicillin and clindamycin and removal of foci of infection, such as intravascular catheters.

Leuconostoc species should be considered potential pathogens in humans, particularly among immunocompromised patients. *Leuconostoc* is frequently misidentified as another species of *Streptococcaceae*. Unless resistance to vancomycin is observed, the clinical spectrum of *Leuconostoc* infection may be much broader than is presently recognized. Therefore, susceptibility testing should be performed on all gram-positive bacteria isolated from normal sterile body sites.

▶ These species are generally found in soil or vegetable matter, although they have been isolated from the vagina and gastric fluid. The name is derived from the small gray-white or colorless colonies formed. Confusion with viridans streptococci, lactobacilli, and enterococci can occur. However, vancomycin resistance distinguishes the former; the arginine hydrolysis and the pyrrolidonylarynlamidase tests rule out the other 2 organisms. Leuconostocs are invariably vancomycin resistant, the exact mechanism of which has not been elucidated.—D.R. Snydman, M.D.

Antimyosin Antibody Cardiac Imaging: Its Role in the Diagnosis of Myocarditis

Dec GW, Palacios I, Yasuda T, Fallon JT, Khaw BA, Strauss HW, Haber E (Massachusetts Gen Hosp, Boston; Harvard Med School)

J Am Coll Cardiol 16:97–104, 1990 12–7

Right ventricular endomyocardial biopsy is the procedure of choice in differentiating patients with left ventricular dysfunction caused by myocarditis from the larger group of patients with idiopathic dilated cardiomyopathy. Despite its specificity, the sensitivity of right ventricular biopsy remains uncertain because of the focal or multifocal nature of this entity. Because myocyte necrosis is an integral component of myocarditis, the use of radiolabeled Fab fragments of monoclonal antimyosin antibodies may prove valuable. The sensitivity, specificity, and predictive value of indium-111 antimyosin antibody cardiac imaging were studied in 82 patients with suspected myocarditis. Antimyosin images were correlated with results of right ventricular biopsy performed within 48 hours of imaging.

In 74 patients, there was dilated cardiomyopathy of less than 1 year's duration with a mean left ventricular ejection fraction of .30; the other 8 patients had normal left ventricular function. Symptoms at presentation included congestive heart failure in 92%, chest pain mimicking myocardial infarction in 6%, and life-threatening ventricular tachyarrhythmias in 2%.

Myocarditis was diagnosed in 18 patients with right ventricular biopsy. Antimyosin scintigraphic imaging was abnormal in 15 and normal in 3 (table). The sensitivity of antimyosin imaging was 83%, specificity was 53%, and predictive value of a normal scan was 92%. Improvement in left ventricular function within 6 months of treatment occurred more

Comparison of Right Ventricular Biopsy Findings and Antimyosin Imaging in 82 Patients With Suspected Myocarditis

Antimyosin Scan Results	Right Ventricular Biopsy Results	
	Myocarditis	Nondiagnostic
Abnormal	15	30
Normal	3	34

Note: The probability that either the 2 columns or the 2 rows of this table were drawn from the same population was .014 by Fischer's test.
(Courtesy of Dec GW, Palacios I, Yasuda T, et al: *J Am Coll Cardiol* 16:97–104, 1990.)

frequently in patients with an abnormal antimyosin scan (54%) than in those with a normal scan (18%).

These data confirm the usefulness of antimyosin scintigraphy in the initial evaluation of patients with dilated and nondilated cardiomyopathy and clinically suspected myocarditis. A normal antimyosin scan is associated with a very low rate of detecting myocarditis on endomyocardial biopsy and thus may obviate the need for biopsy.

13 Miscellaneous

Proposed Mechanism of the Inflammatory Attacks in Familial Mediterranean Fever

Matzner Y, Ayesh SK, Hochner-Celniker D, Ackerman Z, Ferne M (Hadassah Univ Hosp Mount Scopus and Einkarem, Jerusalem, Israel)

Arch Intern Med 150:1289–1291, 1990 13–1

Familial Mediterranean fever (FMF) is an inherited disorder characterized by episodes of nonprovoked inflammation of the joints and the pleural and peritoneal cavities. The attacks of pain and fever can be prevented by colchicine, but their mechanism is not understood. Synovial and peritoneal fluids from patients with FMF lack a protein that inhibits neutrophil chemotaxis by antagonizing C5a.

C5a inhibitor activity was estimated using a C5a binding assay when peritoneal fluid samples were tested for inhibiting recombinant C5a binding to U937 cells induced with dibutyryl cyclic adenosine monophosphate. Unlike normal peritoneal fluids, samples from patients with FMF contained less than 1% of normal C5a inhibitor activity. Gel filtration and ion exchange chromatographic analysis of fluids from these patients failed to yield a fraction that inhibited C5a binding.

Familial Mediterranean fever appears to involve a true deficiency of an inhibitor that neutralizes the complement-derived inflammatory mediator C5a. The disease may reflect inadequate suppression of the inflammatory response to accidentally released C5a. Colchicine suppresses neutrophil motility, making it less likely that sufficient inflammatory cells will migrate to sites of unopposed C5a release.

▶ The etiology of familial Mediterranean fever remains elusive. These authors were the first to describe a deficiency of C5A inhibitor activity in their patients. Their postulate is sound and attractive. I await confirmation from other laboratories.—S.M. Wolff, M.D.

An Outbreak of Toxic Encephalopathy Caused by Eating Mussels Contaminated With Domoic Acid

Perl TM, Bédard L, Kosatsky T, Hockin JC, Todd ECD, Remis RS (Regroupement de départements de santé communautaire du Montréal métropolitain, Montréal; Health and Welfare Canada, Ottawa; Univ of Iowa)

N Engl J Med 322:1775–1780, 1990 13–2

In November and December 1987 a number of persons who had eaten cultivated mussels from Prince Edward Island, Canada, became acutely ill

Symptoms of Illness Among 99 Patients After Consumption of Mussels

Symptom	No. of Yes Responses	Total Responses	%
Nausea	75	98	77
Vomiting *	74	97	76
Abdominal cramps *	48	95	51
Diarrhea *	41	97	42
Headache	40	93	43
Memory loss *	24	96	25

Note: Results were obtained from standardized questionnaires completed for 99 of 107 patients. Total responders do not add up to 99 because not all questions were answered for each person.

*Criterion for inclusion as case.

(Courtesy of Perl TM, Bédard L. Kosatsky T, et al: *N Engl J Med* 322:1775–1780, 1990.)

with gastrointestinal and neurologic symptoms. Reports of the illness made it clear that the disease was different from paralytic shellfish poisoning or any other illnesses previously associated with consumption of mollusks.

The most commonly reported symptoms in the 99 patients who met the case definition and responded to a questionnaire were vomiting, ab-

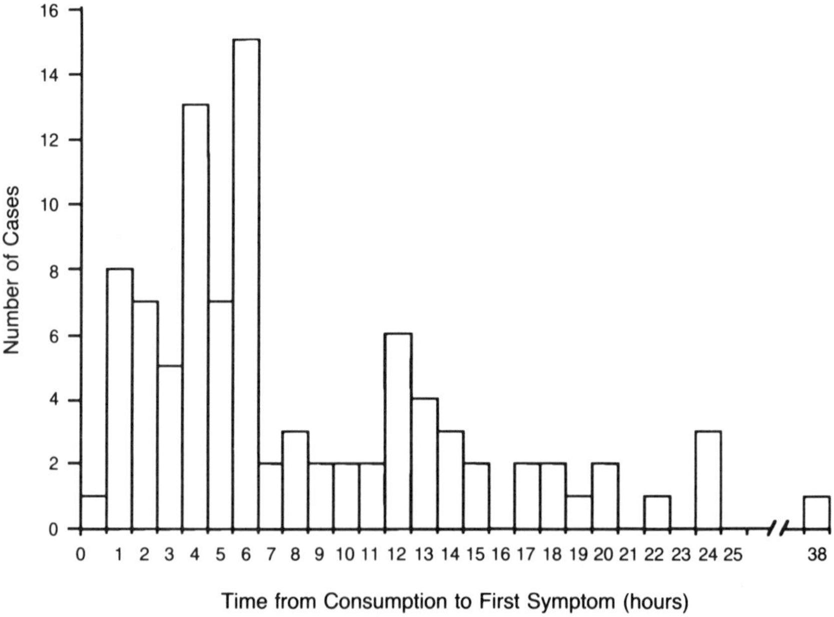

Fig 13–1.—Interval between ingestion of mussels and onset of first symptom (incubation period). Data shown are based on responses to 91 questionnaires. (Courtesy of Perl TM, Bédard L, Kosatsky T, et al: *N Engl J Med* 322:1775–1780, 1990.)

dominal cramps, diarrhea, severe headache, and loss of short-term memory (table). The median time from ingestion of mussels to onset of symptoms was 5.5 hours (Fig 13–1).

Nineteen patients required hospitalization. Older patients and men had a higher risk of hospitalization and of memory loss. The 3 patients who died ranged in age from 71 to 84 years. Brain tissue samples from 2 of these patients and a third who died of acute myocardial infarction 3 months after the outbreak revealed neuronal necrosis or cell loss and astrocytosis. All patients younger than age 65 years who were hospitalized had preexisting illnesses. Younger patients were more likely to have diarrhea.

Laboratory studies identified the toxin as domoic acid, which appeared in mussels left uneaten and in mussels sampled from cultivation beds in 3 river estuaries on the eastern coast of Prince Edward Island. The source of domoic acid, a potent excitatory neurotransmitter, appeared to have been a form of marine vegetation, *Nitzschia pungens.* Mussels are now tested for the presence of domoic acid, and no new cases of the illness have been reported.

▶ As infectious disease specialists we are often called upon to solve complex and puzzling cases, some of which are not infectious in nature. Furthermore, we generally are responsible for analyzing cases of food poisoning. This report marks the description and elucidation of an unusual syndrome caused by domoic acid, a neuroexcitatory amino acid. I was struck by the case report describing the illness which can easily mimic an infectious process. An elderly diabetic, hypertensive man had sudden onset of confusion, leukocytosis of 20,000/mm^3 with neutrophilia, tachycardia, and eventually hypotension. Many of these patients also had diarrhea.

The history of mussel consumption will help in the differential diagnosis. The prompt recognition of this outbreak and control is a tribute to Canadian public health efforts.—D.R. Snydman, M.D.

Chronic Fatigue: A Prospective Clinical and Virologic Study

Gold D, Bowden R, Sixbey J, Riggs R, Katon WJ, Ashley R, Obrigewitch RM, Corey L (Univ of Washington; Fred Hutchinson Cancer Research Ctr, Seattle; St Jude's Children's Research Hosp, Memphis)

JAMA 264:48–53, 1990 13–3

Several recent reports have described elevated Epstein-Barr virus (EBV) titers in some patients with chronic fatigue syndrome. To evaluate the clinical and virological course of patients with chronic fatigue and high titers of antibodies to EBV, 26 such patients were compared with a group of healthy controls.

Both groups underwent clinical and psychiatric evaluations and serologic and viral studies. The mean age of the patients was 34 years; 19 (73%) were women. Nine were unable to work at all, and 13 experienced some degree of functional impairment. Fourteen reported a history of clinical mononucleosis (Table 1). In addition to fatigue, common

TABLE 1.—Demographic and Clinical Characteristics at Enrollment of Patients With Chronic Fatigue

	Patients	Controls	P*
No. of subjects	26	18	...
Age, y†	34.4±7.6	28.5±6.7	<.02‡
Women, No. (%)	19/26 (73)	11/18 (61)	NS§
White, No. (%)	26/26 (100)	18/18 (100)	NS§
Married, No. (%)	11/26 (42)	6/18 (33)	NS§
Heterosexual, No. (%)	20/26 (77)	18/18 (100)	NS
Education, y†	15.5±2.5	17.9±1.7	<.001‡
History of mononucleosis, No. (%)	14/26 (54)	4/18 (22)	.06§
Unable to work, No. (%)	9/24 (38)	0/18	.005§
Able to work part time, No. (%)	4/24 (17)	0/18	NS
Duration of symptoms, y†‖	3.5±2.5	...	...
No. of health care providers before enrollment			
Median	5	0	<.01§
Range	1-16	...	...
Hours of sleep per night			
Median	8.25	7.5	NS
Range	5-12	6-8	...
Sleeping during the day, No. (%)	10/24 (42)	0/18	.002§

*NS indicates not significant.
†Values are means ± standard deviation.
‡Student's t test.
§Fisher's exact test.
‖Number = 24.
(Courtesy of Gold D, Bowden R, Sixbey J, et al: *JAMA* 264:48–53, 1990.)

symptoms included a sensation of enlarged or tender lymph nodes (85%), depression (77%), musculoskeletal complaints (65%), and chest pain or palpitations (50%) (Table 2).

A detailed physical examination found few abnormalities in the patient group. The frequency of isolating EBV in blood and in demonstrating EBV infection by in situ hybridization in blood lymphocytes or saliva was similar in both groups (Table 3). The 2 groups also were similar in the prevalence and titers of antibody to human herpesvirus type 6 (Table 4). However, patients with chronic fatigue had significantly more lifetime episodes of major depression (73%) than controls (22%). Also, higher in vitro natural killer (NK) activity and lower in vitro production of interleukin-2 (IL-2) were observed in patients compared with controls.

At a mean follow-up of 11.3 months, 4 of 21 patients had recovered completely and 8 were significantly improved. However, clinical improvement was not associated with any changes in EBV antibody titer or in EBV in situ hybridization or culture. It was hypothesized that the decreased in vitro production of IL-2 and the elevated NK activity in these patients may have been secondary to their affective disorder. The finding that most patients with chronic fatigue improve over time should be encouraging.

▶ The evidence against any viral etiology for the chronic fatigue syndrome continues to mount. This study excludes an association with EBV infection or in-

TABLE 2.—Signs and Symptoms of Patients With Chronic Fatigue at Enrollment

	Patients, No. (%)
Symptom	
Fatigue	26/26 (100)
Dyslogia	8/9 (89)
Sensation of adenopathy	22/26 (85)
Depression	20/26 (77)
Arthralgias/myalgias	17/26 (65)
Headache	17/25 (68)
Dizziness/paresthesia	16/26 (62)
Sore throat	13/25 (52)
Chest pain/palpitation	13/26 (50)
Upper respiratory tract symptoms	11/25 (44)
Gastrointestinal tract symptoms	11/26 (42)
Rash	9/26 (35)
Low-grade fever (temperature <38°C)	11/26 (42)
Mean ± SD No. of symptoms at enrollment	11.2 ± 4.2
Sign	
Neurologic abnormalities	5/26 (19)
Pharyngitis	2/26 (8)
Temperature >38°C	1/26 (4)
Adenopathy*	1/26 (4)
Hepatic or splenic enlargement	0/26

*Patients were considered to have significant lymphadenopathy if at least 2 nodes 1 cm or more in diameter were present at any site.

(Courtesy of Gold D, Bowden R, Sixbey J, et al: *JAMA* 264:48–53, 1990.)

fection with human herpesvirus type 6. It confirms the close association with depression and other affective disorders, which has been reported previously (1). One of the most interesting findings to emerge in recent years is the abnormal cellular immune responses seen in patients with chronic fatigue syndrome. It is noteworthy that depression alone has a similar association. The good news is that more than 50% of the patients in this study improved markedly within the first year. This finding makes it increasingly difficult to demonstrate that therapeutic intervention has a major effect when more than half of the patients recover spontaneously.—M.S. Klempner, M.D.

TABLE 3.—Comparison of EBV Isolation Rates and Demonstration of EBV DNA in Situ Hybridization in Patients and Controls

	Patients, No. (%)	Controls, No. (%)	P†
EBV isolated from PBLs	2/18 (11)	2/18 (11)	NS
EBV DNA in PBLs by in situ hybridization	1/16 (6)	2/10 (20)	NS
EBV isolated from throat washings	0/10 (0)	0/4 (0)	NS
EBV DNA by in situ hybridization in throat washings	0/23 (0)	1/14 (7)	NS
EBV isolated by culture or in situ hybridization	3/23 (13)	3/18 (17)	NS

Abbreviations: PBLs, peripheral blood lymphocytes; *NS,* not significant.

Note: Isolation of EBV was measured by emergence of transformed cells positive for EBV-associated nuclear antigen.

*Fisher's exact test.

(Courtesy of Gold D, Bowden R, Sixbey J, et al: *JAMA* 264:48–53, 1990.)

TABLE 4.—Laboratory Characteristics of Patients and Controls

	Patients	Controls	P*
Atypical lymph nodes, No. (%)	2/25 (8)	3/18 (17)	NS
Seroprevalence of cytomegalovirus, No. (%)	10/21 (48)	6/17 (35)	NS
Seroprevalence of toxoplasmosis, No. (%)	2/25 (8)	1/18 (6)	NS
Seroprevalence of HHV-6,† No. (%)	19/23 (83)	12/12 (100)	NS
Geometric mean antibody titer of HHV-6	24.66	25.11	NS
Abnormal C1q binding, No. (%)	6/19 (32)	Not done	. . .
Antinuclear antibodies, No. (%)	2/21 (10)	3/17 (18)	NS
T4 cells, %‡	37±3	29±2	.03§
T8 cells, %‡	28±3	24±3	NS
T4/T8 ratio‡	1.6±0.18‖	1.6±0.23	NS
Phytohemagglutinin (stimulation index)‡	228.7±33	281.9±47	NS
Interleukin 2, U/mL‡	301.5±48	509.8±62	0.3§
Natural killer activity, lytic units per 1×10^6 effector cells producing 50% lysis†	11.7±2.3	10.4±3.2	0.3§

*NS indicates not significant.
†HHV-6 indicates human herpesvirus type 6.
‡Values are mean ± standard deviation.
§Wilcoxon rank-sum test.
‖Mean ± standard error of mean.
(Courtesy of Gold D, Bowden R, Sixbey J, et al: *JAMA* 264:48–53, 1990.)

Reference

1. Kroenke K, et al: *JAMA* 260:929, 1988.

A Controlled Trial of Intravenous Immunoglobulin G in Chronic Fatigue Syndrome

Peterson PK, Shepard J, Macres M, Schenck C, Crosson J, Rechtman D, Lurie N (Univ of Minnesota; Hennepin County Med Ctr, Minneapolis; Baxter Health-care Corp, Glendale, Calif)
Am J Med 89:554–560, 1990 13–4

Chronic fatigue syndrome consists of unexplained disabling fatigue and other nonspecific symptoms, usually following an acute viral-like illness. It occurs chiefly in young to middle-aged women. No established therapy is available, but IgG was tried because of suggestions that the syndrome might involve chronic viral infection or an immunoregulatory defect.

Thirty patients with a diagnosis of chronic fatigue syndrome were enrolled in a double-blind, placebo-controlled trial of intravenous IgG. A dose of 1 g/kg was given every 30 days over 6 months; placebo recipients were given 1% albumin solution.

The 28 patients who completed the trial initially described moderate to severe fatigue. Marked impairment was evident on measures of social functioning and perceived health. Many patients had low serum levels of IgG1 or IgG3. No significant symptomatic or functional improvement ensued despite restoration of normal IgG1 levels. Major adverse reactions occurred in 3 patients in each group. Intravenous immunoglobulin G does not appear to provide apparent clinical benefit to patients with chronic fatigue. It is necessary to learn more of the cause and pathogenesis of this disorder.

A Double-Blind, Placebo-Controlled Trial of Intravenous Immunoglobulin Therapy in Patients With Chronic Fatigue Syndrome

Lloyd A, Hickie I, Wakefield D, Boughton C, Dwyer J (Prince Henry and Prince of Wales Hosps, Sydney, Australia)

Am J Med 89:561–568, 1990 13–5

Cell-mediated immunity often is disrupted in patients with chronic fatigue syndrome, and IgG subclass deficiencies have been described. High-dose IgG given intravenously was evaluated in 49 patients with a diagnosis of chronic fatigue syndrome, 40 of whom had abnormalities of cell-mediated immunity. The patients, all adults, had not previously received immunologic therapy. Patients received 3 infusions per month of placebo solution or IgG at a dose of 2 g/kg. The physician and psychiatrist who estimated the severity of symptoms and of disability were unaware of the treatment status.

Ten of 23 patients given immunoglobulin (43%) and 3 of 26 given placebo (12%) were thought to have a substantial reduction in symptoms and were able to resume work and social activity. Psychological and immunologic measures indicated improvement in the responding patients. Phlebitis, constitutional symptoms, and impaired concentration were more frequent in immunoglobulin-treated patients than in placebo recipients. A significant number of patients in this trial responded to intravenous immunoglobulin treatment. Improved physical and psychological well-being correlated with less deranged cell-mediated immune function.

▶ It would seem to me that the chronic fatigue syndrome needs to be better defined as a clinical entity, and objective abnormalities delineated, before one can carry out meaningful therapeutic trials.—S.M. Wolff, M.D.

Double-Blind Placebo-Controlled Study of Three-Month Treatment With Lymecycline in Reactive Arthritis, With Special Reference to *Chlamydia* Arthritis

Lauhio A, Leirisalo-Repo M, Lähdevirta J, Saikku P, Repo H (Aurora Hosp, Helsinki; Univ of Helsinki; Helsinki Univ Central Hosp)

Arthritis Rheum 34:6–14, 1991 13–6

The role of antimicrobial therapy in the treatment of reactive arthritis (ReA) is controversial. In a double-blind, placebo-controlled, randomized study the effects on ReA of 3 months of treatment with lymecycline, a form of tetracycline, were examined. Forty patients with ReA received either lymecycline, 300 mg, or placebo twice daily for 3 months. The trig-

Characteristics of Patients With ReA at Entry Into Study

	All patients (n = 40)		*Chlamydia* arthritis (n = 21)	
	Lymecycline group (n = 21)	Placebo group (n = 19)	Lymecycline group (n = 12)	Placebo group (n = 9)
Age	30.9 ± 2.0	30.7 ± 1.9	28.8 ± 2.0	27.8 ± 2.3
Sex				
Female	8 (38)	4 (21)	4 (33)	2 (22)
Male	13 (62)	15 (79)	8 (67)	7 (78)
Previous ReA	5 (24)	5 (26)	2 (17)	3 (33)
Previous sacroiliitis	0	1 (5)	0	0
Triggering microbe				
Chlamydia	12 (57)	9 (47)	12 (100)	9 (100)
Yersinia	3 (14)	5 (26)		
Campylobacter	2 (10)	1 (5)		
Preceding urethritis? etiology	1 (5)	1 (5)		
Preceding enteritis? etiology	3 (14)	3 (16)		
Weeks of ReA before trial drug	7.7 ± 1.4	6.3 ± 1.1	9.5 ± 2.1	8.2 ± 2.1
No. of swollen joints	4.6 ± 0.7	4.3 ± 0.8	3.6 ± 0.9	3.8 ± 0.9
No. of painful joints	1.2 ± 0.3	1.9 ± 0.7	0.9 ± 0.4	2.0 ± 1.4
Low back pain	11 (52)	11 (58)	6 (50)	6 (67)
Enthesopathy	9 (43)	5 (26)	5 (42)	3 (33)
Extraarticular manifestations	11 (52)	6 (32)	8 (67)	3 (33)
Urethritis	9 (43)	4 (21)	5 (42)	3 (33)
Eye inflammation	2 (10)	3 (16)	2 (17)	2 (22)
Mucocutaneous lesion	3 (14)	2 (11)	3 (25)	0
Fever >37.5°C	9 (43)	11 (58)	4 (33)	4 (44)
ESR, mm/hour	59.3 ± 8.1	66.0 ± 6.3	41.7 ± 9.3	55.6 ± 10.7
CRP, mg/liter	68.6 ± 17.9	67.0 ± 11.4	46.1 ± 12.2	65.4 ± 19.5
WBC, $\times 10^9$/liter	8.5 ± 0.5	10.0 ± 0.7	8.8 ± 0.7	9.4 ± 0.9
Hgb, gm/liter	133.5 ± 3.2	128.5 ± 3.0	138.0 ± 3.9	127.6 ± 4.4
HLA–B27 positive	19 (90)	16 (84)	10 (82)	6 (67)

Abbreviations: ESR, erythrocyte sedimentation rate (Westergren); *WBC*, white blood cells; *Hgb*, hemoglobin.
Note: Values are number of (%) or mean ± standard error of mean.
(Courtesy of Lauhio A, Leirisalo-Repo M, Lähdevirta J, et al: *Arthritis Rheum* 34:6–14, 1991.)

gering microbe was *Chlamydia trachomatis* in 21 patients, *Yersinia* in 8, and *Campylobacter* in 3; 6 patients had a preceding gastroenteritis and 2 had a preceding urethritis, both of unknown etiology (table).

Overall, except for the shorter duration of the elevated level of C-reactive protein (CRP) in the lymecycline group, the clinical and laboratory responses did not differ significantly between the lymecycline-treated and the placebo-treated patients. However, when the patients with *Chlamydia* arthritis were evaluated separately, those treated with lymecycline had a significantly shorter duration of illness, as well as a shorter duration of arthralgia, elevated erythrocyte sedimentation rate, and elevated level of CRP, compared with the placebo group. These effects were not seen in other ReA patients. Adverse effects caused by lymecycline were mild and few. The results suggest that it is important to verify the triggering microbe in ReA before treatment, and that a prolonged course of lymecycline is beneficial in patients with *Chlamydia* arthritis.

► I chose this paper mostly because of the juxtaposition of the name of the antibiotic used (lymecycline) for the treatment of ReA. What a prophetic name, because this tetracycline derivative has been around since the mid-1960s. It is not available in the United States, or I am sure it would have had an instant trial in patients with Lyme disease. If nothing else, the table presents a very nice review of the clinical characteristics of patients with ReA following infection with *Chlamydia, Yersinia,* and *Campylobacter.*—M.S. Klempner, M.D.

Cat-Scratch Disease: Acute Encephalopathy and Other Neurologic Manifestations

Carithers HA, Margileth AM (Univ of Florida; Uniformed Services Univ of the Health Sciences, Bethesda, Md)

Am J Dis Child 145:98–101, 1991 13–7

Cat-scratch disease (CSD) is an infection caused by a gram-negative bacillus, and its most serious clinical feature is an encephalopathy. Data were reviewed on the course and outcome of 76 patients with CSD and its neurologic complications. Encephalopathy was found in 61 of the 76 patients. Those affected were aged 1–66 years (mean, 10.6 years). Encephalopathy occurred in twice as many male as female patients, compared to an almost equal sex ratio among patients with uncomplicated CSD. Fever was not a characteristic feature; only 26% of patients had temperatures higher than 39° C. Convulsions occurred in 46% of patients, and transient combative behavior was seen in 39%. Lethargy with or without coma was accompanied by variable neurologic signs.

Results of laboratory studies, including imaging of the CNS, were often inconsistent and nondiagnostic. All but 1 of the skin tests were positive for cat-scratch antigen. Skin or lymph node biopsy specimens from 14 patients showed pathologic features compatible with CSD, and Warthin-Starry staining showed the "English-Wear" bacillus in 10.

Among the 15 patients with CSD without encephalopathy, 2 children with facial nerve paresis had cranial nerve symptoms or signs, 10 had CSD neuroretinitis, and 3 women had peripheral neuritis.

For the patients with CSD encephalopathy, treatment consisted of control of convulsions and supportive measures. Commonly used antibiotics administered to more than half the patients were apparently not effective. All 76 patients recovered within 12 months, and 78% recovered within 1–12 weeks. No neurologic sequelae were observed during a follow-up period of 3 months to 22 years.

Cat-scratch disease encephalopathy should be considered in a young patient who has the sudden onset of convulsions or coma. Although it is believed that antibiotics do not modify the course of CSD, intravenous injection of gentamicin sulfate is recommended for severely ill patients.

▶ The authors have an impressive experience with CSD. Although a precise denominator is difficult to obtain, they estimate an incidence of encephalopathy in about 2% of the patients with CSD. The interval from the onset of CSD to the onset of neurologic symptoms in this series ranged from a few days to 2 months. The features of headache, malaise, convulsions, coma, and a chacteristic form of combative behavior usually abate spontaneously after a week or so but can also last for many weeks. The authors suggest that CSD encephalopathy should be suspected when young patients present with a sudden onset of coma or convulsions, especially if a history of exposure to cats (particularly young cats) can be obtained or a site of inoculation with regional lymphadenopathy can be found. Although antimicrobial treatment is of uncertain benefit, the authors suggest an aminoglycoside or trimethoprim-sulfamethoxazole. I would raise the additional possibility of ciprofloxacin, as was recently reported in a small series (1).—M.S. Klempner, M.D.

Reference

1. Holley HP: *JAMA* 265:1563, 1991.

Clinical and Pathological Features of Bacillary Peliosis Hepatis in Association With Human Immunodeficiency Virus Infection

Perkocha LA, Geaghan SM, Yen TSB, Nishimura SL, Chan SP, Garcia-Kennedy R, Honda G, Stoloff AC, Klein HZ, Goldman RL, Van Meter S, Ferrell LD, LeBoit PE (Univ of California, San Francisco; Pacific Presbyterian Med Ctr, San Francisco; Inst for Forensic Sciences, Oakland, Calif)

N Engl J Med 323:1581–1586, 1990 13–8

Peliosis hepatis is characterized by cystic, blood-filled spaces in hepatic parenchyma and can occur in patients with chronic infections or advanced cancer or in those who receive therapy with anabolic steroids or other drugs. Data on 8 HIV-infected patients who had peliosis hepatis were reviewed; 2 of the patients were also infected with cutaneous bacillary angiomatosis, a recently described pseudoneoplastic vascular proliferation containing bacteria.

Liver tissue from the 8 patients was examined. For comparison, tissue from 4 patients with peliosis hepatis but without HIV infection also was examined. The histologic features seen in peliosis hepatis associated with

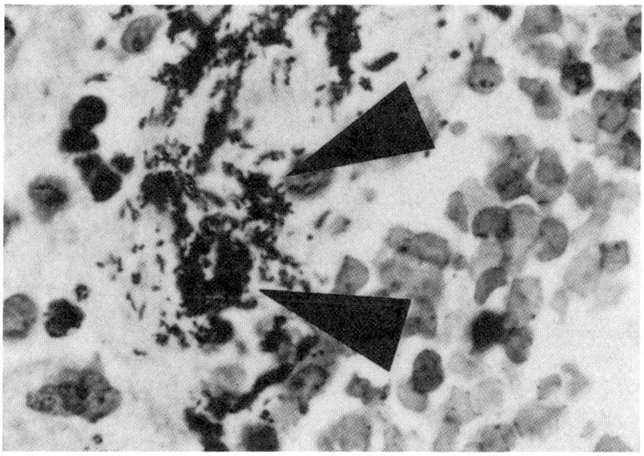

Fig 13–2.—Granular purple material *(arrows)* subsequently identified as bacilli. Note the surrounding myxoid stroma, as well as the erythrocytes in the peliotic space to the left (hematoxylin-eosin, original magnification, ×450; oil immersion). (Courtesy of Perkocha LA, Geaghan SM, Yen TSB, et al: *N Engl J Med* 323:1581–1586, 1990.)

HIV infection were myxoid stroma and clumps of granular purple material (Figs 13–2 and 13–3). The granular material was identified as bacilli morphologically identical to that found in the skin lesions of cutaneous bacillary angiomatosis. The 2 patients with this "bacillary peliosis hepatis" responded to antibiotics. Tissue from the 4 patients with hepatis without HIV infection did not have the same histologic features.

Opportunistic HIV-associated bacillary peliosis hepatis is probably caused by the same organism as cutaneous bacillary angiomatosis and is treatable with antibiotics. In patients with non–HIV-associated peliosis

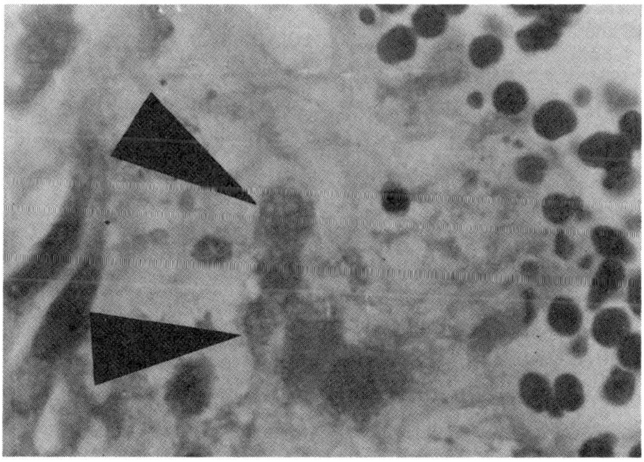

Fig 13–3.—Clumps of bacilli *(arrows)* identified by Warthin-Starry staining of a section of liver. Erythrocytes are present in the adjacent peliotic space to the left (original magnification, ×450; oil immersion). (Courtesy of Perkocha LA, Geaghan SM, Yen TSB, et al: *N Engl J Med* 323:1581–1586, 1990.)

hepatis, the absence of bacilli implies that other pathogenic mechanisms may also be responsible.

▶ The lesions of bartonellosis are similar to cutaneous bacillary angiomatosis. An angiogenic factor has been identified as being elaborated by *Bartonella bacilliformis.* Alternatively, there have been reports linking bacillary peliosis hepatis to the organism implicated in cat-scratch disease. However, erythromycin, which has been reported to be effective in some cases of peliosis hepatis, is not active against the cat-scratch bacillus. Several patients in this series appeared to respond to erythromycin; doxycycline and antituberculous therapy have also been reported to be effective.—D.R. Snydman, M.D.

The Agent of Bacillary Angiomatosis: An Approach to the Identification of Uncultured Pathogens

Relman DA, Loutit JS, Schmidt TM, Falkow S, Tompkins LS (Stanford Univ, Indiana Univ)

N Engl J Med 323:1573–1580, 1990 13–9

Bacillary angiomatosis is a vascular proliferative disorder initially described in the skin and nodes of HIV-seropositive patients. Lesions contain clusters of bacilli that stain positively by the Warthin-Starry technique, resembling those of cat-scratch disease. The histologic findings, however, differ from those of classic cat-scratch disease.

The polymerase chain reaction (PCR) technique was used to analyze tissues from 4 patients with a diagnosis of bacillary angiomatosis. Oligonucleotide primers complementary to the 16S ribosomal RNA genes of eubacteria served to amplify 16S ribosomal gene fragments directly from tissue samples. The target DNA was from a recent case of disseminated bacillary angiomatosis. The DNA sequence of the ribosomal gene fragments was analyzed for phylogenetic relatedness to known organisms.

Tissues from 3 unrelated patients yielded a unique 16S gene sequence, and the sequence from the fourth patient differed at only 4 of 241 base positions. No related 16S gene fragment was found in normal tissues. The sequences found in tissues from bacillary angiomatosis appeared most closely related to *Rochalimaea quintana,* an organism transmitted by the body louse that causes trench fever. This approach may prove helpful in investigating other infectious diseases whose cause is uncertain.

▶ A wonderful example of how modern molecular biological techniques can provide important new information. It is not too much to hope that the etiology of other granulomatous diseases of unknown etiology (e.g., sarcoid) will eventually be found using such technology.—S.M. Wolff, M.D.

Management of Autonomic Dysfunction in Severe Tetanus: The Use of Magnesium Sulphate and Clonidine

Sutton DN, Tremlett MR, Woodcock TE, Nielsen MS (Southampton Gen Hosp, England)
Intensive Care Med 16:75–80, 1990 13–10

Patients with autonomic dysfunction in severe tetanus may experience cardiovascular instability secondary to sympathetic overactivity and elevated catecholamine levels. These patients have a reported mortality exceeding 50%. Recent studies have shown that magnesium sulfate may be an effective treatment for the autonomic dysfunction.

Man, 45, contracted tetanus 3 days after sustaining a compound fracture of his right elbow. The patient was admitted to the intensive care unit and given antibiotic therapy. Human tetanus immunoglobulin was given intramuscularly, and the patient was sedated by diazepam infusion and morphine. Twenty-four hours later the patient required a tracheotomy, ventilation, and increased sedation. By day 2 spasms were under control, but autonomic instability developed. On day 4, a loading dose of magnesium sulfate (70 mg/kg) was followed by continuous infusion at 1–4 g/hr to achieve a therapeutic level of 2.5–4 mmol/L. Levels were easily held within this range. Improvements in heart rate and pulse variation produced by the loading dose were sustained, and blood pressure stability improved. The sedation and neuromuscular blockade were reduced. However, on day 6 cardiovascular function became steadily more unstable despite increased midazolam infusion. Clonidine therapy was started on day 8, and cardiovascular instability improved dramatically over the next 4 days. The patient required reintroduction of neuromuscular blockade and increased sedation on day 13 and responded well thereafter. Cardiovascular stability was restored by day 17, and all sedatives had been discontinued by day 24. He was weaned from the ventilator by day 25, and magnesium infusion was stopped. Gradually reduced doses of clonidine were discontinued before discharge to the ward on day 30. The patient made a full recovery.

Sedation, neuromuscular blockade, and controlled ventilation are the basic treatments for severe tetanus. Magnesium may suppress sympathetic overactivity without hazard, but it may not be adequate as the sole therapeutic agent. In the described case, clonidine provided good control in combination with magnesium, sedation, and paralysis. It would be worthwhile to further investigate clonidine use in a center treating a larger number of tetanus cases.

▶ Tetanus, like cholera, should not kill anybody; it is simply a matter of early diagnosis and proper management, including fluids and respiratory and nutritional support, respectively. Cholera, however, still kills, especially when the well-known principles of management of severe dehydration and shock are not followed. In the case of tetanus, the management principles for autonomic dysfunction and cardiac instability are not established. This review suggests that clonidine should be further investigated as an adjunctive agent. The problem is that too few centers see enough patients to carry out good systematic studies, including a comparison of regimens. The ability to assess the impact of therapy on outcome will be severely compromised. And all of this for a fully preventable disease!—G.T. Keusch, M.D.

Public Health Implications of the Microbial Pesticide *Bacillus thuringiensis:* An Epidemiological Study, Oregon, 1985–86

Green M, Heumann M, Sokolow R, Foster LR, Bryant R, Skeels M (Oregon State Health Div, Portland; Oregon Health Sciences Univ, Portland)

Am J Public Health 80:848–852, 1990 13–11

The microbial pesticide *Bacillus thuringiensis* var. *kurstaki* (B.t.-k) has been widely used for more than 30 years. The bacterium is considered to be harmless to mammals, yet its potential for causing human infection has never been the subject of an epidemiologic study. During 2 seasons of aerial B.t.-k spraying for gypsy moth control, a surveillance for human infections caused by B.t.-k was conducted.

Four clinical laboratories in the study area subcultured routinely obtained cultures that were positive for any *Bacillus* species. Follow-up information was collected for all B.t.-positive specimens. A total of 55 B.t.-positive cultures was identified in cultures that had been taken from 18 different body sites or fluids. All but 3 of the B.t. isolates were assessed to be contaminants and not the cause of the disease that had prompted the culture. In 3 patients, B.t. was a possible pathogen, yet all 3 patients had preexisting medical problems.

The fact that B.t. specimens were from a variety of body sites or fluids suggests that the *Bacillus* is not appearing as a pathogen, for there is no consistent pattern of disease associated with its presence. Although the safety record of B.t.-k has been remarkable, there is now an increased proportion of persons in any community with some degree of immunocompromise. In addition, no bacterium can be labeled as absolutely nonpathogenic to humans. Thus precautions must be taken to prevent B.t.-k and other microorganisms used for pest control from causing disease in exposed persons, particularly those who are immunocompromised on same basis.

▶ B.t.-k is a highly effective biological warfare agent when used against certain insects; it is being applied increasingly. The product is often used in large-scale aerial spraying for gypsy moth, as well as by commercial landscapers and home gardeners. The product I have personally used is called Safer; however, the only comment about how safe it is for humans is the generic, "Keep out of reach of children" and "avoid inhalation or contact with eyes or skin." That's very helpful, right? Bacteriologic surveillance during 2 years of aerial spraying in Oregon, described in this paper, revealed 55 B.t. isolates, of which 52 were classified as probable contaminants.

The 3 patients in whom B.t. could not be ruled out as a pathogen included a 77-year-old with a malignant superior vena cava syndrome and repeated chest drainage procedures in whom pneumonia and effusion developed; a positive blood culture for B.t. grew in 1 of 4 culture bottles. No other relevant cultures were obtained, and when the patient died 13 days later no autopsy was performed. Case 2 was a 32-year-old retarded woman with chronic pyuria who was receiving trimethoprim-sulfamethoxazole prophylaxis. She had experienced several months of intermittent right upper quadrant pain caused by stones; ultimately, acute gangrenous cholecystitis developed with an impacted stone in the cystic duct. The bile grew B.t. in the broth, but not on the agar plates, and no organisms were found on histologic examination of the surgical specimen. Case 3 was a 25-year-old methamphetamine injector in whom an abscess developed 5 days after an injection in the antecubital fossa; B.t. grew from abscess fluid.

These cases are not convincing. In addition, the lack of a definable pattern of infection or site predilection is evidence against the pathogenic role of B.t.-k in humans. Although concluding that the use of B.t. is safe, the authors are appropriately cautious about its potential to cause disease, especially in immunocompromised individuals. Their suggestion to continue surveillance and to advise immunodeficient patients who may live in areas where B.t.-k is being used, or who may use the product themselves, to exert caution is most reasonable but hard to define in specific terms.—G.T. Keusch, M.D.

Reduced Mortality Among Children in Southern India Receiving a Small Weekly Dose of Vitamin A

Rahmathullah L, Underwood BA, Thulasiraj RD, Milton RC, Ramaswamy K, Rahmathullah R, Babu G (Aravind Children's Hosp, Madurai, India; Aravind Eye Hosp, Madurai, India; Natl Eye Inst, Bethesda, Md)

N Engl J Med 323:929–935, 1990 13–12

An estimated 20–40 million children worldwide have at least mild vitamin A deficiency. Several Indonesian studies have reported that high-dose vitamin A supplementation significantly reduces mortality among infants and young children. However, the results of these studies have been questioned in regard to study design and lack of compliance data. To further define the role of vitamin A deficiency and its treatment in children, a 1-year, randomized, placebo-controlled trial was conducted in an economically and environmentally deprived area in southern India.

The study population consisted of 15,419 children between the ages of 6 and 60 months who had been identified by trained enumerators in a house-by-house survey. Medical examination teams then performed ocular examinations, made anthropometric measurements, and obtained a morbidity history. All children with symptoms of xerophthalmia at the baseline examination were treated with a large-dose combination of vitamin A and vitamin E. The remaining children were randomly allocated to either a treatment solution containing 8.7 μmol of vitamin A and 46 μmol of vitamin E or a placebo solution containing 46 μmol of vitamin E alone. This dose of vitamin A could be obtained from foods. Community health volunteers visited each home weekly for 52 weeks to dispense the appropriate liquid supplement directly into the mouth of the study child and to record mortality and morbidity.

TABLE 1.—Mortality According to Age and Study Group

Age and Study Group	No. of Children	No. of Deaths	Cumulative Mortality Rate	Relative Risk*
0–11 Mo				
Control	678	14	0.021	0.28 (0.09, 0.85)†
Treated	689	4	0.006	
12–35 Mo				
Control	3185	52	0.016	0.46 (0.26, 0.81)‡
Treated	3179	24	0.008	
≥36 Mo				
Control	3792	14	0.004	0.63 (0.26, 1.50)
Treated	3896	9	0.002	
Total				
Control	7655	80	0.010	0.46 (0.29, 0.71)‡
Treated	7764	37	0.005	
Age-adjusted total				0.46 (0.30, 0.71)‡

*Relative risk for the treated group, as compared with the control group. Values in parentheses are 95% confidence limits.

†$P = .05$.

‡$P = .01$.

(Courtesy of Rahmathullah L, Underwood BA, Thulasiraj RD, et al: *N Engl J Med* 323:929–935, 1990.)

The baseline prevalence of xerophthalmia was 11%, and 7 children had active corneal involvement. Based on anthropometric measurements, 72% of the children were undernourished. Approximately one third of these children were stunted, 18% were stunted and wasted, and 23% were wated. During the 52-week surveillance period, 117 nonaccidental deaths occurred—80 in the control group and 37 in the treatment group (Table 1). Vitamin A administration reduced the age-adjusted total relative risk (RR) of mortality to .46 compared to nontreated children. Treatment with vitamin A reduced the RR of mortality in both sexes, although the reduction was somewhat greater among girls. The greatest reduction in risk of mortality occurred among children less than 3 years old and among chronically undernourished children (Table 2). The symptom-specific risk of mortality was significantly associated with diarrhea, convulsions, and other infection-related symptoms. The mortality rate among children with xerophthalmia was approximately 50% higher than that among children without this condition.

▶ I have already reviewed this paper in an editorial in the *New England Journal of Medicine* entitled "Vitamin A Supplements–Too Good Not to Be True" (323:985, 1990). The point of the editorial was that this study, in contrast to many before it, was well controlled and produced convincing data. Therefore, it seemed reasonable to take the leap of faith (that's what good data are for) and to implement vitamin A supplements in areas of the world with deficiency states and heavy infectious disease burdens. The question is how to do it and at what cost (and, given the limited health budgets in most developing countries, making the implied choice of doing this instead of something else).

The best means to increase the vitamin A intake is, no doubt, via the diet by developing better national agricultural and nutritional policies (i.e., assuring that vitamin A foods are available to and used by all at risk) and not by medicinal

TABLE 2.—Mortality According to Nutritional Status

Nutritional Status and Study Group	No. of Children	No. of Deaths	Cumulative Mortality Rate	Relative Risk *
Unknown				
Control	201	6	0.030	0.13 (0.01, 1.14)
Treated	268	1	0.004	
Stunted				
Control	2385	27	0.011	0.11 (0.03, 0.36) †
Treated	2418	3	0.001	
Wasted				
Control	1806	14	0.008	0.72 (0.30, 1.72)
Treated	1798	10	0.006	
Stunted and wasted				
Control	1373	22	0.016	0.65 (0.30, 1.41)
Treated	1340	14	0.010	
Normal				
Control	1890	11	0.006	0.80 (0.32, 2.00)
Treated	1940	9	0.005	

*Relative risk for the treated group, as compared with the control group. Values in parentheses are 95% confidence limits.

†$P = .01$.

(Courtesy of Rahmathullah L, Underwood BA, Thulasiraj RD, et al: *N Engl J Med* 323:929–935, 1990)

means. At the same time, good evidence has been presented for the efficacy of bolus vitamin A administration to children with measles in Africa to reduce inhospital mortality (1). This is a separate issue—acute pharmacologic doses in the course of a serious infection vs. chronic increased intake over prolonged periods of time, as in the present study. Both approaches may be valid and both need to be given priority by the public health establishment, using cost-benefit and cost-effectiveness methods. Considering some of the discussions of prioritizing health care expenditures in this country, we may be in need of the same sort of prioritizing as the rest of the world.—G.T. Keusch, M.D.

Reference

1. Hussey GD, et al: *N Engl J Med* 323:160, 1990.-

Subject Index

A

C

I

K

L

N

O

P

Q

R

S

T

U

V

W

Y

Z

Author Index

A

B

C

H

I

J

K

L

M

S

T

U

V

W

Y

Z